Understanding Hormones, Enzymes & Cell Receptors

Improve Your Health

By David W. Brown

P53 Publishing

Understanding Hormones, Enzymes & Cell Receptors

First Printing, 2024

This book is dedicated to my wonderful mother who always believed in me. You are deeply missed!

INTRODUCTION

In the intricate symphony of life, our bodies rely on a complex interplay of biological molecules to maintain health, regulate functions, and adapt to ever-changing environments. Among these molecules, hormones, enzymes, and cell receptors play pivotal roles. Their harmonious interactions ensure that our physiological processes operate seamlessly, from the simplest cellular functions to the most intricate systems governing growth, metabolism, and immunity. In ***"Understanding Hormones, Enzymes & Cell Receptors,"*** you will embark on a journey to demystify these fundamental components of life, exploring their functions, production, and regulation.

Hormones, often described as the body's chemical messengers, are crucial in orchestrating a myriad of physiological activities. They travel through the bloodstream, delivering signals to organs and tissues, and guiding them in performing specific functions. From regulating metabolism and growth to controlling mood and reproductive processes, hormones are indispensable. Each hormone has a unique role, and the delicate balance among them is essential for maintaining health. An imbalance can lead to disorders ranging from diabetes and thyroid issues to hormonal imbalances in men and women.

Enzymes, on the other hand, are the catalysts of life. These remarkable proteins accelerate biochemical reactions, enabling the myriad processes that sustain life. Whether it's digesting food, replicating DNA, or facilitating cellular repair, enzymes are at the heart of these activities. They work with precision and efficiency, ensuring that reactions occur at the right time and place. The importance of enzymes cannot be overstated; without them, the chemical reactions necessary for life would proceed too slowly to sustain us. "The human body contains a vast array of hormones, and enzymes, far too many to list comprehensively here. Therefore, I have chosen to focus on the top 50 most significant hormones and enzymes."

Cell receptors are equally vital, serving as the body's communication hubs. These specialized proteins are embedded in cell membranes and act as binding sites for hormones, neurotransmitters, and other signaling molecules. When a molecule binds to its corresponding receptor, it triggers a cascade of events within the cell, leading to a specific response. This interaction is crucial for processes such as immune response, cellular growth, and the regulation of metabolic pathways. Understanding how cell receptors function and how they can be modulated offers insights into developing targeted therapies for various diseases.

This book delves deep into the intricacies of these biological marvels, providing a comprehensive overview of over 80 hormones, enzymes, and receptors. Each chapter is dedicated to a specific molecule or a group of molecules, detailing their discovery, structure, and function. You will explore how these molecules are produced within the body, the regulatory mechanisms that control their activity, and the consequences of their dysregulation.

A unique aspect of this book is its holistic approach, emphasizing the interconnectedness of these molecules within the broader context of human health. You will learn how lifestyle factors, such as diet and exercise, can influence hormone levels, enzyme activity, and receptor function. Special attention is given to the role of a plant-based diet, highlighting its potential to promote hormonal balance, enhance enzymatic efficiency, and optimize receptor function.

"Understanding Hormones, Enzymes & Cell Receptors" is designed to be accessible to both healthcare professionals and curious readers. It combines scientific rigor with clear, engaging writing, making complex topics understandable and relevant. Through this book, I aim to empower readers with knowledge, fostering a deeper appreciation for the biochemical wonders within us and inspiring informed decisions about health and wellness.

As you navigate through the chapters, you will uncover the secrets of these vital molecules, gaining insights into their roles in health and disease. This journey promises to be enlightening, offering a new perspective on the biological foundations of life and the potential for harnessing this knowledge to improve health outcomes. Welcome to a deeper understanding of hormones, enzymes, and cell receptors—a journey into the very essence of life itself.

If you are looking for the references used in the creation of this book, I have chosen to post them online to save space. To access these references, please email your name, email address, and proof of purchase to dave@thep53.com, and I will provide you with a login. I apologize for any inconvenience this may cause. Additionally, I invite you to explore my other books at thep53.com.

Thank You,
David W. Brown

TABLE OF CONTENTS

Chapter 14 Other Important Hormones

Chapter 15 Digestive Enzymes

Chapter 16 DNA/RNA Processing Enzymes

Chapter 17 Energy Production Enzymes

Chapter 18 Gluconeogenesis/Glycogen Metabolism Enzymes

Chapter 19 Fatty Acid Metabolism Enzymes

Chapter 20 Krebs Cycle Enzymes

Chapter 26 Amino Acid Metabolism Enzymes

Chapter 27 Neurotransmitter Metabolism Enzymes

Chapter 28 G-Protein-Coupled Receptors (GPCRs)

Chapter 29 Receptor Tyrosine Kinases (RTKs)

Chapter 30 Ion Channel-Linked Receptors

Chapter 31 Nuclear Receptors

Chapter 32 Cytokine Receptors

1

Pituitary Gland Hormones

Understanding Hormones

Hormones are vital chemical messengers that facilitate communication between different parts of the body, regulating various physiological and behavioral processes. They play a crucial role in maintaining homeostasis, growth, metabolism, reproduction, and mood regulation. Understanding hormones involves delving into their production, function, regulation, and the intricate systems they interact within the human body. This book will cover the basic concepts of hormones, their classification, major endocrine glands, significant hormones and their functions, regulatory mechanisms, and the impact of lifestyle and diet on hormonal balance.

Basic Concepts of Hormones

Hormones are biochemical substances produced by endocrine glands and released directly into the bloodstream. From there, they travel to target organs or tissues to elicit specific physiological responses. Unlike neurotransmitters, which communicate between nerve cells, hormones can affect distant cells throughout the body.

Endocrine System

The endocrine system is a network of glands that produce and secrete hormones. It works closely with the nervous system to regulate bodily functions. Key endocrine glands include the hypothalamus, pituitary gland, thyroid gland, parathyroid glands, adrenal glands, pancreas, ovaries in females, and testes in males.

Hormonal Classification

Hormones can be classified based on their chemical structure, solubility, and mode of action:

1. **Peptide Hormones**: These are chains of amino acids, such as insulin and growth hormone. They are water-soluble and cannot pass through cell membranes, thus binding to surface receptors.
2. **Steroid Hormones**: Derived from cholesterol, these include cortisol and sex hormones (estrogen and testosterone). They are lipid-soluble and can pass through cell membranes to bind to intracellular receptors.
3. **Amine Hormones**: Derived from amino acids, such as thyroid hormones and catecholamines (epinephrine and norepinephrine). They can be either water-soluble or lipid-soluble.

Major Endocrine Glands and Their Hormones

Hypothalamus

The hypothalamus, located in the brain, is the control center for the endocrine system. It produces releasing and inhibiting hormones that regulate the pituitary gland. Key hormones include:

- **Thyrotropin-releasing Hormone (TRH)**: Stimulates the release of thyroid-stimulating hormone (TSH) from the pituitary.
- **Corticotropin-releasing Hormone (CRH)**: Stimulates the release of adrenocorticotropic hormone (ACTH) from the pituitary.
- **Gonadotropin-releasing Hormone (GnRH)**: Stimulates the release of luteinizing hormone (LH) and follicle-stimulating hormone (FSH) from the pituitary.

Pituitary Gland

Often referred to as the "master gland," the pituitary gland is divided into the anterior and posterior lobes, each secreting different hormones:

- **Anterior Pituitary**:
    - **Growth Hormone (GH)**: Stimulates growth and cell reproduction.
    - **Prolactin (PRL)**: Promotes milk production.
    - **Adrenocorticotropic Hormone (ACTH)**: Stimulates the adrenal glands to produce cortisol.
    - **Thyroid-stimulating Hormone (TSH)**: Stimulates the thyroid gland to produce thyroid hormones.
    - **Luteinizing Hormone (LH) and Follicle-stimulating Hormone (FSH)**: Regulate reproductive processes.
- **Posterior Pituitary**:
    - **Oxytocin**: Stimulates uterine contractions during childbirth and milk ejection during breastfeeding.
    - **Antidiuretic Hormone (ADH)**: Regulates water balance by promoting water reabsorption in the kidneys.

Thyroid Gland

Located in the neck, the thyroid gland produces hormones that regulate metabolism:

- **Thyroxine (T4) and Triiodothyronine (T3)**: Increase metabolic rate, oxygen consumption, and energy production.
- **Calcitonin**: Lowers blood calcium levels by inhibiting osteoclast activity and promoting calcium excretion by the kidneys.

Parathyroid Glands

These small glands located behind the thyroid produce parathyroid hormone (PTH), which regulates calcium levels in the blood by:

- Increasing calcium absorption in the intestines.
- Promoting calcium reabsorption in the kidneys.
- Stimulating the release of calcium from bones.

Adrenal Glands

Situated atop the kidneys, the adrenal glands consist of the cortex and medulla, each producing different hormones:

- **Adrenal Cortex:**
    - **Cortisol:** Regulates metabolism, stress response, and immune function.
    - **Aldosterone:** Regulates sodium and potassium balance, affecting blood pressure.
    - **Androgens:** Contribute to sex characteristics and reproductive function.
- **Adrenal Medulla:**
    - **Epinephrine (Adrenaline) and Norepinephrine (Noradrenaline):** Increase heart rate, blood pressure, and energy availability during stress (fight-or-flight response).

Pancreas

The pancreas has both endocrine and exocrine functions. Its endocrine function involves the production of hormones that regulate blood glucose levels:

- **Insulin:** Lowers blood glucose levels by promoting glucose uptake by cells.
- **Glucagon:** Raises blood glucose levels by stimulating glycogen breakdown in the liver.
- **Somatostatin:** Inhibits the release of insulin and glucagon, regulating their balance.

Gonads

The ovaries and testes produce sex hormones that regulate reproductive functions and secondary sexual characteristics:

- **Ovaries:**
    - **Estrogen**: Regulates female reproductive development, menstrual cycle, and secondary sexual characteristics.
    - **Progesterone**: Prepares the uterus for pregnancy and maintains pregnancy.
- **Testes:**
    - **Testosterone**: Regulates male reproductive development, sperm production, and secondary sexual characteristics.

Hormonal Regulation Mechanisms

Hormonal regulation involves intricate feedback mechanisms to maintain balance within the body. These mechanisms include:

Negative Feedback

The most common regulatory mechanism, negative feedback, involves the inhibition of hormone production when levels reach a certain threshold. For example, high levels of thyroid hormones inhibit the release of TRH and TSH, reducing thyroid hormone production.

Positive Feedback

Less common, positive feedback amplifies the response until a specific event occurs. For instance, during childbirth, oxytocin release stimulates uterine contractions, which in turn increase oxytocin release until delivery.

Hormonal Interactions

Hormones can interact synergistically, antagonistically, or permissively:

- **Synergistic Effects**: Two or more hormones work together to produce a stronger effect, such as glucagon and epinephrine increasing blood glucose levels.
- **Antagonistic Effects**: Hormones have opposing effects, such as insulin lowering and glucagon raising blood glucose levels.
- **Permissive Effects**: One hormone enhances the effect of another, such as thyroid hormones increasing the sensitivity of cells to epinephrine.

Impact of Lifestyle and Diet on Hormonal Balance

Hormonal balance is crucial for overall health, and lifestyle and dietary choices can significantly influence this balance.

Diet and Hormones

Certain foods and nutrients play vital roles in hormone production and regulation:

- **Healthy Fats**: Essential for the production of steroid hormones. Sources include avocados, nuts, seeds, and olive oil.
- **Proteins**: Provide amino acids necessary for the synthesis of peptide hormones. Sources include legumes, beans, lentils, and tofu.
- **Fiber**: Helps regulate insulin and estrogen levels by promoting healthy digestion and excretion. Sources include whole grains, fruits, and vegetables.
- **Micronutrients**: Vitamins and minerals such as vitamin D, B vitamins, magnesium, and zinc are crucial for hormone production and function. Sources include leafy greens, nuts, seeds, and fortified foods.

Exercise and Hormones

Regular physical activity has numerous benefits for hormonal balance:

- **Reduces Insulin Resistance**: Exercise enhances the sensitivity of cells to insulin, helping regulate blood glucose levels.
- **Increases Endorphins**: Physical activity stimulates the release of endorphins, which improve mood and reduce stress.
- **Balances Sex Hormones**: Regular exercise can help regulate estrogen and testosterone levels, improving reproductive health.

Sleep and Hormones
Quality sleep is essential for hormonal balance:

- **Melatonin**: Regulates sleep-wake cycles. Poor sleep can disrupt melatonin production.
- **Growth Hormone**: Released during deep sleep, it is crucial for growth, cell repair, and metabolism.
- **Cortisol**: Regulates stress response. Lack of sleep can elevate cortisol levels, leading to various health issues.

Stress Management and Hormones
Chronic stress can significantly impact hormonal balance:

- **Cortisol**: Prolonged stress increases cortisol levels, which can lead to weight gain, immune suppression, and other health problems.
- **Adrenaline**: Chronic stress keeps adrenaline levels elevated, leading to cardiovascular issues.
- **Mindfulness and Relaxation Techniques**: Practices like meditation, yoga, and deep breathing can help reduce stress and balance cortisol levels.

Hormonal Imbalances and Disorders
Hormonal imbalances can lead to various disorders, affecting different systems in the body. Some common hormonal disorders include:

Diabetes Mellitus

Characterized by high blood glucose levels due to insulin deficiency (Type 1) or insulin resistance (Type 2). Management involves lifestyle changes and medication.

Hypothyroidism

An underactive thyroid gland produces insufficient thyroid hormones, leading to symptoms like fatigue, weight gain, and depression. Treatment typically involves hormone replacement therapy.

Hyperthyroidism

An overactive thyroid gland produces excessive thyroid hormones, causing symptoms like weight loss, anxiety, and rapid heartbeat. Treatment options include medication, radioactive iodine therapy, or surgery.

Polycystic Ovary Syndrome (PCOS)

A hormonal disorder in women characterized by irregular menstrual cycles, excess androgens, and polycystic ovaries. Management includes lifestyle changes, medication, and hormone therapy.

Addison's Disease

A rare disorder where the adrenal glands produce insufficient cortisol and aldosterone, leading to fatigue, weight loss, and low blood pressure. Treatment involves hormone replacement therapy.

Cushing's Syndrome

Caused by prolonged exposure to high cortisol levels, leading to symptoms like weight gain, high blood pressure, and skin changes. Treatment options include medication, surgery, or radiation.

Plant-Based Diet and Hormonal Health

A plant-based diet can have a positive impact on hormonal health, providing essential nutrients and reducing the risk of hormonal imbalances:

Phytoestrogens

Found in foods like soy, flaxseeds, and legumes, phytoestrogens are plant compounds that mimic estrogen in the body. They can help balance estrogen levels, reducing symptoms of menopause and lowering the risk of hormone-dependent cancers.

Antioxidants

Rich in fruits, vegetables, and whole grains, antioxidants protect cells from oxidative stress, which can disrupt hormone production and function.

Fiber

High-fiber diets promote healthy digestion and excretion, helping to regulate insulin and estrogen levels.

Healthy Fats

Plant-based sources of healthy fats, such as avocados, nuts, and seeds, support the production of steroid hormones.

Understanding hormones and their functions is fundamental to appreciating how the body maintains homeostasis and responds to internal and external stimuli. Hormones regulate vital processes, from growth and metabolism to mood and reproductive health. Maintaining hormonal balance through a healthy lifestyle, balanced diet, regular exercise, quality sleep, and stress management is crucial for overall well-being. As research continues to uncover the complexities of hormonal interactions and their impact on health, individuals can make informed choices to support their endocrine health and enhance their quality of life.

Growth Hormone (GH)

Growth hormone (GH), also known as somatotropin, is a peptide hormone that plays a crucial role in growth, metabolism, and overall health. Its impact spans from childhood development to maintaining tissues and organs throughout life. This comprehensive analysis will delve into the function, production, and regulation of GH, particularly from a plant-based viewpoint, highlighting dietary influences on its activity and balance.

Function of Growth Hormone

Growth hormone's primary function is to stimulate growth, cell reproduction, and regeneration. It achieves this by:

1. **Promoting Growth**: GH stimulates the liver to produce insulin-like growth factor 1 (IGF-1), which plays a significant role in bone and muscle growth. In children and adolescents, GH drives the longitudinal growth of bones, leading to increased height.
2. **Metabolic Effects**: GH influences various metabolic processes. It promotes protein synthesis, increases muscle mass, and enhances the breakdown of fats (lipolysis) for energy. GH also helps regulate carbohydrate metabolism by reducing the sensitivity of insulin receptors, thereby increasing blood glucose levels.
3. **Cell Regeneration**: GH supports the repair and regeneration of tissues. It stimulates the production of new cells, particularly in the skin and other connective tissues, contributing to overall tissue health and longevity.
4. **Bone Health**: GH and IGF-1 are critical for bone remodeling and density. They stimulate the activity of osteoblasts (cells responsible for bone formation) and osteoclasts (cells responsible for bone resorption), maintaining a balance in bone turnover.
5. **Cognitive Function**: Research suggests that GH may have a role in brain function, influencing mood, cognitive abilities, and overall mental health.

Production of Growth Hormone

Growth hormone is produced by the pituitary gland, a pea-sized gland located at the base of the brain. The production process involves several steps:

1. **Synthesis**: GH is synthesized and secreted by somatotropic cells in the anterior pituitary gland. The gene responsible for GH production is located on chromosome 17 in humans.
2. **Regulation by Hypothalamus**: The hypothalamus, a region of the brain that controls various physiological processes, regulates GH production through two main hormones:
    - **Growth Hormone-Releasing Hormone (GHRH)**: Stimulates the release of GH.
    - **Somatostatin**: Inhibits GH release.
3. **Pulsatile Secretion**: GH is secreted in a pulsatile manner, with several peaks throughout the day. The most significant peak occurs shortly after the onset of deep sleep.
4. **Influencing Factors**: Several factors influence GH production, including:
    - **Age**: GH levels peak during puberty and decline with age.
    - **Gender**: Males typically have higher baseline GH levels than females.
    - **Exercise**: Physical activity, particularly high-intensity exercise, stimulates GH secretion.
    - **Nutrition**: Diet, especially protein intake, plays a role in GH production.

Regulation of Growth Hormone

The regulation of GH is a complex process involving feedback mechanisms and external factors:

1. **Feedback Loops**: GH and IGF-1 levels are regulated through negative feedback loops. High levels of GH and IGF-1 inhibit the release of GHRH and stimulate the release of somatostatin from the hypothalamus, reducing GH secretion.
2. **Sleep**: Sleep is a critical regulator of GH production. Deep sleep stages (slow-wave sleep) are associated with the highest peaks

of GH secretion. Disrupted sleep patterns can lead to altered GH levels.

3. **Exercise**: Regular physical activity, particularly resistance and high-intensity interval training, significantly boosts GH secretion. Exercise-induced GH release is thought to be mediated by increased GHRH and reduced somatostatin levels.
4. **Nutritional Status**: Fasting and hypoglycemia increase GH secretion, while hyperglycemia and high-fat diets can suppress it. Amino acids, especially arginine, stimulate GH release.
5. **Hormones**: Other hormones, such as ghrelin (the "hunger hormone") and sex steroids (testosterone and estrogen), also influence GH production. Ghrelin stimulates GH release, while sex steroids modulate its levels during puberty and adulthood.

Plant-Based Diet and Growth Hormone Regulation

A plant-based diet, rich in fruits, vegetables, whole grains, nuts, and seeds, can have a profound impact on GH regulation through various mechanisms:

1. **Nutrient Density**: Plant-based diets are typically high in essential nutrients, vitamins, and minerals that support overall health and hormonal balance. For example, vitamin D, found in fortified plant milks and mushrooms, is crucial for bone health and GH activity.
2. **Amino Acids**: Certain amino acids, such as arginine and glutamine, found in plant foods like nuts, seeds, and legumes, are known to stimulate GH release. These amino acids play a role in protein synthesis and muscle growth, indirectly supporting GH function.
3. **Antioxidants**: Fruits and vegetables are rich in antioxidants, which help reduce oxidative stress. Lower oxidative stress levels

are associated with improved GH secretion and overall endocrine function.

4. **Healthy Fats**: Plant-based sources of fats, such as avocados, nuts, and seeds, provide essential fatty acids that support hormone production and regulation. Omega-3 fatty acids, in particular, have anti-inflammatory properties that can enhance GH activity.
5. **Fiber**: High-fiber diets, common in plant-based eating, support gut health and hormone regulation. A healthy gut microbiome can influence GH levels through the production of short-chain fatty acids and other metabolites.
6. **Caloric Balance**: Maintaining a healthy weight through a balanced plant-based diet can prevent obesity-related suppression of GH. Excess body fat, particularly visceral fat, is linked to lower GH levels due to increased production of somatostatin.
7. **Glycemic Control**: Plant-based diets, which are low in refined sugars and high in complex carbohydrates, help maintain stable blood glucose levels. This stability prevents hyperglycemia-induced suppression of GH secretion.

Plant-Based Diet on Growth Hormone-Related Health Outcomes

1. **Muscle Mass and Strength**: Contrary to the misconception that plant-based diets lack sufficient protein for muscle building, numerous studies show that plant-based proteins can support muscle growth and strength when combined with resistance training. Foods like beans, lentils, quinoa, and tofu provide high-quality protein that stimulates GH release and muscle protein synthesis.
2. **Bone Health**: Plant-based diets rich in calcium, magnesium, and vitamin K support bone health. Leafy greens, fortified plant milk, and nuts are excellent sources of these nutrients, which work

synergistically with GH to maintain bone density and reduce the risk of osteoporosis.

3. **Weight Management**: Plant-based diets are effective for weight management, reducing body fat, and improving insulin sensitivity. Lower body fat and better glycemic control enhance GH secretion and overall metabolic health.
4. **Anti-Aging Effects**: The antioxidant-rich nature of plant-based diets helps combat oxidative stress, a key factor in aging. Improved GH levels, coupled with reduced oxidative damage, contribute to healthier aging and better maintenance of lean body mass.
5. **Mental Health**: Emerging evidence suggests that plant-based diets may benefit mental health by reducing inflammation and oxidative stress, which are linked to mood disorders. Improved GH levels also support cognitive function and emotional well-being.

Growth hormone plays a pivotal role in growth, metabolism, and overall health throughout life. Its production and regulation are influenced by various factors, including age, sleep, exercise, and diet. A plant-based diet, rich in essential nutrients, amino acids, antioxidants, and healthy fats, supports optimal GH function and balance.

By promoting muscle growth, bone health, weight management, and mental well-being, a plant-based diet can enhance the benefits of GH and contribute to a healthier, more vibrant life. As research continues to uncover the intricate relationships between diet and hormonal health, it becomes increasingly clear that plant-based nutrition offers a powerful tool for optimizing growth hormone levels and overall health.

Adrenocorticotropic Hormone (ACTH)

Adrenocorticotropic hormone (ACTH), also known as corticotropin, is a polypeptide hormone produced and secreted by the anterior pituitary gland. It plays a crucial role in the body's response to stress and regulates various physiological processes, including metabolism, immune response, and energy balance. This analysis will delve into the function, production, and regulation of ACTH, particularly from a plant-based viewpoint, highlighting dietary influences on its activity and balance.

Function of Adrenocorticotropic Hormone

ACTH's primary function is to stimulate the adrenal cortex to secrete glucocorticoids, mainly cortisol. Cortisol is essential for various bodily functions, including:

1. **Stress Response:** ACTH is released in response to stress, triggering the adrenal glands to produce cortisol. Cortisol helps the body manage stress by increasing blood sugar levels, enhancing brain function, and reducing inflammation.
2. **Metabolism Regulation:** Cortisol, stimulated by ACTH, influences metabolism by promoting gluconeogenesis (the production of glucose from non-carbohydrate sources), increasing protein breakdown, and mobilizing fat stores for energy.
3. **Immune Function:** ACTH-induced cortisol production modulates the immune system, reducing inflammation and suppressing immune responses to prevent overactivity, which can lead to autoimmune diseases.
4. **Energy Balance:** ACTH helps regulate the balance of energy production and consumption, ensuring the body has sufficient resources to handle physical and mental demands.

Production of Adrenocorticotropic Hormone

ACTH is produced by the corticotroph cells in the anterior pituitary gland. The production process involves several steps:

1. **Synthesis:** ACTH is synthesized as part of a larger precursor molecule called proopiomelanocortin (POMC). Enzymes cleave POMC to produce ACTH along with other peptides.
2. **Regulation by Hypothalamus:** The hypothalamus regulates ACTH production through the release of corticotropin-releasing hormone (CRH). CRH stimulates the pituitary gland to secrete ACTH.
3. **Circadian Rhythm:** ACTH is secreted in a pulsatile manner, following a circadian rhythm. Levels peak in the early morning and decline throughout the day, with the lowest levels occurring at night.

Regulation of Adrenocorticotropic Hormone

The regulation of ACTH is a complex process involving feedback mechanisms and external factors:

1. **Feedback Loops:** Cortisol levels regulate ACTH secretion through a negative feedback loop. High cortisol levels inhibit CRH and ACTH release, while low cortisol levels stimulate their production.
2. **Stress:** Physical and psychological stressors increase CRH and ACTH secretion, leading to elevated cortisol levels to manage the stress response.
3. **Sleep-Wake Cycle:** The circadian rhythm plays a crucial role in ACTH regulation. Sleep disorders and disruptions in the sleep-wake cycle can alter ACTH secretion patterns.
4. **Nutrition:** Diet influences ACTH levels. Certain nutrients and dietary patterns can modulate the hypothalamic-pituitary-adrenal (HPA) axis, affecting ACTH and cortisol production.

Plant-Based Diet and ACTH Regulation

A plant-based diet, rich in fruits, vegetables, whole grains, nuts, and seeds, can have a profound impact on ACTH regulation through various mechanisms:

1. **Nutrient Density:** Plant-based diets are high in essential nutrients, vitamins, and minerals that support overall health and hormonal balance. For example, vitamin C, found in abundance in fruits and vegetables, is crucial for adrenal function and ACTH activity.
2. **Antioxidants:** Fruits and vegetables are rich in antioxidants, which help reduce oxidative stress. Lower oxidative stress levels are associated with improved HPA axis function and balanced ACTH secretion.
3. **Healthy Fats:** Plant-based sources of fats, such as avocados, nuts, and seeds, provide essential fatty acids that support hormone production and regulation. Omega-3 fatty acids, in particular, have anti-inflammatory properties that can enhance ACTH activity.
4. **Fiber:** High-fiber diets, common in plant-based eating, support gut health and hormone regulation. A healthy gut microbiome can influence ACTH levels through the production of short-chain fatty acids and other metabolites.
5. **Glycemic Control:** Plant-based diets, which are low in refined sugars and high in complex carbohydrates, help maintain stable blood glucose levels. This stability prevents hyperglycemia-induced suppression of ACTH secretion.

Impact of Plant-Based Diet on ACTH-Related Health Outcomes

1. **Stress Management:** A plant-based diet rich in antioxidants and anti-inflammatory compounds can help manage stress by

reducing oxidative stress and inflammation, supporting balanced ACTH and cortisol levels.

2. **Metabolic Health:** Plant-based diets are effective for weight management, reducing body fat, and improving insulin sensitivity. Lower body fat and better glycemic control enhance ACTH secretion and overall metabolic health.
3. **Immune Function:** The anti-inflammatory properties of a plant-based diet can support a balanced immune response. Reduced inflammation and oxidative stress can enhance ACTH activity and improve immune function.
4. **Mental Health:** Emerging evidence suggests that plant-based diets may benefit mental health by reducing inflammation and oxidative stress, which are linked to mood disorders. Improved ACTH levels also support cognitive function and emotional well-being.

Adrenocorticotropic hormone plays a pivotal role in the body's response to stress, metabolism, immune function, and energy balance. Its production and regulation are influenced by various factors, including stress, sleep, and diet. A plant-based diet, rich in essential nutrients, antioxidants, healthy fats, and fiber, supports optimal ACTH function and balance. By promoting stress management, metabolic health, immune function, and mental well-being, a plant-based diet can enhance the benefits of ACTH and contribute to a healthier, more vibrant life.

Thyroid-stimulating Hormone (TSH)

Thyroid-stimulating hormone (TSH), also known as thyrotropin, is a critical hormone in the endocrine system. It regulates the function of the thyroid gland, influencing metabolism, growth, and development.

Function of Thyroid-Stimulating Hormone (TSH)

TSH plays a crucial role in the regulation of thyroid hormone production, which in turn affects numerous physiological processes:

1. **Regulation of Thyroid Hormones**: TSH stimulates the thyroid gland to produce and release thyroxine (T4) and triiodothyronine (T3). These hormones regulate metabolism, energy production, and overall metabolic rate.
2. **Metabolic Effects**: TSH indirectly influences various metabolic processes by regulating T3 and T4 levels. These thyroid hormones increase basal metabolic rate, enhance oxygen consumption, and stimulate the breakdown of fats (lipolysis).
3. **Growth and Development**: During childhood and adolescence, TSH plays a significant role in growth and development. Adequate thyroid hormone levels are essential for proper brain development and skeletal growth.
4. **Thermoregulation**: TSH, through its regulation of thyroid hormones, helps maintain body temperature by influencing heat production and energy expenditure.
5. **Cardiovascular Health**: TSH indirectly affects heart rate, cardiac output, and blood pressure by regulating thyroid hormone levels. T3 and T4 enhance the heart's contractility and influence the vascular tone.
6. **Mood and Cognitive Function**: Thyroid hormones, regulated by TSH, play a role in brain function, influencing mood, cognitive abilities, and overall mental health.

Production of Thyroid-Stimulating Hormone (TSH)

TSH is produced by the pituitary gland, specifically the anterior pituitary. The production process involves several steps:

1. **Synthesis**: TSH is synthesized and secreted by thyrotrope cells in the anterior pituitary gland. The gene responsible for TSH production is located on chromosome 1 in humans.
2. **Regulation by Hypothalamus**: The hypothalamus, a region of the brain that controls various physiological processes, regulates TSH production through thyrotropin-releasing hormone (TRH). TRH stimulates the release of TSH from the anterior pituitary.
3. **Feedback Mechanism**: TSH production is regulated by a negative feedback loop involving thyroid hormones. High levels of T3 and T4 inhibit TRH and TSH release, while low levels stimulate their production.
4. **Influencing Factors**: Several factors influence TSH production, including:
    - **Age**: TSH levels vary with age, peaking during infancy and adolescence, then stabilizing in adulthood.
    - **Gender**: Females typically have slightly higher TSH levels compared to males.
    - **Nutritional Status**: Adequate iodine intake is essential for thyroid hormone synthesis, influencing TSH levels. Deficiency can lead to increased TSH production.
    - **Stress and Illness**: Chronic stress and certain illnesses can affect TSH production.

Regulation of Thyroid-Stimulating Hormone (TSH)

The regulation of TSH is a complex process involving feedback mechanisms and external factors:

1. **Feedback Loops**: TSH levels are regulated through negative feedback loops involving thyroid hormones. High levels of T3 and T4 inhibit the release of TRH from the hypothalamus and TSH from the anterior pituitary, reducing TSH secretion.

2. **Sleep**: Sleep patterns can influence TSH secretion. Research indicates that TSH levels peak during the night and are lowest in the late afternoon and evening. Disrupted sleep can alter this pattern.
3. **Nutritional Status**: Adequate nutrition, particularly iodine intake, is crucial for TSH regulation. Iodine is a key component of thyroid hormones, and its deficiency can lead to increased TSH production.
4. **Hormones**: Other hormones, such as cortisol and estrogen, can influence TSH levels. Cortisol, produced during stress, can suppress TSH secretion, while estrogen can increase TSH levels.
5. **Environmental Factors**: Exposure to certain environmental toxins and pollutants can disrupt thyroid function and TSH regulation.

Plant-Based Diet and Thyroid-Stimulating Hormone (TSH) Regulation

A plant-based diet, rich in fruits, vegetables, whole grains, nuts, and seeds, can have a significant impact on TSH regulation through various mechanisms:

1. **Iodine-Rich Foods**: Plant-based sources of iodine, such as sea vegetables (kelp, nori), iodized salt, and some fruits and vegetables, are crucial for thyroid hormone synthesis and TSH regulation. Adequate iodine intake ensures proper thyroid function and prevents TSH elevation due to iodine deficiency.
2. **Antioxidants**: Fruits and vegetables are rich in antioxidants, which help reduce oxidative stress. Lower oxidative stress levels are associated with improved thyroid function and TSH regulation. Foods like berries, citrus fruits, and leafy greens are particularly beneficial.
3. **Selenium**: Selenium is an essential trace element that plays a role in thyroid hormone metabolism. Plant-based sources of selenium

include Brazil nuts, sunflower seeds, and brown rice. Adequate selenium intake supports thyroid health and helps regulate TSH levels.

4. **Fiber**: High-fiber diets, common in plant-based eating, support gut health and hormone regulation. A healthy gut microbiome can influence thyroid function and TSH levels through the production of short-chain fatty acids and other metabolites.
5. **Healthy Fats**: Plant-based sources of fats, such as avocados, nuts, and seeds, provide essential fatty acids that support hormone production and regulation. Omega-3 fatty acids, in particular, have anti-inflammatory properties that can enhance thyroid function and TSH regulation.
6. **Phytochemicals**: Phytochemicals found in plant foods, such as flavonoids and polyphenols, have anti-inflammatory and antioxidant properties. These compounds can support thyroid health and TSH regulation by reducing inflammation and oxidative stress.

Impact of Plant-Based Diet on TSH-Related Health Outcomes

1. **Hypothyroidism**: A well-planned plant-based diet can help manage hypothyroidism by providing adequate iodine and selenium, essential for thyroid hormone synthesis and TSH regulation. Avoiding goitrogens (substances that can interfere with thyroid function) found in high amounts in certain raw cruciferous vegetables is also important.
2. **Hyperthyroidism**: For individuals with hyperthyroidism, a plant-based diet can offer benefits through its anti-inflammatory properties. Foods rich in antioxidants and omega-3 fatty acids can help reduce inflammation and support overall thyroid health.
3. **Weight Management**: A plant-based diet is effective for weight management, reducing body fat and improving insulin sensitivity.

Maintaining a healthy weight can prevent obesity-related suppression of thyroid function and TSH regulation.

4. **Cardiovascular Health**: Plant-based diets are associated with improved cardiovascular health, which can indirectly benefit thyroid function. Reduced inflammation and better lipid profiles support overall endocrine health, including TSH regulation.
5. **Mental Health**: Emerging evidence suggests that plant-based diets may benefit mental health by reducing inflammation and oxidative stress, which are linked to mood disorders. Improved thyroid function and TSH levels also support cognitive function and emotional well-being.

Plant-Based Foods Beneficial for TSH Regulation

1. **Sea Vegetables**: Sea vegetables like kelp and nori are excellent sources of iodine, essential for thyroid hormone production and TSH regulation.
2. **Brazil Nuts**: Rich in selenium, Brazil nuts support thyroid health and help regulate TSH levels.
3. **Berries**: Berries are high in antioxidants, which reduce oxidative stress and support thyroid function.
4. **Leafy Greens**: Leafy greens like spinach and kale provide essential nutrients and antioxidants that support thyroid health and TSH regulation.
5. **Whole Grains**: Whole grains such as quinoa, brown rice, and oats provide fiber and essential nutrients that support overall endocrine health.
6. **Nuts and Seeds**: Nuts and seeds, such as flaxseeds, chia seeds, and walnuts, provide healthy fats and omega-3 fatty acids that support hormone production and regulation.
7. **Legumes**: Legumes like lentils, chickpeas, and beans are rich in protein, fiber, and essential nutrients that support thyroid health.

Thyroid-stimulating hormone (TSH) plays a pivotal role in the regulation of thyroid function, influencing metabolism, growth, and overall health. Its production and regulation are influenced by various factors, including age, sleep, nutritional status, and environmental factors. A plant-based diet, rich in essential nutrients, antioxidants, and healthy fats, supports optimal TSH function and balance.

By providing adequate iodine, selenium, and other essential nutrients, a plant-based diet can help manage thyroid-related conditions such as hypothyroidism and hyperthyroidism. Additionally, the anti-inflammatory and antioxidant properties of plant-based foods support overall endocrine health, including TSH regulation.

Luteinizing Hormone (LH)

Luteinizing hormone (LH) is a crucial hormone in the reproductive system, responsible for regulating the function of gonads in both males and females. It plays a significant role in the production of sex hormones, ovulation, and spermatogenesis. This comprehensive analysis delves into the function, production, and regulation of LH from a plant-based viewpoint, highlighting dietary influences on its activity and balance.

Function of Luteinizing Hormone

Luteinizing hormone has distinct roles in males and females, which are vital for reproductive health and overall endocrine function.

In Females

1. **Ovulation**: LH is essential for triggering ovulation. During the menstrual cycle, a surge in LH levels causes the mature follicle in the ovary to release an egg, a process known as ovulation.

2. **Corpus Luteum Formation**: After ovulation, LH supports the formation and maintenance of the corpus luteum, which produces progesterone necessary for maintaining the uterine lining for potential pregnancy.
3. **Hormone Production**: LH stimulates the theca cells in the ovaries to produce androgens, which are then converted to estrogen by the granulosa cells. Estrogen is crucial for regulating the menstrual cycle and supporting reproductive health.

In Males

1. **Testosterone Production**: LH stimulates the Leydig cells in the testes to produce testosterone, which is critical for the development of male secondary sexual characteristics, spermatogenesis, and overall reproductive function.
2. **Spermatogenesis**: Testosterone produced under the influence of LH supports the process of spermatogenesis, the production of sperm cells.

Additional Roles

1. **Puberty**: LH plays a key role in the onset of puberty by initiating the production of sex hormones that lead to the development of secondary sexual characteristics.
2. **Bone Health**: LH indirectly supports bone health by regulating sex hormones, which are essential for maintaining bone density and strength.

Production of Luteinizing Hormone

Luteinizing hormone is produced by the anterior pituitary gland through a complex interaction of signaling pathways.

Synthesis

1. **Gene Encoding**: The gene responsible for LH production is located on chromosome 19. It encodes the beta subunit of LH, which combines with the common alpha subunit to form the active hormone.
2. **Glycoprotein Hormone**: LH is a glycoprotein hormone, consisting of alpha and beta subunits. The alpha subunit is common to other pituitary hormones like FSH (follicle-stimulating hormone) and TSH (thyroid-stimulating hormone), while the beta subunit is unique to LH, conferring its specific biological activity.

Regulation by Hypothalamus

1. **Gonadotropin-Releasing Hormone (GnRH)**: The hypothalamus regulates LH production through the release of GnRH. Pulsatile secretion of GnRH stimulates the anterior pituitary to produce and release LH.
2. **Feedback Mechanisms**: Sex hormones like estrogen, progesterone, and testosterone provide feedback to the hypothalamus and pituitary gland to regulate LH levels. High levels of these hormones typically inhibit LH release, while low levels stimulate its production.

Pulsatile Secretion

LH is secreted in a pulsatile manner, with frequency and amplitude of pulses varying throughout the menstrual cycle in females and maintaining a relatively steady state in males.

Influencing Factors

1. **Age**: LH levels vary with age, peaking during puberty and fluctuating with reproductive cycles in females.
2. **Gender**: LH levels and patterns of secretion differ between males and females, reflecting their distinct reproductive roles.
3. **Exercise and Stress**: Physical activity and stress can influence LH secretion. Intense exercise and chronic stress may disrupt normal LH patterns.
4. **Nutrition**: Nutritional status, including dietary intake and overall health, affects LH production.

Regulation of Luteinizing Hormone

The regulation of LH involves a complex interplay of feedback mechanisms, external factors, and physiological states.

Feedback Loops

1. **Negative Feedback**: High levels of sex hormones (estrogen, progesterone, testosterone) inhibit GnRH and LH secretion. For example, high estrogen levels during the luteal phase of the menstrual cycle inhibit further LH production.
2. **Positive Feedback**: During the late follicular phase, rising estrogen levels stimulate a surge in LH through positive feedback, leading to ovulation.

Sleep

Sleep patterns significantly influence LH secretion. Disrupted sleep can alter the pulsatile release of GnRH and subsequently affect LH levels.

Exercise

Regular physical activity, particularly moderate exercise, supports healthy LH levels. However, excessive or high-intensity exercise can disrupt LH secretion due to increased stress and energy demands.

Nutritional Status

1. **Fasting and Malnutrition**: Low energy availability, as seen in fasting or malnutrition, can suppress LH secretion. This suppression is a protective mechanism to prevent reproduction during times of inadequate nutritional support.
2. **High-Fat Diets**: Diets high in saturated fats may negatively impact LH levels by disrupting overall hormonal balance.
3. **Plant-Based Nutrients**: Certain nutrients found in plant-based diets can support LH production and overall reproductive health.

Hormones

Other hormones, such as insulin, leptin, and thyroid hormones, interact with the reproductive axis and influence LH production.

Plant-Based Diet and Luteinizing Hormone Regulation

A plant-based diet, rich in fruits, vegetables, whole grains, nuts, and seeds, can positively influence LH regulation through various mechanisms.

Nutrient Density

Plant-based diets provide a wealth of essential nutrients, vitamins, and minerals that support overall health and hormonal balance. For example, vitamin D, found in fortified plant milks and mushrooms, is crucial for reproductive health and LH activity.

Amino Acids

Certain amino acids, such as arginine and glutamine, found in plant foods like nuts, seeds, and legumes, support hormone production. These amino acids play a role in protein synthesis and overall endocrine function.

Antioxidants

Fruits and vegetables are rich in antioxidants, which help reduce oxidative stress. Lower oxidative stress levels are associated with improved hormonal balance, including LH secretion.

Healthy Fats

Plant-based sources of fats, such as avocados, nuts, and seeds, provide essential fatty acids that support hormone production and regulation. Omega-3 fatty acids, in particular, have anti-inflammatory properties that can enhance endocrine function.

Fiber

High-fiber diets, common in plant-based eating, support gut health and hormone regulation. A healthy gut microbiome can influence hormonal balance through the production of short-chain fatty acids and other metabolites.

Caloric Balance

Maintaining a healthy weight through a balanced plant-based diet can prevent obesity-related hormonal imbalances. Excess body fat, particularly visceral fat, is linked to disrupted LH levels due to increased production of inflammatory markers.

Glycemic Control

Plant-based diets, which are low in refined sugars and high in complex carbohydrates, help maintain stable blood glucose levels. This stability prevents insulin resistance, which can negatively impact reproductive hormones, including LH.

Impact of Plant-Based Diet on LH-Related Health Outcomes

Reproductive Health

1. **Fertility**: A plant-based diet can support fertility by providing essential nutrients and maintaining hormonal balance. For instance, antioxidants in fruits and vegetables protect reproductive tissues from oxidative damage, supporting healthy ovulation and sperm production.

2. **Menstrual Health**: Women following a plant-based diet may experience more regular menstrual cycles and reduced symptoms of conditions like polycystic ovary syndrome (PCOS) due to improved hormonal regulation.
3. **Pregnancy Outcomes**: Adequate intake of nutrients like folate, iron, and omega-3 fatty acids from plant sources supports a healthy pregnancy and reduces the risk of complications.

Bone Health

Plant-based diets rich in calcium, magnesium, and vitamin K support bone health. Leafy greens, fortified plant milk, and nuts are excellent sources of these nutrients, which work synergistically with LH and sex hormones to maintain bone density and reduce the risk of osteoporosis.

Weight Management

Plant-based diets are effective for weight management, reducing body fat, and improving insulin sensitivity. Lower body fat and better glycemic control enhance overall hormonal balance, including LH secretion.

Mental Health

Emerging evidence suggests that plant-based diets may benefit mental health by reducing inflammation and oxidative stress, which are linked to mood disorders. Improved hormonal balance, including LH levels, supports cognitive function and emotional well-being.

Anti-Aging Effects

The antioxidant-rich nature of plant-based diets helps combat oxidative stress, a key factor in aging. Improved hormonal balance, coupled with reduced oxidative damage, contributes to healthier aging and better maintenance of reproductive health.

Luteinizing hormone plays a pivotal role in reproductive health, regulating functions from ovulation and testosterone production to overall endocrine balance. Its production and regulation are influenced by various factors, including age, sleep, exercise, and diet. A plant-based diet, rich in essential nutrients, amino acids, antioxidants, and healthy fats, supports optimal LH function and balance.

By promoting reproductive health, bone density, weight management, and mental well-being, a plant-based diet can enhance the benefits of LH and contribute to a healthier, more vibrant life.

Follicle-stimulating Hormone (FSH)

Follicle-stimulating hormone (FSH) is a critical hormone in the regulation of reproductive processes in both males and females. It plays a vital role in the development of germ cells and the regulation of reproductive organs. This comprehensive analysis delves into the function, production, and regulation of FSH, particularly from a plant-based viewpoint, highlighting dietary influences on its activity and balance.

Function of Follicle-Stimulating Hormone

FSH is essential for the proper functioning of the reproductive system. Its primary functions include:

Ovarian Follicle Development in Females:

- FSH stimulates the growth and maturation of ovarian follicles, which contain the eggs. It promotes the granulosa cells within the follicles to proliferate and produce estradiol, a form of estrogen.

- The maturation of these follicles is crucial for ovulation and fertility.

Spermatogenesis in Males:

- In males, FSH acts on the Sertoli cells in the testes to support the production and maturation of sperm. It plays a significant role in the early stages of spermatogenesis by facilitating the proliferation and differentiation of spermatogonia.

Regulation of Gonadal Function:

- FSH works in concert with luteinizing hormone (LH) to regulate the functions of the gonads (ovaries in females and testes in males). This regulation ensures the proper production of sex steroids (estrogens and androgens) and gametes (eggs and sperm).

Hormonal Balance:

- FSH is involved in maintaining the balance of sex hormones in the body. It helps regulate the menstrual cycle in females and supports the hormonal environment necessary for spermatogenesis in males.

Production of Follicle-Stimulating Hormone

FSH is produced by the anterior pituitary gland, a small gland located at the base of the brain. The production process involves several steps:

Synthesis and Secretion:

- FSH is synthesized and secreted by gonadotroph cells in the anterior pituitary gland. The gene responsible for FSH production is located on chromosome 11 in humans.

Regulation by Hypothalamus:

- The hypothalamus, a region of the brain that controls various physiological processes, regulates FSH production through the release of gonadotropin-releasing hormone (GnRH). GnRH stimulates the anterior pituitary to release both FSH and LH.

Feedback Mechanisms:

- The levels of FSH are regulated through feedback mechanisms involving sex steroids (estrogens and androgens) and inhibin, a hormone produced by the gonads. High levels of estrogens and inhibin inhibit the release of FSH, while low levels stimulate its production.

Influencing Factors:

- Several factors influence FSH production, including age, sex, and hormonal status. For example, FSH levels fluctuate throughout the menstrual cycle in females and vary with age and pubertal status in both sexes.

Regulation of Follicle-Stimulating Hormone

The regulation of FSH involves complex interactions between the hypothalamus, pituitary gland, and gonads. Key regulatory mechanisms include:

GnRH Pulsatility:

- GnRH is released in a pulsatile manner from the hypothalamus, and this pulsatility is crucial for the proper release of FSH and LH. The frequency and amplitude of GnRH pulses influence the levels of FSH.

Negative Feedback Loops:

- Estrogens and inhibin produced by the ovaries in females, and inhibin produced by the testes in males, provide negative feedback to the hypothalamus and pituitary gland to regulate FSH levels. High levels of these hormones inhibit the release of FSH to prevent overstimulation of the gonads.

Reproductive Cycle:

- In females, FSH levels vary throughout the menstrual cycle. During the follicular phase, FSH levels rise to stimulate follicle development. As estradiol levels increase, they exert negative feedback on FSH release. During the luteal phase, inhibin produced by the corpus luteum further suppresses FSH levels.

Puberty and Aging:

- During puberty, increased pulsatile release of GnRH leads to a rise in FSH and LH levels, initiating the maturation of the reproductive system. In aging, especially in women approaching menopause, FSH levels increase due to decreased ovarian function and reduced negative feedback.

Plant-Based Diet and Follicle-Stimulating Hormone Regulation

A plant-based diet can have a profound impact on the regulation of FSH through various mechanisms:

Nutrient Density:

- Plant-based diets are typically rich in essential nutrients, vitamins, and minerals that support overall health and hormonal balance. For example, vitamins such as vitamin D, found in fortified plant milk and mushrooms, play a crucial role in reproductive health and FSH regulation.

Phytoestrogens:

- Phytoestrogens are plant-derived compounds found in foods like soy, flaxseeds, and legumes that have estrogen-like activity. They can modulate estrogen levels and influence FSH secretion through feedback mechanisms. Studies have shown that phytoestrogens can help balance hormone levels, particularly in menopausal women.

Antioxidants:

- Fruits and vegetables are rich in antioxidants, which help reduce oxidative stress. Lower oxidative stress levels are associated with improved reproductive health and hormone balance. Antioxidants support the overall function of the hypothalamus and pituitary gland, aiding in the proper regulation of FSH.

Healthy Fats:

- Plant-based sources of fats, such as avocados, nuts, and seeds, provide essential fatty acids that support hormone production and regulation. Omega-3 fatty acids, in particular, have anti-inflammatory properties that can enhance reproductive health and FSH activity.

Fiber:

- High-fiber diets, common in plant-based eating, support gut health and hormone regulation. A healthy gut microbiome can influence hormone levels, including FSH, through the production of short-chain fatty acids and other metabolites.

Caloric Balance:

- Maintaining a healthy weight through a balanced plant-based diet can prevent obesity-related suppression of FSH. Excess body fat is linked to hormonal imbalances, including altered FSH levels. Weight management is crucial for maintaining reproductive health.

Glycemic Control:

- Plant-based diets, which are low in refined sugars and high in complex carbohydrates, help maintain stable blood glucose levels. This stability prevents hyperglycemia-induced hormonal imbalances, supporting proper FSH regulation.

Plant-Based Diet on Follicle-Stimulating Hormone-Related Health Outcomes

Reproductive Health in Females:

- A plant-based diet can support reproductive health in females by providing essential nutrients and phytoestrogens that help balance hormone levels. Improved FSH regulation can enhance ovarian function, support regular menstrual cycles, and increase fertility.

Spermatogenesis in Males:

- Plant-based diets rich in antioxidants and healthy fats can improve sperm quality and support spermatogenesis. Proper FSH regulation is crucial for the early stages of sperm production, and a diet that promotes hormonal balance can enhance male fertility.

Menopausal Health:

- Phytoestrogens in plant-based foods can help alleviate menopausal symptoms by modulating estrogen levels and supporting FSH regulation. This can lead to improved quality of life and reduced risk of menopausal health issues such as osteoporosis and cardiovascular disease.

Bone Health:

- FSH and estrogen play significant roles in bone health. A plant-based diet rich in calcium, magnesium, and vitamin K supports bone density and strength. Leafy greens, fortified plant milk, and nuts are excellent sources of these nutrients, which work synergistically with FSH to maintain bone health.

Weight Management and Metabolic Health:

- Plant-based diets are effective for weight management and improving insulin sensitivity. Maintaining a healthy weight through a balanced diet can prevent obesity-related hormonal imbalances and support proper FSH regulation.

Follicle-stimulating hormone plays a pivotal role in the regulation of reproductive processes and overall hormonal balance. Its production and regulation are influenced by various factors, including age, sex, and dietary habits. A plant-based diet, rich in essential nutrients, phytoestrogens, antioxidants, and healthy fats, supports optimal FSH function and balance.

By promoting reproductive health, bone density, weight management, and overall metabolic health, a plant-based diet can enhance the benefits of FSH and contribute to a healthier, more vibrant life.

Prolactin (PRL)

Prolactin (PRL) is a peptide hormone primarily associated with lactation, but its functions extend to various physiological processes including reproduction, metabolism, and immune regulation. This comprehensive analysis will delve into the function, production, and regulation of prolactin from a plant-based viewpoint, highlighting dietary influences on its activity and balance.

Function of Prolactin

Prolactin plays multiple roles in the body, and its functions can be categorized into several key areas:

1. **Lactation**: The most well-known function of prolactin is its role in milk production. It stimulates the mammary glands to produce milk after childbirth. During pregnancy, prolactin levels rise, preparing the breasts for lactation. After childbirth, the hormone helps maintain milk production.
2. **Reproductive Health**: Prolactin influences reproductive health in both males and females. In females, it helps regulate the menstrual cycle by inhibiting gonadotropin-releasing hormone (GnRH), which in turn reduces the levels of luteinizing hormone (LH) and follicle-stimulating hormone (FSH). This can prevent ovulation during periods of high prolactin levels, such as breastfeeding. In males, prolactin influences the production of testosterone and sperm.
3. **Metabolism**: Prolactin affects metabolism by regulating fat and carbohydrate metabolism. It has been shown to promote the storage of fat and influence insulin sensitivity.
4. **Immune System**: Prolactin has immunomodulatory effects, meaning it can modulate the immune response. It has been implicated in enhancing the body's defense mechanisms against pathogens.
5. **Behavior and Neurogenesis**: Prolactin influences behavior and has been associated with maternal behavior in animals. It also

plays a role in neurogenesis, the process by which new neurons are formed in the brain.

6. **Fluid Balance**: Prolactin helps regulate fluid balance in the body by influencing renal function.

Production of Prolactin

Prolactin is produced by the anterior pituitary gland, a pea-sized gland located at the base of the brain. The production process involves several steps:

Synthesis: Prolactin is synthesized and secreted by lactotrophic cells in the anterior pituitary gland. The PRL gene, responsible for prolactin production, is located on chromosome 6 in humans.

Regulation by Hypothalamus: The hypothalamus regulates prolactin production through several hormones:

- **Dopamine**: Acts as a prolactin-inhibiting hormone (PIH). It inhibits the release of prolactin.
- **Thyrotropin-Releasing Hormone (TRH)**: Stimulates the release of prolactin.
- **Estrogen**: Enhances prolactin production, particularly during pregnancy.

Circadian Rhythm: Prolactin secretion follows a circadian rhythm, with the highest levels occurring during sleep.

Influencing Factors: Several factors influence prolactin production, including:

- **Pregnancy and Lactation**: Prolactin levels increase significantly during pregnancy and peak shortly after childbirth to facilitate lactation.

- **Stress**: Physical and emotional stress can elevate prolactin levels.
- **Exercise**: Intense physical activity can transiently increase prolactin levels.

Regulation of Prolactin

The regulation of prolactin involves complex feedback mechanisms and external factors:

1. **Feedback Loops**: Prolactin regulation involves feedback loops with dopamine and estrogen. High levels of prolactin stimulate the release of dopamine from the hypothalamus, which in turn inhibits further prolactin release.
2. **Sleep**: Sleep, particularly in the early stages of sleep, is associated with increased prolactin secretion. Disrupted sleep patterns can lead to altered prolactin levels.
3. **Stress**: Stressful conditions can lead to elevated prolactin levels, as the body responds to stress by increasing the production of this hormone.
4. **Exercise**: Physical activity, especially high-intensity exercise, can temporarily raise prolactin levels. This is thought to be a result of the body's physiological response to exercise-induced stress.
5. **Nutritional Status**: Diet and nutritional status can influence prolactin levels. Certain dietary components can either enhance or suppress prolactin secretion.

Plant-Based Diet and Prolactin Regulation

A plant-based diet, rich in fruits, vegetables, whole grains, nuts, and seeds, can impact prolactin regulation through various mechanisms:

1. **Phytoestrogens**: Plant-based diets often contain phytoestrogens, compounds found in soy products, flaxseeds, and whole grains that mimic estrogen in the body. These phytoestrogens can influence prolactin levels by modulating the estrogen pathways. For instance, they may help balance estrogen levels, thus indirectly affecting prolactin production and release.
2. **Nutrient Density**: Plant-based diets are high in essential nutrients, vitamins, and minerals that support overall hormonal balance. Nutrients such as vitamin B6, found in bananas, chickpeas, and potatoes, play a role in prolactin regulation by influencing dopamine levels, which in turn affect prolactin secretion.
3. **Antioxidants**: Fruits and vegetables are rich in antioxidants, which help reduce oxidative stress. Lower oxidative stress levels are associated with improved hormonal balance, including prolactin regulation.
4. **Healthy Fats**: Plant-based sources of fats, such as avocados, nuts, and seeds, provide essential fatty acids that support hormone production and regulation. Omega-3 fatty acids, in particular, have anti-inflammatory properties that can positively influence prolactin levels.
5. **Fiber**: High-fiber diets, common in plant-based eating, support gut health and hormone regulation. A healthy gut microbiome can influence prolactin levels through the production of short-chain fatty acids and other metabolites.
6. **Caloric Balance**: Maintaining a healthy weight through a balanced plant-based diet can prevent obesity-related hormonal imbalances. Excess body fat can alter estrogen levels, which in turn affects prolactin production. By promoting a healthy weight, a plant-based diet helps maintain optimal prolactin levels.
7. **Glycemic Control**: Plant-based diets, which are low in refined sugars and high in complex carbohydrates, help maintain stable blood glucose levels. This stability prevents hyperglycemia-

induced hormonal imbalances, including those affecting prolactin secretion.

Plant-Based Diet on Prolactin-Related Health Outcomes

1. **Reproductive Health**: A balanced plant-based diet can support reproductive health by maintaining optimal prolactin levels. For instance, high levels of dietary fiber and phytoestrogens from plants can help regulate menstrual cycles and support fertility in women.
2. **Lactation**: While prolactin is crucial for lactation, the quality and quantity of breast milk are also influenced by maternal nutrition. A nutrient-dense plant-based diet can ensure that breastfeeding mothers get the necessary vitamins and minerals to support both their own health and that of their infants.
3. **Metabolic Health**: Prolactin plays a role in metabolism, and a plant-based diet supports metabolic health by providing a balanced intake of macronutrients and micronutrients. This can help in maintaining a healthy body weight and preventing metabolic disorders.
4. **Immune Function**: Prolactin has immunomodulatory effects, and a diet rich in plant-based foods can enhance immune function through high levels of antioxidants and anti-inflammatory compounds.
5. **Mental Health**: Emerging evidence suggests that plant-based diets may benefit mental health by reducing inflammation and oxidative stress, which are linked to mood disorders. Improved prolactin levels, supported by a nutrient-rich diet, can also contribute to better mental well-being.

Prolactin is a multifunctional hormone with significant roles in lactation, reproductive health, metabolism, immune function, and behavior. Its production and regulation are influenced by a variety of factors, including hormonal feedback mechanisms, stress, sleep, and nutrition.

A plant-based diet, rich in phytoestrogens, essential nutrients, antioxidants, healthy fats, and fiber, supports optimal prolactin function and balance. By promoting reproductive health, lactation, metabolic health, immune function, and mental well-being, a plant-based diet can enhance the benefits of prolactin and contribute to overall health.

Antidiuretic Hormone (ADH)

Antidiuretic hormone (ADH), also known as vasopressin, is a peptide hormone that plays a critical role in maintaining water balance, blood pressure, and overall homeostasis in the body.

Function of Antidiuretic Hormone

ADH's primary functions include regulating water balance, influencing blood pressure, and impacting social and behavioral functions. Its actions are primarily mediated through its effects on the kidneys and blood vessels.

1. Water Balance

ADH is crucial for maintaining water homeostasis in the body. It acts on the kidneys to promote water reabsorption, thereby reducing urine output and conserving body water. This process involves:

- **Increased Water Reabsorption:** ADH binds to receptors on the cells of the kidney's collecting ducts, leading to the insertion of water channels called aquaporins into the cell membranes. This increases water reabsorption from the filtrate back into the bloodstream.

- **Concentration of Urine:** By promoting water reabsorption, ADH helps concentrate urine, reducing the volume of water lost from the body.

2. Blood Pressure Regulation

ADH plays a role in regulating blood pressure through its vasoconstrictive properties:

- **Vasoconstriction:** ADH can cause blood vessels to constrict, increasing peripheral resistance and thereby raising blood pressure. This effect is particularly important during situations of significant blood loss or dehydration.

3. Social and Behavioral Functions

Recent research has highlighted ADH's role in social and behavioral processes:

- **Social Bonding and Stress Response:** ADH is involved in social behaviors, such as bonding and aggression. It also plays a role in the body's stress response, influencing the release of other stress hormones like cortisol.

Production of Antidiuretic Hormone

ADH is produced in the hypothalamus and released from the posterior pituitary gland. The production process involves several steps:

1. Synthesis in the Hypothalamus

- **Neurosecretory Cells:** ADH is synthesized by neurosecretory cells in the supraoptic and paraventricular nuclei of the hypothalamus. These cells produce ADH as a precursor protein, which is then transported down the axons to the posterior pituitary gland.

2. Transport and Storage

- **Axonal Transport:** The precursor protein is transported along the axons of the neurosecretory cells to the posterior pituitary, where it is stored in vesicles until needed.
- **Conversion to Active Form:** During transport, the precursor is processed into the active form of ADH.

3. Release from the Posterior Pituitary

- **Stimulus-Driven Release:** ADH is released into the bloodstream in response to specific physiological stimuli, such as increased plasma osmolality (a measure of solute concentration in the blood) or decreased blood volume and pressure.

Regulation of Antidiuretic Hormone

The regulation of ADH is a complex process involving feedback mechanisms and external factors:

1. Osmoregulation

- **Osmoreceptors:** Specialized cells in the hypothalamus, known as osmoreceptors, detect changes in plasma osmolality. When osmolality increases (indicating dehydration), osmoreceptors stimulate the release of ADH.
- **Feedback Mechanism:** Once ADH has acted to reabsorb water and dilute the plasma, osmoreceptors signal to reduce ADH release, maintaining homeostasis.

2. Volume and Pressure Regulation

- **Baroreceptors:** These receptors, located in the heart and blood vessels, detect changes in blood volume and pressure. A decrease in blood volume or pressure triggers the release of ADH to conserve water and increase blood pressure.

- **Renin-Angiotensin-Aldosterone System (RAAS):** ADH interacts with other hormones in the RAAS to regulate blood pressure and fluid balance. Activation of RAAS can stimulate ADH release, enhancing its effects on water reabsorption and vasoconstriction.

3. Other Influencing Factors

- **Stress and Pain:** Physical or emotional stress, as well as pain, can increase ADH release through the activation of the hypothalamic-pituitary-adrenal (HPA) axis.
- **Drugs and Substances:** Certain medications, alcohol, and other substances can influence ADH levels. For example, alcohol inhibits ADH release, leading to increased urine production and potential dehydration.

Plant-Based Diet and Antidiuretic Hormone Regulation

A plant-based diet, rich in fruits, vegetables, whole grains, nuts, and seeds, can have a significant impact on ADH regulation through various mechanisms:

1. Hydration and Electrolyte Balance

- **High Water Content Foods:** Plant-based diets typically include foods with high water content, such as fruits and vegetables. These foods help maintain adequate hydration levels, reducing the need for excessive ADH release.
- **Electrolyte Balance:** Many plant-based foods are rich in potassium and magnesium, which support electrolyte balance and proper kidney function, aiding in optimal ADH activity.

2. Antioxidants and Anti-Inflammatory Compounds

- **Oxidative Stress Reduction:** Antioxidant-rich foods, such as berries, leafy greens, and nuts, help reduce oxidative stress, which can influence ADH regulation and overall endocrine function.
- **Anti-Inflammatory Effects:** Plant-based diets are known for their anti-inflammatory properties, which can positively impact ADH levels by reducing inflammation-related disruptions in hormonal balance.

3. Weight Management and Insulin Sensitivity

- **Healthy Weight Maintenance:** A plant-based diet supports healthy weight management, reducing the risk of obesity-related conditions that can affect ADH levels, such as sleep apnea and hypertension.
- **Improved Insulin Sensitivity:** Plant-based eating can enhance insulin sensitivity, which is associated with better hydration status and more stable ADH levels.

4. Impact on Blood Pressure

- **Blood Pressure Regulation:** Plant-based diets are effective in lowering blood pressure, which can influence ADH regulation. Foods high in nitrates, like leafy greens and beets, help dilate blood vessels, potentially reducing the need for ADH-mediated vasoconstriction.

5. Stress and Mental Health

- **Stress Reduction:** A plant-based diet can improve mental health and reduce stress levels, impacting the HPA axis and subsequently

ADH release. Nutrients like omega-3 fatty acids, found in flaxseeds and walnuts, play a role in mental well-being.

- **Mood Stabilization:** Foods rich in tryptophan, such as seeds and nuts, can enhance serotonin production, promoting a balanced mood and potentially influencing ADH regulation.

Impact of Plant-Based Diet on Antidiuretic Hormone-Related Health Outcomes

1. Hydration Status

A plant-based diet supports optimal hydration status through high water content foods and electrolyte balance. This can lead to more stable ADH levels and improved overall hydration.

2. Kidney Health

Plant-based diets are beneficial for kidney health, reducing the risk of kidney stones and chronic kidney disease. Improved kidney function supports the effective action of ADH in maintaining water balance.

3. Blood Pressure Control

The blood pressure-lowering effects of plant-based diets can reduce the need for ADH-mediated vasoconstriction, promoting cardiovascular health and reducing the risk of hypertension-related complications.

4. Weight Management

Maintaining a healthy weight through a plant-based diet can prevent obesity-related suppression of ADH. Excess body fat, particularly visceral fat, is linked to altered ADH levels due to increased production of stress hormones and inflammatory markers.

5. Mental Health and Stress Management

Improved mental health and stress management through a plant-based diet can positively influence ADH levels, reducing stress-induced disruptions in hormone balance and promoting overall endocrine health.

Antidiuretic hormone plays a pivotal role in water balance, blood pressure regulation, and social behaviors. Its production and regulation are influenced by various factors, including hydration status, blood pressure, stress, and diet. A plant-based diet, rich in essential nutrients, antioxidants, and anti-inflammatory compounds, supports optimal ADH function and balance.

Oxytocin

Oxytocin, often referred to as the "love hormone" or "cuddle hormone," plays a significant role in social bonding, reproduction, childbirth, and the period following childbirth. This comprehensive analysis delves into the function, production, and regulation of oxytocin, particularly from a plant-based viewpoint, highlighting dietary influences on its activity and balance.

Function of Oxytocin

Oxytocin's primary functions encompass various physiological and psychological processes:

1. Social Bonding and Emotional Regulation

Oxytocin is crucial for forming social bonds and emotional connections. It enhances trust, empathy, and social recognition, fostering healthy interpersonal relationships. The hormone is also associated with the ability to read emotional cues and respond appropriately, promoting social cohesion.

2. Reproductive Functions

Oxytocin is vital in several reproductive processes:

- **Labor and Delivery:** It stimulates uterine contractions during labor, facilitating childbirth. The hormone is often administered medically to induce labor or strengthen contractions.

- **Breastfeeding:** Postpartum, oxytocin triggers milk ejection from the mammary glands, essential for breastfeeding.

3. Stress Reduction

Oxytocin can mitigate the effects of stress by reducing levels of cortisol, the primary stress hormone. Its anxiolytic effects contribute to emotional stability and reduce stress-related disorders.

4. Healing and Growth

Oxytocin promotes healing and regeneration by influencing cell growth and reducing inflammation. It enhances wound healing processes and may improve muscle recovery post-injury.

Production of Oxytocin

Oxytocin is synthesized and released through a complex interplay of neural and hormonal signals:

1. Synthesis and Secretion

Oxytocin is produced by the hypothalamus and secreted by the posterior pituitary gland. The hormone is synthesized in magnocellular neurosecretory cells of the hypothalamus and then transported down axons to the posterior pituitary for storage and release into the bloodstream.

2. Stimuli for Release

Various stimuli trigger oxytocin release:

- **Social Interactions:** Positive social interactions, such as hugging, touching, and other forms of physical contact, stimulate oxytocin release.
- **Childbirth and Nursing:** Stretching of the cervix and uterus during labor and stimulation of the nipples during breastfeeding are potent triggers.
- **Stress Response:** In some cases, mild stress can prompt oxytocin release as part of the body's effort to mitigate stress effects.

Regulation of Oxytocin

Oxytocin regulation involves multiple feedback mechanisms and external factors:

1. Positive Feedback Loops

Oxytocin operates primarily through positive feedback mechanisms. For example, during childbirth, oxytocin-induced uterine contractions stimulate more oxytocin release, intensifying contractions until delivery is achieved.

2. External Influences

Several external factors influence oxytocin levels:

- **Social Environment:** A supportive social environment enhances oxytocin release, while social isolation can reduce it.
- **Physical Touch:** Physical touch, such as massages and affectionate gestures, directly increases oxytocin levels.
- **Dietary Factors:** Nutrients and dietary patterns can modulate oxytocin levels, impacting its production and release.

Plant-Based Diet and Oxytocin Regulation

A plant-based diet can profoundly impact oxytocin regulation through various mechanisms:

1. Nutrient Density

Plant-based diets are rich in essential nutrients, vitamins, and minerals that support overall health and hormonal balance. For instance, magnesium, found abundantly in leafy greens and nuts, is crucial for nerve function and can influence oxytocin production.

2. Amino Acids

Certain amino acids, such as tryptophan and phenylalanine, are precursors to neurotransmitters that interact with oxytocin. Foods like legumes, nuts, and seeds provide these essential amino acids, supporting neurotransmitter synthesis and hormonal balance.

3. Antioxidants

Fruits and vegetables are rich in antioxidants, which help reduce oxidative stress and inflammation. Lower oxidative stress levels are associated with improved hormonal balance, including oxytocin production.

4. Healthy Fats

Plant-based sources of fats, such as avocados, nuts, and seeds, provide essential fatty acids that support hormone production and regulation. Omega-3 fatty acids, in particular, have anti-inflammatory properties that can enhance oxytocin activity.

5. Fiber

High-fiber diets, common in plant-based eating, support gut health and hormone regulation. A healthy gut microbiome can influence oxytocin levels through the production of short-chain fatty acids and other metabolites.

6. Caloric Balance

Maintaining a healthy weight through a balanced plant-based diet can prevent obesity-related suppression of oxytocin. Excess body fat, particularly visceral fat, is linked to lower oxytocin levels due to increased inflammation and hormonal imbalances.

7. Glycemic Control

Plant-based diets, which are low in refined sugars and high in complex carbohydrates, help maintain stable blood glucose levels. This stability prevents hyperglycemia-induced suppression of oxytocin secretion.

Impact of Plant-Based Diet on Oxytocin-Related Health Outcomes

1. Mental Health and Emotional Well-being

Plant-based diets are associated with improved mental health outcomes. The rich supply of antioxidants, vitamins, and minerals found in plant foods can reduce oxidative stress and inflammation, which are linked to mood disorders. Improved oxytocin levels support emotional well-being and social interactions.

2. Reproductive Health

A nutrient-dense plant-based diet supports reproductive health by providing essential vitamins and minerals necessary for hormonal balance. For instance, folate, found in leafy greens, is crucial for fertility and pregnancy health.

3. Stress Reduction

Plant-based diets can enhance stress resilience through various mechanisms, including improved gut health and reduced inflammation. These factors support a more balanced hormonal environment, promoting better stress management and higher oxytocin levels.

4. Cardiovascular Health

Oxytocin has cardioprotective effects, including reducing blood pressure and promoting heart health. Plant-based diets, known for their cardiovascular benefits, support oxytocin's protective roles by providing heart-healthy nutrients like fiber, antioxidants, and healthy fats.

Oxytocin plays a pivotal role in social bonding, reproductive health, stress reduction, and healing processes. Its production and regulation are influenced by various factors, including social interactions, physical touch, stress, and diet. A plant-based diet, rich in essential nutrients, amino acids, antioxidants, and healthy fats, supports optimal oxytocin function and balance.

2

Thyroid Gland Hormones

Thyroxine (T4)

Thyroxine (T4) is one of the primary hormones produced by the thyroid gland, playing a crucial role in regulating metabolism, growth, and development.

Function of Thyroxine (T4)
Thyroxine is essential for several physiological processes, including:

1. **Metabolism Regulation**: T4 significantly impacts the body's metabolic rate. It increases the basal metabolic rate (BMR), influencing how the body converts nutrients into energy. This hormone stimulates the production of proteins and the breakdown of fats and carbohydrates.
2. **Growth and Development**: T4 is vital for normal growth and development, especially in children. It ensures proper development of the brain and nervous system during fetal life and early childhood.
3. **Thermoregulation**: Thyroxine helps regulate body temperature by influencing metabolic processes. An increase in T4 levels boosts heat production, helping maintain body temperature.

4. **Cardiovascular Function**: T4 increases heart rate and strengthens the force of heart contractions. It also enhances blood flow by dilating blood vessels.
5. **Mood and Cognitive Function**: T4 affects mood and cognitive functions. Adequate levels are necessary for maintaining mental health, while imbalances can lead to mood disorders and cognitive impairments.

Production of Thyroxine (T4)

The production of thyroxine involves several steps and regulatory mechanisms:

1. **Synthesis**: T4 is synthesized in the thyroid gland, located at the base of the neck. The process begins with the uptake of iodine from the bloodstream by thyroid cells. Iodine is essential for the synthesis of thyroid hormones.
2. **Iodination and Coupling**: Inside the thyroid gland, iodine atoms attach to the amino acid tyrosine in a process called iodination. Two molecules of iodinated tyrosine combine to form thyroxine (T4).
3. **Storage and Release**: T4 is stored in the thyroid gland as part of a larger protein called thyroglobulin. When the body needs T4, it is cleaved from thyroglobulin and released into the bloodstream.
4. **Regulation by Hypothalamus and Pituitary**: The production of T4 is regulated by the hypothalamus and pituitary gland. The hypothalamus releases thyrotropin-releasing hormone (TRH), which stimulates the pituitary gland to release thyroid-stimulating hormone (TSH). TSH then stimulates the thyroid gland to produce and release T4.

Regulation of Thyroxine (T4)

The regulation of T4 involves complex feedback mechanisms and external factors:

1. **Feedback Loops**: T4 levels are regulated through negative feedback loops. High levels of T4 inhibit the release of TRH and TSH, reducing the production of T4. Conversely, low levels of T4 stimulate the release of TRH and TSH, increasing T4 production.
2. **Iodine Levels**: Adequate iodine intake is crucial for T4 production. Iodine deficiency can lead to reduced T4 synthesis and hypothyroidism, while excess iodine can also disrupt thyroid function.
3. **Nutritional Status**: Various nutrients influence T4 production and regulation. Selenium, zinc, and iron are essential for thyroid hormone synthesis and metabolism.
4. **Environmental Factors**: Exposure to certain environmental toxins and pollutants can interfere with thyroid function and T4 production. For example, substances like perchlorate and certain pesticides can disrupt iodine uptake by the thyroid gland.
5. **Lifestyle Factors**: Stress, physical activity, and sleep patterns can impact thyroid function. Chronic stress and lack of sleep can disrupt the hypothalamic-pituitary-thyroid (HPT) axis, affecting T4 levels.

Plant-Based Diet and Thyroxine (T4) Regulation

A plant-based diet can have a significant impact on the regulation of T4 through various mechanisms:

1. **Nutrient Density**: Plant-based diets are rich in essential nutrients, including vitamins and minerals that support thyroid health. Foods like seaweed, nuts, seeds, and legumes provide iodine, selenium, and zinc, which are crucial for T4 production and regulation.
2. **Antioxidants**: Fruits and vegetables are high in antioxidants, which help reduce oxidative stress. Lower oxidative stress levels are associated with improved thyroid function and T4 production.
3. **Healthy Fats**: Plant-based sources of fats, such as avocados, nuts, and seeds, provide essential fatty acids that support hormone production and regulation. Omega-3 fatty acids, in particular, have anti-inflammatory properties that can enhance thyroid function.
4. **Fiber**: High-fiber diets support gut health and hormone regulation. A healthy gut microbiome can influence thyroid function through the production of short-chain fatty acids and other metabolites.
5. **Glycemic Control**: Plant-based diets, which are low in refined sugars and high in complex carbohydrates, help maintain stable blood glucose levels. Stable blood glucose prevents hyperglycemia-induced suppression of T4 secretion.

Impact of Plant-Based Diet on Thyroxine-Related Health Outcomes

1. **Hypothyroidism Management**: Hypothyroidism, characterized by low T4 levels, can benefit from a plant-based diet. Foods rich in iodine, selenium, and zinc support thyroid function and T4 production. Additionally, anti-inflammatory foods like berries, leafy greens, and turmeric can help reduce thyroid inflammation.
2. **Weight Management**: Maintaining a healthy weight through a balanced plant-based diet can prevent obesity-related suppression of thyroid function. Excess body fat, particularly visceral fat, is

linked to lower T4 levels due to increased production of inflammatory cytokines.

3. **Cardiovascular Health**: A plant-based diet can improve cardiovascular health by lowering cholesterol levels and reducing inflammation. Improved heart health supports overall metabolic function, including thyroid activity.
4. **Cognitive Function and Mood**: Plant-based diets rich in antioxidants and anti-inflammatory compounds support brain health and cognitive function. Adequate T4 levels are necessary for mental health, and a diet that supports thyroid function can help prevent mood disorders and cognitive impairments.
5. **Bone Health**: Plant-based diets provide essential nutrients like calcium, magnesium, and vitamin K, which support bone health. Proper thyroid function and T4 levels are crucial for maintaining bone density and reducing the risk of osteoporosis.

Thyroxine (T4) plays a pivotal role in regulating metabolism, growth, and development. Its production and regulation are influenced by various factors, including iodine levels, nutritional status, environmental toxins, and lifestyle factors. A plant-based diet, rich in essential nutrients, antioxidants, healthy fats, and fiber, supports optimal thyroid function and T4 balance.

Triiodothyronine (T3)

Triiodothyronine (T3) is one of the primary hormones produced by the thyroid gland, playing a vital role in regulating metabolism, growth, and development. This comprehensive analysis will explore the function, production, and regulation of T3, emphasizing how a plant-based diet can influence its activity and balance.

Function of Triiodothyronine (T3)
T3 is crucial for various physiological processes, including:

1. **Metabolic Regulation:** T3 significantly impacts basal metabolic rate (BMR), influencing how the body utilizes energy. It enhances oxygen consumption and heat production in tissues, thereby increasing energy expenditure.
2. **Protein Synthesis and Degradation:** T3 stimulates the synthesis of proteins and the breakdown of fats and carbohydrates. It promotes the growth and development of tissues by enhancing protein production while facilitating the mobilization of fat stores for energy.
3. **Growth and Development:** T3 is essential for normal growth and development, particularly in the central nervous system. It supports neuronal differentiation, myelination, and synaptic connectivity, which are crucial during fetal development and early childhood.
4. **Cardiovascular Health:** T3 influences heart rate, cardiac output, and blood pressure. It increases the responsiveness of the heart to catecholamines (e.g., adrenaline) and enhances the force of myocardial contractions, contributing to overall cardiovascular health.
5. **Thermoregulation:** By stimulating thermogenesis, T3 helps maintain body temperature. It achieves this by increasing the activity of uncoupling proteins in brown adipose tissue, which dissipate energy as heat.
6. **Mental Health:** Adequate T3 levels are associated with cognitive function, mood regulation, and emotional well-being. Imbalances in T3 can lead to mood disorders, including depression and anxiety.

Production of Triiodothyronine (T3)

The production of T3 involves several key steps:

1. **Synthesis in the Thyroid Gland:** T3 is synthesized in the thyroid gland, located in the neck, through the iodination of the amino acid tyrosine. The process involves the incorporation of iodine into the thyroglobulin protein, forming T3 and thyroxine (T4).
2. **Regulation by Thyroid-Stimulating Hormone (TSH):** The pituitary gland secretes TSH, which stimulates the thyroid gland to produce and release T3 and T4. TSH levels are regulated by the hypothalamus through thyrotropin-releasing hormone (TRH).
3. **Conversion from T4:** While a small amount of T3 is directly secreted by the thyroid gland, the majority of T3 is derived from the peripheral conversion of T4. This conversion occurs mainly in the liver and kidneys through the action of deiodinase enzymes.

Regulation of Triiodothyronine (T3)

The regulation of T3 involves complex feedback mechanisms and external factors:

1. **Feedback Loops:** T3 levels are regulated through negative feedback loops. High levels of T3 and T4 inhibit the release of TRH and TSH, reducing thyroid hormone production. Conversely, low levels of T3 stimulate the release of TRH and TSH, increasing hormone production.
2. **Dietary Iodine:** Iodine is a crucial component of T3, and adequate dietary intake is essential for thyroid hormone synthesis. Sources of iodine include sea vegetables (e.g., seaweed), iodized salt, and certain fruits and vegetables grown in iodine-rich soil.
3. **Nutritional Status:** Overall nutritional status, including protein and micronutrient intake, affects T3 production and metabolism.

Nutrients such as selenium, zinc, and iron are vital for thyroid function and hormone synthesis.

4. **Hormonal Interactions:** Other hormones, including cortisol and estrogen, influence T3 levels. Elevated cortisol levels (e.g., during stress) can suppress T3 production, while estrogen levels can modulate the availability of thyroid-binding proteins.
5. **Environmental Factors:** Exposure to environmental toxins, such as heavy metals and endocrine-disrupting chemicals, can interfere with thyroid function and T3 production. Reducing exposure to these toxins supports optimal thyroid health.

Plant-Based Diet and Triiodothyronine (T3) Regulation

A plant-based diet can significantly impact T3 regulation through various mechanisms:

1. **Nutrient Density:** Plant-based diets are rich in essential nutrients, including vitamins, minerals, and antioxidants, which support thyroid function. For example, selenium, found in Brazil nuts, and zinc, found in legumes and whole grains, are crucial for the conversion of T4 to T3.
2. **Iodine Sources:** Sea vegetables such as nori, dulse, and kelp are excellent sources of iodine, essential for T3 synthesis. Ensuring adequate iodine intake from plant-based sources supports thyroid hormone production.
3. **Antioxidants:** Fruits and vegetables are rich in antioxidants, which help reduce oxidative stress and inflammation. Lower oxidative stress levels are associated with improved thyroid function and T3 production.
4. **Healthy Fats:** Plant-based sources of fats, such as avocados, nuts, and seeds, provide essential fatty acids that support hormone production and regulation. Omega-3 fatty acids, in particular, have anti-inflammatory properties that can enhance thyroid health.

5. **Fiber:** High-fiber diets, common in plant-based eating, support gut health and hormone regulation. A healthy gut microbiome can influence thyroid function and T3 levels through the production of short-chain fatty acids and other metabolites.
6. **Glycemic Control:** Plant-based diets, which are low in refined sugars and high in complex carbohydrates, help maintain stable blood glucose levels. This stability prevents hyperglycemia-induced suppression of T3 secretion.

Impact of Plant-Based Diet on T3-Related Health Outcomes

1. **Metabolism and Weight Management:** A plant-based diet can support healthy metabolism and weight management. Studies have shown that plant-based diets are effective for weight loss and improving insulin sensitivity, which can enhance T3 levels and metabolic health.
2. **Cardiovascular Health:** Plant-based diets are associated with improved cardiovascular health, including lower blood pressure, cholesterol levels, and reduced risk of heart disease. These benefits are partly mediated by optimal T3 levels, which support cardiovascular function.
3. **Cognitive Function:** Emerging evidence suggests that plant-based diets may benefit cognitive function and mental health by reducing inflammation and oxidative stress, which are linked to mood disorders. Improved T3 levels also support cognitive function and emotional well-being.
4. **Thyroid Health:** A well-balanced plant-based diet can support overall thyroid health by providing essential nutrients and reducing exposure to environmental toxins. This dietary approach helps maintain optimal T3 levels and prevents thyroid disorders such as hypothyroidism.

Triiodothyronine (T3) plays a pivotal role in regulating metabolism, growth, and overall health. Its production and regulation are influenced by various factors, including dietary intake, nutritional status, and environmental exposures. A plant-based diet, rich in essential nutrients, iodine sources, antioxidants, and healthy fats, supports optimal T3 function and balance.

3

Parathyrold Gland Hormones

Parathyroid Hormone (PTH)

Parathyroid hormone (PTH), also known as parathormone, is a critical peptide hormone secreted by the parathyroid glands. It plays a vital role in regulating calcium levels in the blood and bone metabolism.

Function of Parathyroid Hormone

Parathyroid hormone serves several key functions in maintaining calcium homeostasis and bone health:

Regulation of Blood Calcium Levels: PTH is the primary hormone responsible for maintaining adequate calcium levels in the blood. When calcium levels drop, PTH is released to restore balance by:

- Stimulating osteoclasts to break down bone tissue, releasing calcium into the bloodstream.
- Increasing calcium reabsorption in the kidneys, reducing calcium loss through urine.
- Enhancing the activation of vitamin D in the kidneys increases calcium absorption from the intestines.

Bone Remodeling: PTH plays a crucial role in bone remodeling, a continuous process where old bone is replaced by new bone tissue.

PTH stimulates osteoclast activity, leading to bone resorption, which releases calcium into the blood. This process is balanced by osteoblast activity, which forms new bone.

Phosphate Regulation: PTH helps regulate phosphate metabolism by reducing phosphate reabsorption in the kidneys, leading to increased excretion of phosphate in the urine. This action helps prevent hyperphosphatemia (high phosphate levels in the blood), which can disrupt calcium balance.

Magnesium Homeostasis: PTH also influences magnesium levels in the body. It increases magnesium reabsorption in the kidneys, which helps maintain adequate magnesium levels essential for various physiological processes, including enzyme function and muscle contraction.

Production of Parathyroid Hormone

Parathyroid hormone is produced by the parathyroid glands, four small glands located on the posterior surface of the thyroid gland. The production process involves several steps:

1. **Synthesis**: PTH is synthesized as a preprohormone, preproparathyroid hormone, in the ribosomes of the parathyroid gland cells. It undergoes cleavage to form proparathyroid hormone, which is further processed to produce the active hormone, PTH.
2. **Storage and Secretion**: The active PTH is stored in secretory granules within the parathyroid cells. When calcium levels in the blood fall below a certain threshold, these cells rapidly release PTH into the bloodstream.
3. **Regulation by Calcium-Sensing Receptors (CaSRs)**: The activity of the parathyroid glands is regulated by calcium-sensing receptors located on the surface of the parathyroid cells. These receptors detect changes in blood calcium levels and modulate PTH secretion accordingly. When calcium levels are low, CaSRs trigger the release of PTH, and when calcium levels are high, they inhibit PTH secretion.

Regulation of Parathyroid Hormone

The regulation of PTH involves complex feedback mechanisms and various factors:

1. **Negative Feedback Loop**: PTH secretion is primarily regulated through a negative feedback loop involving blood calcium levels. High calcium levels inhibit PTH release, while low calcium levels stimulate it. This feedback mechanism ensures that calcium levels remain within a narrow physiological range.
2. **Vitamin D**: Active vitamin D (calcitriol) plays a significant role in regulating PTH. Increased levels of calcitriol suppress PTH synthesis and release. This regulation is crucial for maintaining calcium balance, as calcitriol enhances calcium absorption from the intestines.
3. **Phosphate Levels**: Elevated phosphate levels in the blood can stimulate PTH secretion. This response helps increase phosphate excretion by the kidneys, thereby reducing phosphate levels and maintaining calcium-phosphate balance.
4. **Magnesium Levels**: Magnesium deficiency can lead to impaired PTH secretion and action. Adequate magnesium levels are necessary for the proper function of the calcium-sensing receptors and PTH release.

Plant-Based Diet and Parathyroid Hormone Regulation

A plant-based diet, rich in fruits, vegetables, whole grains, nuts, and seeds, can significantly influence PTH regulation through various mechanisms:

1. **Calcium Intake**: Plant-based diets provide an adequate amount of calcium through leafy greens, fortified plant milks, tofu, almonds, and sesame seeds. Maintaining adequate calcium intake

helps regulate PTH secretion by preventing hypocalcemia (low blood calcium levels).

2. **Vitamin D**: Plant-based sources of vitamin D, such as fortified plant milks and exposure to sunlight, are essential for calcium absorption and PTH regulation. Adequate vitamin D levels help suppress excessive PTH secretion and support calcium homeostasis.
3. **Phytates and Oxalates**: Certain plant compounds, such as phytates and oxalates, can interfere with calcium absorption. However, a well-planned plant-based diet that includes a variety of foods can mitigate these effects. For example, soaking and cooking beans and grains can reduce phytate content, and consuming calcium-rich foods along with vitamin C-rich foods can enhance calcium absorption.
4. **Magnesium**: Plant-based diets are typically high in magnesium, found in foods like spinach, nuts, seeds, and whole grains. Adequate magnesium intake supports PTH secretion and action, contributing to calcium homeostasis.
5. **Protein Intake**: Adequate protein intake from plant sources, such as legumes, nuts, and seeds, is crucial for bone health. Protein supports bone matrix formation and can influence calcium metabolism, indirectly affecting PTH regulation.

Plant-Based Diet on Parathyroid Hormone-Related Health Outcomes

1. **Bone Health**: A plant-based diet rich in calcium, magnesium, and vitamin K supports bone health. Leafy greens, fortified plant milk, nuts, and seeds are excellent sources of these nutrients, which work synergistically with PTH to maintain bone density and reduce the risk of osteoporosis.
2. **Calcium Homeostasis**: Consuming a variety of plant-based calcium sources helps maintain stable calcium levels in the blood,

preventing hypocalcemia and excessive PTH secretion. This balance is essential for bone health and overall metabolic functions.

3. **Kidney Health**: Plant-based diets are generally lower in phosphorus compared to animal-based diets. This lower phosphorus intake helps regulate phosphate levels and prevents hyperphosphatemia, reducing the burden on the kidneys and lowering PTH levels.
4. **Cardiovascular Health**: High PTH levels are associated with cardiovascular risk factors such as hypertension and vascular calcification. A plant-based diet, rich in antioxidants and anti-inflammatory compounds, can help reduce these risks by maintaining optimal PTH levels and supporting cardiovascular health.
5. **Weight Management**: Plant-based diets are effective for weight management, reducing body fat and improving insulin sensitivity. Lower body fat can enhance calcium metabolism and reduce PTH levels, contributing to better metabolic health.

Parathyroid hormone plays a pivotal role in maintaining calcium homeostasis, bone health, and overall metabolic functions. Its production and regulation are influenced by various factors, including blood calcium levels, vitamin D, phosphate, and magnesium. A plant-based diet, rich in essential nutrients, vitamins, and minerals, supports optimal PTH function and balance.

4

Adrenal Gland Hormones

Cortisol

Cortisol, often referred to as the "stress hormone," is a steroid hormone that plays a crucial role in various bodily functions, including metabolism, immune response, and stress regulation. This comprehensive analysis will delve into the function, production, and regulation of cortisol, particularly from a plant-based viewpoint, highlighting dietary influences on its activity and balance.

Function of Cortisol

Cortisol's primary functions are to help the body respond to stress, regulate metabolism, and maintain homeostasis. It achieves these by:

1. Stress Response

Cortisol is pivotal in the body's response to stress. It is part of the hypothalamic-pituitary-adrenal (HPA) axis and is released in response to stressors such as physical injury, emotional stress, or infection.

- **Fight-or-Flight Response**: During stressful situations, cortisol prepares the body for a fight-or-flight response by increasing heart rate, blood pressure, and energy supplies. It achieves this by:
    - **Increasing glucose availability**: Cortisol stimulates gluconeogenesis, the production of glucose from non-carbohydrate sources, in the liver to ensure adequate energy supply.

  - **Enhancing fat and protein metabolism**: It promotes the breakdown of fats and proteins to provide energy and repair tissues.
- **Immune Response Modulation**: Cortisol has immunosuppressive properties that help reduce inflammation and modulate the immune response during stress, preventing overactivation of the immune system.

2. Metabolic Effects

Cortisol plays a significant role in metabolism, influencing how the body uses carbohydrates, fats, and proteins.

- **Blood Sugar Regulation**: It helps maintain blood glucose levels by stimulating gluconeogenesis and inhibiting insulin's effects, ensuring a constant energy supply.
- **Fat Metabolism**: Cortisol promotes lipolysis, the breakdown of fat stores in adipose tissue, releasing fatty acids into the bloodstream for energy.
- **Protein Metabolism**: It stimulates protein catabolism in muscles, releasing amino acids for gluconeogenesis and tissue repair.

3. Maintenance of Homeostasis

Cortisol helps maintain homeostasis by regulating various physiological processes.

- **Blood Pressure Regulation**: It supports vascular tone and fluid balance, contributing to blood pressure regulation.
- **Electrolyte Balance**: Cortisol influences sodium and potassium balance in the kidneys, affecting fluid retention and blood pressure.
- **Circadian Rhythm**: Cortisol levels follow a diurnal pattern, peaking in the morning and declining throughout the day, helping regulate sleep-wake cycles.

Production of Cortisol

Cortisol is produced by the adrenal glands, small glands located on top of each kidney. The production process involves several steps:

1. Synthesis

Cortisol is synthesized from cholesterol in the adrenal cortex, specifically in the zona fasciculata. The process involves multiple enzymatic steps, including the conversion of cholesterol to pregnenolone and subsequently to cortisol.

2. Regulation by the Hypothalamus and Pituitary Gland

The production of cortisol is regulated by the HPA axis, involving the hypothalamus, pituitary gland, and adrenal glands.

- **Hypothalamus**: The hypothalamus releases corticotropin-releasing hormone (CRH) in response to stress or low cortisol levels.
- **Pituitary Gland**: CRH stimulates the anterior pituitary gland to release adrenocorticotropic hormone (ACTH).
- **Adrenal Glands:** ACTH stimulates the adrenal cortex to synthesize and release cortisol.

3. Feedback Mechanisms

Cortisol production is regulated through negative feedback loops. High levels of cortisol inhibit the release of CRH and ACTH, reducing cortisol synthesis. Conversely, low cortisol levels stimulate CRH and ACTH release, increasing cortisol production.

4. Influencing Factors

Several factors influence cortisol production, including:

- **Stress**: Physical, emotional, and psychological stressors significantly increase cortisol levels.
- **Circadian Rhythm**: Cortisol follows a daily pattern, peaking in the early morning and declining in the evening.

- **Nutritional Status**: Diet and nutritional status can impact cortisol production. For instance, hypoglycemia can stimulate cortisol release.

Regulation of Cortisol

The regulation of cortisol involves complex feedback mechanisms and external factors:

1. Feedback Loops

Cortisol levels are primarily regulated through negative feedback loops involving the HPA axis. High cortisol levels inhibit CRH and ACTH release, reducing cortisol synthesis, while low levels stimulate their release, increasing cortisol production.

2. Stress Response

Acute and chronic stress significantly impact cortisol levels. Acute stress triggers a rapid increase in cortisol to prepare the body for immediate challenges, while chronic stress can lead to prolonged elevated cortisol levels, potentially causing adverse health effects.

3. Sleep and Circadian Rhythms

Cortisol follows a circadian rhythm, with levels peaking in the early morning and declining throughout the day. Disrupted sleep patterns or poor sleep quality can alter this rhythm, leading to dysregulated cortisol levels.

4. Physical Activity

Exercise influences cortisol levels, with intensity and duration playing key roles. Moderate exercise can increase cortisol transiently, supporting energy demands and recovery, while chronic overtraining may lead to persistently elevated cortisol levels.

5. Nutrition and Diet

Diet significantly affects cortisol regulation. Balanced nutrition supports optimal cortisol levels, while certain dietary patterns, such as high sugar intake, can disrupt cortisol balance.

Plant-Based Diet and Cortisol Regulation

A plant-based diet, rich in fruits, vegetables, whole grains, nuts, and seeds, can profoundly impact cortisol regulation through various mechanisms:

1. Nutrient Density

Plant-based diets are typically high in essential nutrients, vitamins, and minerals that support overall health and hormonal balance.

- **Vitamin C**: Found in citrus fruits, berries, and leafy greens, vitamin C plays a crucial role in adrenal function and cortisol synthesis. It helps reduce cortisol levels during stress by supporting the adrenal glands.
- **Magnesium**: Present in nuts, seeds, and leafy greens, magnesium helps regulate the HPA axis and reduces cortisol production during stress.

2. Antioxidants

Fruits and vegetables are rich in antioxidants, which help reduce oxidative stress. Lower oxidative stress levels are associated with improved cortisol regulation and overall endocrine function.

- **Polyphenols**: Found in foods like berries, tea, and dark chocolate, polyphenols have anti-inflammatory and antioxidant properties that help modulate cortisol levels and reduce stress.

3. Fiber

High-fiber diets, common in plant-based eating, support gut health and hormone regulation. A healthy gut microbiome can influence cortisol levels through the production of short-chain fatty acids and other metabolites.

- **Prebiotics**: Foods like garlic, onions, and bananas contain prebiotics that support gut health and can positively impact cortisol levels by promoting a healthy gut microbiome.

4. Healthy Fats

Plant-based sources of fats, such as avocados, nuts, and seeds, provide essential fatty acids that support hormone production and regulation. Omega-3 fatty acids, in particular, have anti-inflammatory properties that can enhance cortisol activity.

- **Omega-3 Fatty Acids**: Found in flaxseeds, chia seeds, and walnuts, omega-3 fatty acids help reduce inflammation and cortisol levels, promoting stress resilienc.

5. Glycemic Control

Plant-based diets, which are low in refined sugars and high in complex carbohydrates, help maintain stable blood glucose levels. This stability prevents hyperglycemia-induced suppression of cortisol secretion.

- **Low Glycemic Index Foods**: Whole grains, legumes, and vegetables have a low glycemic index, which helps maintain stable blood sugar levels and prevent cortisol spikes.

6. Phytochemicals

Plant foods are rich in phytochemicals, which have various health benefits, including stress reduction and cortisol regulation.

- **Adaptogens**: Certain plant-based adaptogens, such as ashwagandha and Rhodiola, have been shown to reduce cortisol levels and improve stress response.

Plant-Based Diet on Cortisol-Related Health Outcomes

1. Stress and Mental Health

Plant-based diets may positively impact mental health by reducing inflammation and oxidative stress, which are linked to mood disorders. Improved cortisol levels also support cognitive function and emotional well-being.

- **Reduced Inflammation**: Anti-inflammatory compounds in plant foods, such as flavonoids, can help reduce systemic inflammation and cortisol levels, improving stress resilience.
- **Enhanced Mood**: Nutrients like magnesium and omega-3 fatty acids found in plant foods support neurotransmitter function and mood regulation, contributing to lower cortisol levels and better mental health.

2. Immune Function

A balanced cortisol level is essential for proper immune function. Plant-based diets, rich in vitamins and minerals, support immune health and cortisol balance.

- **Vitamin D**: Found in fortified plant milks and mushrooms, vitamin D is crucial for immune function and can help modulate cortisol levels.

3. Weight Management

Plant-based diets are effective for weight management, reducing body fat, and improving insulin sensitivity. Lower body fat and better glycemic control enhance cortisol regulation and overall metabolic health.

- **Reduced Visceral Fat**: High-fiber, low-calorie plant foods help reduce visceral fat, which is associated with lower cortisol levels.

4. Cardiovascular Health

Cortisol plays a role in blood pressure regulation and cardiovascular health. A plant-based diet can support heart health and improve cortisol balance.

- **Potassium-Rich Foods**: Bananas, sweet potatoes, and spinach are high in potassium, which helps regulate blood pressure and reduce the cardiovascular strain associated with high cortisol levels.

5. Anti-Aging Effects

The antioxidant-rich nature of plant-based diets helps combat oxidative stress, a key factor in aging. Improved cortisol levels, coupled with reduced oxidative damage, contribute to healthier aging and better maintenance of overall health.

- **Reduced Oxidative Stress**: Antioxidants in plant foods help neutralize free radicals and reduce oxidative stress, supporting healthy cortisol levels and slowing the aging process.

6. Bone Health

Cortisol can affect bone health by influencing calcium metabolism. Plant-based diets rich in calcium, magnesium, and vitamin K support bone health and mitigate the negative effects of cortisol on bones.

- **Calcium-Rich Foods**: Leafy greens, fortified plant milk, and tofu provide calcium, which is essential for bone health and can counteract the bone-resorptive effects of high cortisol levels.

Cortisol plays a pivotal role in stress response, metabolism, and maintaining homeostasis throughout life. Its production and regulation are influenced by various factors, including stress, sleep, exercise, and diet.

Aldosterone

Aldosterone, a mineralocorticoid hormone, plays a critical role in maintaining blood pressure, electrolyte balance, and fluid homeostasis. This comprehensive analysis will delve into the function, production, and regulation of aldosterone, highlighting the dietary influences on its activity and balance, particularly from a plant-based viewpoint.

Function of Aldosterone

Aldosterone primarily functions to regulate sodium and potassium levels in the body, thereby controlling blood pressure and fluid balance. Its major functions include:

1. Sodium Retention

Aldosterone promotes the reabsorption of sodium ions (Na^+) in the distal tubules and collecting ducts of the kidneys. This process increases sodium retention, which in turn helps to maintain blood volume and pressure.

2. Potassium Excretion

Simultaneously, aldosterone facilitates the excretion of potassium ions (K^+) through the urine. This balance is crucial for normal cellular function, particularly in muscle and nerve cells.

3. Water Balance

By enhancing sodium reabsorption, aldosterone indirectly promotes water retention through osmosis. This helps maintain adequate blood volume and pressure, essential for proper cardiovascular function.

4. Acid-Base Balance

Aldosterone also plays a role in maintaining acid-base balance by promoting the excretion of hydrogen ions (H^+), which helps regulate blood pH levels.

Production of Aldosterone

Aldosterone is synthesized and secreted by the adrenal glands, specifically the zona glomerulosa of the adrenal cortex. The production process involves several steps:

1. Synthesis

The synthesis of aldosterone begins with cholesterol, which is converted into pregnenolone by the enzyme cholesterol side-chain cleavage enzyme (P450scc). This is the first step in the steroidogenesis pathway.

2. Conversion to Aldosterone

Pregnenolone undergoes a series of enzymatic reactions to form aldosterone. Key enzymes involved in this process include:

- 3β-Hydroxysteroid dehydrogenase (3β-HSD)
- 21-Hydroxylase (CYP21A2)
- 11β-Hydroxylase (CYP11B2)

3. Regulation by the Renin-Angiotensin-Aldosterone System (RAAS)

The RAAS plays a pivotal role in regulating aldosterone production. The system involves:

- **Renin**: Secreted by the juxtaglomerular cells of the kidneys in response to low blood pressure, low sodium levels, or sympathetic nervous system stimulation.
- **Angiotensin II**: Formed from angiotensin I by the action of angiotensin-converting enzyme (ACE). Angiotensin II stimulates the adrenal cortex to produce aldosterone.

4. Influencing Factors

Several factors influence aldosterone production, including:

- **Blood Pressure**: Low blood pressure triggers renin release, leading to increased aldosterone production.
- **Sodium Levels**: Low sodium levels stimulate renin release, enhancing aldosterone synthesis.
- **Potassium Levels**: High potassium levels directly stimulate aldosterone secretion.

Regulation of Aldosterone

The regulation of aldosterone involves a complex interplay of feedback mechanisms and external factors:

1. Feedback Loops

Aldosterone levels are regulated through negative feedback loops. High levels of aldosterone and increased blood pressure inhibit renin release, thereby reducing aldosterone production.

2. Renin-Angiotensin-Aldosterone System (RAAS)

The RAAS is a key regulatory pathway for aldosterone. Renin release is stimulated by low blood pressure, low sodium levels, and sympathetic nervous system activation. Angiotensin II, a product of this system, directly stimulates aldosterone synthesis.

3. Potassium Levels

Elevated potassium levels in the blood directly stimulate the adrenal cortex to secrete aldosterone, ensuring proper potassium excretion and balance.

4. Adrenocorticotropic Hormone (ACTH)

ACTH, released by the pituitary gland, can also influence aldosterone production, although its effect is less significant compared to the RAAS.

Plant-Based Diet and Aldosterone Regulation

A plant-based diet, rich in fruits, vegetables, whole grains, nuts, and seeds, can significantly impact aldosterone regulation through various mechanisms:

1. Nutrient Density

Plant-based diets are high in essential nutrients, vitamins, and minerals that support overall health and hormonal balance. For example, potassium-rich foods like bananas, potatoes, and spinach can help regulate aldosterone levels by maintaining electrolyte balance.

2. Antioxidants

Fruits and vegetables are rich in antioxidants, which help reduce oxidative stress. Lower oxidative stress levels are associated with improved adrenal function and optimal aldosterone regulation.

3. Healthy Fats

Plant-based sources of fats, such as avocados, nuts, and seeds, provide essential fatty acids that support hormone production and regulation. Omega-3 fatty acids, in particular, have anti-inflammatory properties that can enhance adrenal function.

4. Fiber

High-fiber diets, common in plant-based eating, support gut health and hormone regulation. A healthy gut microbiome can influence aldosterone levels through the production of short-chain fatty acids and other metabolites.

5. Caloric Balance

Maintaining a healthy weight through a balanced plant-based diet can prevent obesity-related suppression of aldosterone. Excess body fat is linked to altered adrenal function and dysregulated hormone levels.

6. Glycemic Control

Plant-based diets, which are low in refined sugars and high in complex carbohydrates, help maintain stable blood glucose levels. This stability prevents hyperglycemia-induced hormonal imbalances that can affect aldosterone production.

Plant-Based Diet on Aldosterone-Related Health Outcomes

1. Blood Pressure Management

A plant-based diet can help regulate blood pressure by providing potassium-rich foods that counteract the effects of sodium. This balance is crucial for maintaining healthy aldosterone levels and preventing hypertension.

2. Electrolyte Balance

Consuming a variety of fruits and vegetables ensures an adequate intake of essential electrolytes like potassium and magnesium. These minerals play a significant role in aldosterone regulation and overall electrolyte balance.

3. Kidney Health

Plant-based diets support kidney health by reducing the risk of kidney stones and promoting proper kidney function. This can enhance the kidneys' ability to regulate aldosterone and maintain fluid balance.

4. Cardiovascular Health

By promoting a healthy balance of electrolytes and reducing oxidative stress, a plant-based diet supports cardiovascular health. Proper aldosterone regulation is essential for maintaining blood pressure and preventing cardiovascular diseases.

5. Anti-Inflammatory Effects

The anti-inflammatory properties of a plant-based diet can help reduce chronic inflammation, which is associated with various hormonal imbalances, including those affecting aldosterone production.

6. Weight Management

A plant-based diet is effective for weight management, reducing body fat, and improving insulin sensitivity. Lower body fat and better glycemic control enhance adrenal function and optimal aldosterone regulation.

Aldosterone plays a crucial role in regulating blood pressure, electrolyte balance, and fluid homeostasis. Its production and regulation are influenced by various factors, including the renin-angiotensin-aldosterone system, blood pressure, electrolyte levels, and hormonal feedback mechanisms.

Epinephrine

Epinephrine, commonly known as adrenaline, is a critical hormone and neurotransmitter involved in the body's response to stress, often referred to as the "fight or flight" response.

Function of Epinephrine

Epinephrine serves several vital roles in the body, particularly in response to stress and danger:

1. Cardiovascular Effects

Epinephrine increases heart rate, contracts blood vessels, and dilates air passages. This is crucial for the immediate physical readiness required in stressful situations. By stimulating β1-adrenergic receptors in the heart, it increases cardiac output and blood flow to essential organs.

2. Metabolic Effects

Epinephrine stimulates glycogenolysis in the liver and muscles, converting glycogen to glucose, thus providing a rapid energy source. It also promotes lipolysis, breaking down fat stores into free fatty acids and glycerol, which can be used for energy.

3. Respiratory Effects

Epinephrine causes bronchodilation, expanding the airways and improving oxygen intake. This is particularly beneficial during physical exertion or in conditions like asthma.

4. Nervous System Effects

As a neurotransmitter, epinephrine enhances alertness, arousal, and focus. It prepares the brain and body to react quickly to a threat by improving cognitive functions and sensory perception.

5. Muscular Effects

Epinephrine increases blood flow to skeletal muscles, preparing them for rapid and intense activity. This effect is crucial for physical performance and endurance.

6. Immune System Modulation

Epinephrine can modulate the immune response, reducing inflammation and the release of certain cytokines. This helps in managing acute stress responses without triggering excessive immune activity.

Production of Epinephrine

Epinephrine is produced mainly in the adrenal medulla, the inner part of the adrenal glands located on top of the kidneys. The production process involves several steps:

1. Synthesis

Epinephrine is synthesized from the amino acid tyrosine through a series of enzymatic reactions:

- **Tyrosine Hydroxylase:** Converts tyrosine to L-DOPA.
- **Aromatic L-Amino Acid Decarboxylase:** Converts L-DOPA to dopamine.
- **Dopamine β-Hydroxylase:** Converts dopamine to norepinephrine.
- **Phenylethanolamine N-Methyltransferase (PNMT):** Converts norepinephrine to epinephrine, predominantly in the adrenal medulla.

2. Storage and Release

Epinephrine is stored in chromaffin cells within the adrenal medulla. Upon stimulation by the sympathetic nervous system (SNS), it is released into the bloodstream, typically in response to stressors such as physical danger, emotional stress, or intense exercise.

3. Regulation by Hypothalamus and Pituitary

The hypothalamus and pituitary gland play a crucial role in regulating epinephrine production. The hypothalamus releases corticotropin-releasing hormone (CRH), stimulating the pituitary gland to release adrenocorticotropic hormone (ACTH), which in turn stimulates the adrenal medulla to produce epinephrine.

Regulation of Epinephrine

The regulation of epinephrine involves complex feedback mechanisms and external factors:

1. Sympathetic Nervous System (SNS)

The SNS directly controls the release of epinephrine. In response to stress, SNS activation leads to the release of acetylcholine, which stimulates chromaffin cells in the adrenal medulla to secrete epinephrine.

2. Feedback Loops

Negative feedback mechanisms ensure that epinephrine levels remain balanced. High levels of circulating epinephrine inhibit further release by reducing SNS activity and through feedback inhibition at the hypothalamic and pituitary levels.

3. Circadian Rhythms

Epinephrine levels exhibit diurnal variation, typically peaking in the morning and declining throughout the day. This pattern aligns with the body's circadian rhythm, preparing the body for daily activities and stressors.

4. Stress Response

Acute stress triggers a rapid increase in epinephrine production. Chronic stress, however, can lead to dysregulation, either through sustained high levels or eventual depletion, contributing to stress-related disorders.

5. Diet and Nutrition

Dietary factors can influence epinephrine production and regulation. Nutrient intake, particularly of amino acids like tyrosine, plays a role in synthesizing epinephrine.

Plant-Based Diet and Epinephrine Regulation

A plant-based diet, rich in fruits, vegetables, whole grains, nuts, and seeds, can profoundly impact epinephrine regulation through various mechanisms:

1. Nutrient Density

Plant-based diets are typically high in essential nutrients, vitamins, and minerals that support overall health and hormonal balance. For example, vitamins C and B6, found in various fruits and vegetables, are crucial for synthesizing neurotransmitters, including epinephrine.

2. Amino Acids

Certain amino acids, such as tyrosine, found in plant foods like nuts, seeds, legumes, and soy products, are precursors to epinephrine. Adequate intake of these amino acids ensures proper synthesis and balance of this hormone.

3. Antioxidants

Fruits and vegetables are rich in antioxidants, which help reduce oxidative stress. Lower oxidative stress levels are associated with better regulation of the stress response and epinephrine levels.

4. Healthy Fats

Plant-based sources of fats, such as avocados, nuts, and seeds, provide essential fatty acids that support hormone production and regulation. Omega-3 fatty acids, in particular, have anti-inflammatory properties that can enhance epinephrine activity.

5. Fiber

High-fiber diets, common in plant-based eating, support gut health and hormone regulation. A healthy gut microbiome can influence epinephrine levels through the production of short-chain fatty acids and other metabolites.

6. Glycemic Control

Plant-based diets, which are low in refined sugars and high in complex carbohydrates, help maintain stable blood glucose levels. This stability prevents hypoglycemia-induced epinephrine release and supports overall hormonal balance.

7. Anti-Inflammatory Effects

Plant-based diets are known for their anti-inflammatory properties. Chronic inflammation can disrupt hormonal balance, including epinephrine regulation. Reducing inflammation through diet can help maintain optimal epinephrine levels.

Plant-Based Diet on Epinephrine-Related Health Outcomes

1. Stress Management

A plant-based diet can help manage stress by supporting overall health and reducing the physiological impact of stress. Nutrient-dense foods, antioxidants, and healthy fats all contribute to better stress resilience and epinephrine regulation.

2. Cardiovascular Health

By promoting heart health and reducing the risk of hypertension and atherosclerosis, a plant-based diet indirectly supports the proper functioning of epinephrine in cardiovascular regulation. Foods rich in potassium, magnesium, and antioxidants are particularly beneficial.

3. Metabolic Health

A balanced plant-based diet supports metabolic health by improving insulin sensitivity and reducing the risk of metabolic syndrome. This helps regulate epinephrine's role in glucose metabolism and energy production.

4. Respiratory Health

Anti-inflammatory properties of plant-based diets can benefit respiratory health, potentially reducing the severity of conditions like asthma, where epinephrine is used as a treatment for bronchodilator.

5. Cognitive Function

Improved cognitive function and mental health are associated with plant-based diets, partly due to reduced inflammation and better nutrient profiles. Epinephrine, as a neurotransmitter, plays a role in cognitive alertness and focus, which can be supported by a healthy diet.

6. Weight Management

Maintaining a healthy weight through a plant-based diet can prevent obesity-related dysregulation of epinephrine. Excess body fat, particularly visceral fat, is linked to hormonal imbalances, including those affecting epinephrine.

7. Immune Function

The immune-modulating effects of a plant-based diet can help maintain a balanced stress response and optimal epinephrine levels. Nutrient-rich foods support overall immune health, reducing the burden on the body's stress response systems.

Epinephrine plays a critical role in the body's response to stress and danger, affecting various physiological systems including cardiovascular, metabolic, respiratory, and nervous systems. Its production and regulation are complex processes influenced by the sympathetic nervous system, feedback mechanisms, circadian rhythms, and diet.

Norepinephrine

Norepinephrine, also known as noradrenaline, is a critical hormone and neurotransmitter that plays a significant role in the body's fight-or-flight response, mood regulation, attention, and overall physiological balance. This comprehensive analysis delves into the function, production, and regulation of norepinephrine, particularly from a plant-based viewpoint, highlighting dietary influences on its activity and balance.

Function of Norepinephrine

Norepinephrine's primary functions include:

Fight-or-Flight Response: Norepinephrine is a key player in the body's acute stress response. It prepares the body to react to stressful situations by:

- Increasing heart rate and blood pressure.
- Expanding air passages in the lungs.
- Dilating the pupils.

- Redirecting blood flow to essential organs and muscles.

Mood Regulation: Norepinephrine has a substantial impact on mood and emotional stability. It is involved in the modulation of:

- **Arousal and Alertness**: Enhancing wakefulness and alertness, is crucial for responding to environmental stimuli.
- **Mood**: Low levels of norepinephrine are associated with depression and anxiety disorders.

Cognitive Function: Norepinephrine contributes to various cognitive processes, such as:

- **Attention**: Improving focus and concentration.
- **Memory Formation**: Enhancing the consolidation of memories.

Metabolic Effects: Norepinephrine influences metabolic processes by:

- **Energy Mobilization**: Stimulating the breakdown of fat (lipolysis) and glycogen in the liver to release glucose.
- **Thermogenesis**: Increasing body heat production by activating brown adipose tissue.

Production of Norepinephrine

Norepinephrine is synthesized and secreted by neurons in the central and peripheral nervous systems and by chromaffin cells in the adrenal medulla. The production process involves several steps:

Synthesis: Norepinephrine is synthesized from the amino acid tyrosine through a series of enzymatic reactions:

- ◦ **Tyrosine Hydroxylation**: Tyrosine is converted into L-DOPA by the enzyme tyrosine hydroxylase.
- ◦ **Decarboxylation**: L-DOPA is converted into dopamine by aromatic L-amino acid decarboxylase.
- ◦ **Hydroxylation**: Dopamine is then converted into norepinephrine by dopamine β-hydroxylase.

Storage and Release: Norepinephrine is stored in synaptic vesicles and adrenal medulla granules. Upon stimulation, it is released into the synaptic cleft or bloodstream.

Regulation by Autonomic Nervous System: The autonomic nervous system, particularly the sympathetic division, regulates norepinephrine production and release.

Regulation of Norepinephrine

The regulation of norepinephrine involves complex mechanisms including feedback loops and external factors:

- ◦ **Autoreceptors**: Presynaptic receptors (α2-adrenoceptors) that inhibit norepinephrine release when activated by high levels of the hormone.
- ◦ **Metabolic Inactivation**: Enzymes like monoamine oxidase (MAO) and catechol-O-methyltransferase (COMT) degrade norepinephrine to maintain balance.

Neuronal Activity: Norepinephrine release is influenced by neuronal firing rates. Increased neuronal activity in the locus coeruleus (a brainstem nucleus) enhances norepinephrine release.

Stress and Environmental Stimuli: Acute and chronic stress, as well as various environmental stimuli, can significantly affect norepinephrine levels.

Diet and Nutrition: Nutritional status, particularly the intake of amino acids and certain vitamins, plays a role in norepinephrine synthesis.

Plant-Based Diet and Norepinephrine Regulation

A plant-based diet can have a profound impact on norepinephrine regulation through various mechanisms:

Nutrient Density: Plant-based diets are rich in essential nutrients that support overall health and hormonal balance. For example:

- **Tyrosine**: Found in foods like soy products, nuts, seeds, and legumes, is the precursor for norepinephrine synthesis.
- **Vitamins and Minerals**: Vitamins B6, and C, and minerals such as iron and copper are cofactors in norepinephrine synthesis. These nutrients are abundant in fruits, vegetables, and whole grains.

Antioxidants: Fruits and vegetables are rich in antioxidants, which help reduce oxidative stress. Lower oxidative stress levels are associated with improved norepinephrine function and overall endocrine health.

Healthy Fats: Plant-based sources of fats, such as avocados, nuts, and seeds, provide essential fatty acids that support hormone production and regulation. Omega-3 fatty acids, in particular, have anti-inflammatory properties that can enhance norepinephrine activity.

Fiber: High-fiber diets, common in plant-based eating, support gut health and hormone regulation. A healthy gut microbiome can influence norepinephrine levels through the production of short-chain fatty acids and other metabolites.

Caloric Balance: Maintaining a healthy weight through a balanced plant-based diet can prevent obesity-related suppression of norepinephrine. Excess body fat, particularly visceral fat, is linked to lower norepinephrine levels due to increased production of inhibitory hormones like insulin.

Glycemic Control: Plant-based diets, which are low in refined sugars and high in complex carbohydrates, help maintain stable blood glucose levels. This stability prevents hyperglycemia-induced suppression of norepinephrine secretion.

Plant-Based Diet on Norepinephrine-Related Health Outcomes

1. **Mental Health**: Numerous studies show that plant-based diets can benefit mental health by reducing inflammation and oxidative stress, which are linked to mood disorders. Improved norepinephrine levels support emotional well-being and cognitive function.
2. **Stress Management**: Plant-based diets are associated with lower stress levels. The abundance of antioxidants and anti-inflammatory compounds helps mitigate the effects of chronic stress on norepinephrine regulation.
3. **Energy Levels and Metabolism**: A plant-based diet rich in nutrients supports optimal energy metabolism. Adequate norepinephrine levels enhance fat mobilization and glucose utilization, leading to sustained energy levels.
4. **Cardiovascular Health**: Norepinephrine plays a role in cardiovascular function. Plant-based diets, known for their cardiovascular benefits, can help regulate norepinephrine levels, contributing to better heart health and blood pressure management.
5. **Cognitive Function**: The cognitive benefits of a plant-based diet are linked to its positive effects on norepinephrine. Enhanced norepinephrine activity supports attention, memory, and overall cognitive performance.

Nutrient Sources and Their Impact on Norepinephrine
Tyrosine-Rich Foods:

- **Soy Products**: Tofu, tempeh, and edamame.
- **Nuts and Seeds**: Almonds, pumpkin seeds, and sesame seeds.
- **Legumes**: Lentils, chickpeas, and black beans.

Vitamin B6:

- **Whole Grains**: Brown rice, oats, and quinoa.
- **Bananas**: A rich source of vitamin B6 and other essential nutrients.
- **Avocados**: Also provide healthy fats beneficial for hormone production.

Vitamin C:

- **Citrus Fruits**: Oranges, lemons, and grapefruits.
- **Berries**: Strawberries, blueberries, and raspberries.
- **Leafy Greens**: Spinach, kale, and broccoli.

Iron and Copper:

- **Legumes**: Beans, lentils, and peas.
- **Nuts and Seeds**: Cashews, sunflower seeds, and chia seeds.
- **Dark Chocolate**: A plant-based source of iron and copper.

Benefits of a Plant-Based Diet on Norepinephrine Function

1. Mood and Cognitive Enhancement

Plant-based diets can support mental health by providing a steady supply of nutrients required for norepinephrine synthesis and function. The anti-inflammatory properties of plant foods help maintain brain health and protect against mood disorders.

2. Stress Reduction

The high antioxidant content in plant-based diets reduces oxidative stress, which can otherwise impair norepinephrine production and regulation. Lower stress levels contribute to balanced norepinephrine activity and overall well-being.

3. Metabolic Support

A diet rich in plant-based foods supports metabolic health by providing the necessary cofactors for norepinephrine synthesis. This helps in maintaining optimal energy levels and preventing metabolic disorders.

Norepinephrine plays a pivotal role in the body's stress response, mood regulation, cognitive function, and metabolism. Its production and regulation are influenced by various factors, including diet and nutritional status.

5

Pancreatic Hormones

Insulin

Insulin, a hormone produced by the pancreas, is pivotal for regulating blood glucose levels and metabolic processes within the body.

Function of Insulin

Insulin's primary role is to regulate blood glucose levels, but its functions extend beyond this to various metabolic processes:

1. Glucose Regulation

Insulin facilitates the uptake of glucose by cells, particularly in muscle and fat tissues, allowing it to be used for energy or stored as glycogen in the liver and muscles. This process is crucial for maintaining stable blood glucose levels and preventing hyperglycemia (high blood sugar) and hypoglycemia (low blood sugar).

2. Metabolic Effects

Insulin plays a significant role in lipid metabolism by inhibiting the breakdown of fat (lipolysis) and promoting fat storage. It also promotes protein synthesis by enhancing the uptake of amino acids by cells, thus supporting muscle growth and repair.

3. Cell Growth and Division

Insulin stimulates cell proliferation and differentiation, contributing to tissue growth and regeneration. This function is particularly important in healing processes and maintaining healthy tissues.

4. Regulation of Enzyme Activity

Insulin influences the activity of various enzymes involved in metabolism. For example, it activates glycogen synthase, an enzyme responsible for glycogen synthesis, and inhibits glycogen phosphorylase, which breaks down glycogen.

5. Electrolyte Balance

Insulin helps regulate electrolyte balance by promoting the uptake of potassium into cells. This process is crucial for maintaining normal cellular function and preventing hyperkalemia (high potassium levels in the blood).

Production of Insulin

Insulin is produced by the beta cells of the pancreatic islets (also known as the islets of Langerhans). The production process involves several key steps:

1. Synthesis

Insulin is synthesized as a precursor molecule called preproinsulin, which is then converted to proinsulin in the endoplasmic reticulum of the beta cells. Proinsulin is further processed in the Golgi apparatus, where it is cleaved to form mature insulin and C-peptide.

2. Storage and Release

Insulin is stored in secretory granules within the beta cells. Upon stimulation, these granules fuse with the cell membrane to release insulin into the bloodstream. This process is tightly regulated to ensure that insulin is released in response to rising blood glucose levels.

3. Regulation by Glucose Levels

The primary stimulus for insulin secretion is an increase in blood glucose levels. Glucose enters the beta cells through glucose transporters (GLUT2), leading to a series of metabolic events that result in insulin release. This feedback mechanism ensures that insulin secretion is closely matched to the body's metabolic needs.

4. Other Influencing Factors

Insulin production and release are also influenced by various other factors, including:

- **Hormones**: Incretin hormones (such as GLP-1 and GIP) released from the gut enhance insulin secretion in response to food intake.
- **Nervous System**: The autonomic nervous system modulates insulin secretion, with parasympathetic stimulation promoting and sympathetic stimulation inhibiting release.
- **Nutrients**: Amino acids (particularly leucine and arginine) and fatty acids can stimulate insulin secretion.

Regulation of Insulin

The regulation of insulin involves complex feedback mechanisms and interactions with other hormones and metabolic factors:

1. Feedback Loops

Insulin secretion is regulated through negative feedback loops. High levels of insulin in the blood inhibit further insulin release, while low levels stimulate its production. This ensures that insulin levels remain within an optimal range.

2. Counter-Regulatory Hormones

Several hormones counteract the effects of insulin to maintain glucose homeostasis. These include glucagon (produced by the alpha cells of the pancreas), cortisol, epinephrine, and growth hormone. These hormones increase blood glucose levels by promoting glycogenolysis (breakdown of glycogen) and gluconeogenesis (production of glucose from non-carbohydrate sources).

3. Nutritional Status

Fasting and low-carbohydrate diets reduce insulin secretion, while high-carbohydrate meals stimulate its release. This adaptive response ensures that insulin is available when needed to process dietary glucose.

4. Physical Activity

Exercise enhances insulin sensitivity, allowing cells to respond more effectively to insulin. This effect is beneficial for glucose regulation and overall metabolic health. Regular physical activity is associated with improved insulin sensitivity and lower insulin levels.

5. Stress

Chronic stress can impact insulin regulation through the release of stress hormones like cortisol and adrenaline, which raise blood glucose levels and can lead to insulin resistance over time.

Plant-Based Diet and Insulin Regulation

A plant-based diet, rich in fruits, vegetables, whole grains, nuts, and seeds, has a significant impact on insulin regulation through various mechanisms:

1. Nutrient Density

Plant-based diets are typically high in essential nutrients, vitamins, and minerals that support overall health and insulin sensitivity. For example, magnesium, found in leafy greens, nuts, and seeds, plays a crucial role in insulin action and glucose metabolism.

2. Fiber

High-fiber diets, common in plant-based eating, improve insulin sensitivity and help maintain stable blood glucose levels. Soluble fiber, found in foods like oats, beans, and fruits, slows the absorption of glucose, preventing rapid spikes in blood sugar and reducing the insulin response.

3. Phytochemicals

Plant-based diets are rich in phytochemicals, such as polyphenols and flavonoids, which have antioxidant and anti-inflammatory properties. These compounds help reduce oxidative stress and inflammation, both of which are linked to insulin resistance.

4. Healthy Fats

Plant-based sources of fats, such as avocados, nuts, and seeds, provide essential fatty acids that support insulin sensitivity. Omega-3 fatty acids, in particular, have anti-inflammatory properties that can enhance insulin function.

5. Glycemic Control

Plant-based diets, which are low in refined sugars and high in complex carbohydrates, help maintain stable blood glucose levels. This stability prevents hyperglycemia-induced insulin resistance and promotes better glycemic control.

6. Weight Management

Maintaining a healthy weight through a balanced plant-based diet can prevent obesity-related insulin resistance. Excess body fat, particularly visceral fat, is linked to lower insulin sensitivity and increased risk of type 2 diabetes.

Plant-Based Diet on Insulin-Related Health Outcomes

1. Type 2 Diabetes

Numerous studies have shown that plant-based diets can significantly reduce the risk of developing type 2 diabetes. The combination of high fiber intake, low glycemic load, and nutrient density helps improve insulin sensitivity and glycemic control.

2. Cardiovascular Health

Insulin resistance is closely linked to cardiovascular disease. A plant-based diet, with its high content of antioxidants, fiber, and healthy fats, supports cardiovascular health by improving insulin sensitivity, reducing inflammation, and promoting healthy lipid profiles.

3. Weight Management

A plant-based diet is effective for weight management, which is crucial for preventing and managing insulin resistance. The high fiber content promotes satiety, reducing overall calorie intake and supporting healthy body weight.

4. Anti-Inflammatory Effects

The anti-inflammatory properties of a plant-based diet, attributed to its rich content of antioxidants and phytochemicals, help reduce chronic inflammation, a key factor in the development of insulin resistance and metabolic syndrome.

5. Metabolic Health

Improved insulin sensitivity and glycemic control, along with the nutrient density of a plant-based diet, contribute to overall metabolic health. This includes better lipid profiles, lower blood pressure, and reduced risk of metabolic syndrome.

Insulin is a vital hormone that regulates blood glucose levels and various metabolic processes. Its production and regulation are influenced by multiple factors, including diet, physical activity, and hormonal interactions.

Glucagon

Glucagon is a critical hormone in maintaining glucose homeostasis, produced by the pancreas, and playing an essential role in blood sugar regulation, metabolism, and energy balance. This comprehensive analysis will delve into the function, production, and regulation of glucagon, particularly from a plant-based viewpoint, highlighting dietary influences on its activity and balance.

Function of Glucagon

Glucagon's primary function is to raise blood glucose levels, especially during fasting or between meals, to ensure a continuous supply of energy. It achieves this through several mechanisms:

1. **Glycogenolysis:** Glucagon stimulates the liver to break down glycogen into glucose, which is then released into the bloodstream. This process is crucial during periods of low blood sugar, such as between meals or during physical activity.
2. **Gluconeogenesis:** Glucagon promotes the production of glucose from non-carbohydrate sources, such as amino acids and glycerol, in the liver. This pathway ensures glucose availability during prolonged fasting or intense exercise.
3. **Lipolysis:** Glucagon enhances the breakdown of triglycerides into free fatty acids and glycerol in adipose tissue. These free fatty acids can be used as an alternative energy source, sparing glucose for use by the brain and other glucose-dependent tissues.
4. **Ketogenesis:** Glucagon stimulates the liver to convert free fatty acids into ketone bodies, which can be used as an energy source by the brain and other tissues during prolonged fasting or low carbohydrate intake.

Production of Glucagon

Glucagon is produced by the alpha cells (α-cells) of the islets of Langerhans in the pancreas. The production process involves several steps:

1. **Synthesis:** Glucagon is synthesized as proglucagon, a precursor protein. Proglucagon is then cleaved by prohormone convertase 2 to produce mature glucagon.
2. **Storage and Release:** Mature glucagon is stored in secretory granules within the α-cells and released into the bloodstream in response to specific stimuli, such as low blood glucose levels.
3. **Regulation by Blood Glucose Levels:** The primary regulator of glucagon secretion is blood glucose concentration. Low blood glucose levels stimulate glucagon release, while high blood glucose levels inhibit its secretion.

Regulation of Glucagon

The regulation of glucagon involves a complex interplay of various factors, including blood glucose levels, hormones, and neural signals:

1. **Blood Glucose Levels:** As mentioned, low blood glucose levels are the primary trigger for glucagon secretion. Conversely, high blood glucose levels suppress glucagon release through a negative feedback mechanism.
2. **Insulin:** Insulin, produced by the beta cells (β-cells) of the pancreas, plays a critical role in regulating glucagon secretion. High insulin levels inhibit glucagon release, while low insulin levels facilitate its secretion.
3. **Amino Acids:** Elevated levels of certain amino acids, such as alanine and arginine, can stimulate glucagon secretion. This mechanism ensures that protein-rich meals do not cause hypoglycemia by stimulating gluconeogenesis.
4. **Neural and Hormonal Signals:** The autonomic nervous system and other hormones, such as adrenaline and cortisol, also influence glucagon secretion. Sympathetic stimulation and stress hormones typically promote glucagon release, preparing the body to meet increased energy demands.

Plant-Based Diet and Glucagon Regulation

A plant-based diet, rich in fruits, vegetables, whole grains, nuts, and seeds, can significantly impact glucagon regulation through various mechanisms:

1. **Low Glycemic Index Foods:** Plant-based diets often include foods with a low glycemic index, which results in slower, more stable increases in blood glucose levels. This stability can help

maintain balanced glucagon secretion without causing drastic spikes or drops in blood glucose.

2. **Fiber-Rich Foods:** High fiber intake, common in plant-based diets, slows the absorption of carbohydrates, leading to a gradual release of glucose into the bloodstream. This gradual release helps prevent rapid blood glucose fluctuations and supports steady glucagon regulation.
3. **Healthy Fats:** Plant-based sources of fats, such as avocados, nuts, and seeds, provide essential fatty acids that support metabolic health and energy balance. These healthy fats can influence glucagon activity by providing an alternative energy source and promoting lipolysis.
4. **Antioxidants and Phytochemicals:** Fruits and vegetables are rich in antioxidants and phytochemicals, which help reduce oxidative stress and inflammation. Lower oxidative stress levels are associated with improved endocrine function, including glucagon regulation.
5. **Protein from Plant Sources:** Plant-based proteins, such as those from beans, lentils, quinoa, and tofu, provide essential amino acids that can stimulate glucagon secretion when necessary. These proteins support gluconeogenesis and overall metabolic health.

Plant-Based Diet on Glucagon-Related Health Outcomes

1. **Blood Sugar Control:** A plant-based diet can enhance blood sugar control by providing a steady supply of low glycemic index carbohydrates and fiber. Improved blood sugar control reduces the risk of diabetes and metabolic syndrome, conditions often associated with dysregulated glucagon activity.
2. **Weight Management:** Plant-based diets are effective for weight management due to their high fiber content and lower calorie

density. Maintaining a healthy weight reduces the burden on the pancreas and supports balanced glucagon and insulin levels.

3. **Cardiovascular Health:** By promoting healthy blood lipid profiles and reducing oxidative stress, plant-based diets can support cardiovascular health. Balanced glucagon levels contribute to lipid metabolism and energy balance, further enhancing cardiovascular outcomes.
4. **Reduced Risk of Chronic Diseases:** The anti-inflammatory and antioxidant properties of plant-based diets help reduce the risk of chronic diseases, such as cardiovascular disease, cancer, and neurodegenerative disorders. These benefits are partly mediated through improved glucagon and overall hormonal regulation.
5. **Energy and Metabolism:** A plant-based diet supports overall energy and metabolic health by providing essential nutrients, fiber, and healthy fats. These dietary components work synergistically to maintain balanced glucagon activity, promoting optimal energy utilization and metabolic function.

Glucagon and Exercise

Exercise is a critical factor in glucagon regulation and overall metabolic health. Both aerobic and resistance exercise have specific effects on glucagon secretion and activity:

1. **Aerobic Exercise:** During aerobic exercise, such as running or cycling, glucagon levels increase to maintain blood glucose levels. This rise in glucagon stimulates glycogenolysis and gluconeogenesis, ensuring a continuous supply of glucose for energy.
2. **Resistance Exercise:** Resistance exercise, such as weight lifting, also elevates glucagon levels. The increased glucagon activity supports muscle repair and growth by providing the necessary energy substrates through gluconeogenesis and lipolysis.

3. **Post-Exercise Recovery:** After exercise, a balanced plant-based meal can support recovery by replenishing glycogen stores and providing essential nutrients. The low glycemic index carbohydrates and plant proteins help stabilize blood glucose levels and support glucagon regulation during recovery.

Glucagon and Sleep

Sleep plays a vital role in hormonal regulation, including glucagon:

1. **Deep Sleep and Glucagon:** Deep sleep stages are associated with stable blood glucose levels and balanced glucagon secretion. Adequate sleep supports overall endocrine function and metabolic health.
2. **Sleep Deprivation:** Chronic sleep deprivation can disrupt glucagon regulation, leading to impaired glucose metabolism and an increased risk of metabolic disorders. A plant-based diet, rich in nutrients that support sleep quality, such as magnesium and tryptophan, can help improve sleep patterns and hormonal balance.

Glucagon and Stress

Stress and the associated hormonal responses can influence glucagon activity:

1. **Acute Stress:** Acute stress triggers the release of adrenaline and cortisol, which in turn stimulate glucagon secretion. This response provides a rapid increase in blood glucose levels to meet the body's immediate energy needs.
2. **Chronic Stress:** Prolonged stress can lead to dysregulated glucagon and insulin levels, contributing to metabolic imbalances and increased risk of diabetes and cardiovascular disease. A plant-based diet, rich in anti-inflammatory and antioxidant compounds, can

help mitigate the negative effects of chronic stress on glucagon regulation.

Glucagon is a crucial hormone in maintaining glucose homeostasis and overall metabolic health. Its production and regulation are influenced by various factors, including blood glucose levels, insulin, amino acids, neural signals, and hormones.

Somatostatin

Somatostatin, also known as growth hormone-inhibiting hormone (GHIH), is a peptide hormone that plays a pivotal role in regulating the endocrine system, particularly in inhibiting the secretion of other hormones.

Function of Somatostatin

Somatostatin's primary functions are to inhibit the release of several other hormones and to regulate the digestive system. Its functions can be categorized as follows:

1. **Inhibition of Growth Hormone Secretion**: Somatostatin inhibits the release of growth hormone (GH) from the anterior pituitary gland. This action is crucial in regulating growth and metabolism in the body.
2. **Regulation of Pancreatic Hormones**: Somatostatin suppresses the release of insulin and glucagon from the pancreas. Insulin lowers blood glucose levels, while glucagon increases them; thus, somatostatin helps maintain glucose homeostasis.

3. **Digestive Functions**: Somatostatin inhibits the secretion of gastric acid, digestive enzymes, and bile. It slows down gastric emptying and reduces smooth muscle contractions and blood flow within the intestine.
4. **Neurotransmitter Modulation**: In the central nervous system, somatostatin functions as a neurotransmitter and neuromodulator. It influences motor control, mood, and cognitive functions.

Production of Somatostatin

Somatostatin is produced in various locations within the body, including:

1. **Hypothalamus**: The hypothalamus produces somatostatin, which then acts on the anterior pituitary gland to inhibit the release of GH.
2. **Pancreas**: In the pancreas, somatostatin is produced by the delta cells of the islets of Langerhans. It plays a key role in regulating the secretion of insulin and glucagon.
3. **Gastrointestinal Tract**: Somatostatin is also produced in the gastrointestinal tract, particularly in the stomach and intestines, where it regulates digestive processes.
4. **Central Nervous System**: Neurons in various parts of the brain produce somatostatin, influencing a range of neural activities.

Regulation of Somatostatin

The regulation of somatostatin involves complex feedback mechanisms and various influencing factors:

1. **Feedback Inhibition**: The secretion of somatostatin is regulated through negative feedback mechanisms. High levels of GH,

insulin, and glucagon stimulate the release of somatostatin to inhibit further secretion of these hormones.
2. **Nutrient Levels**: Blood glucose levels influence somatostatin secretion. High glucose levels stimulate its release to inhibit insulin and glucagon secretion, maintaining glucose balance.
3. **Gastrointestinal Hormones**: The presence of certain gastrointestinal hormones, such as gastrin, secretin, and cholecystokinin (CCK), can stimulate the release of somatostatin to modulate digestive processes.
4. **Neural Regulation**: Neural inputs from the central nervous system also regulate somatostatin secretion, particularly in response to stress, exercise, and other physiological states.

Plant-Based Diet and Somatostatin Regulation

A plant-based diet, rich in fruits, vegetables, whole grains, nuts, and seeds, can significantly influence the regulation of somatostatin through various mechanisms:

1. **Nutrient Density**: Plant-based diets are typically high in essential nutrients, vitamins, and minerals that support overall health and hormonal balance. For instance, magnesium and potassium found in leafy greens and nuts play crucial roles in cellular functions and hormone regulation.
2. **Glycemic Control**: A diet low in refined sugars and high in complex carbohydrates helps maintain stable blood glucose levels. This stability can prevent excessive fluctuations in insulin and glucagon, thereby reducing the need for somatostatin-mediated inhibition.
3. **Fiber**: High-fiber diets support gut health and slow the absorption of carbohydrates, which helps in maintaining stable blood sugar levels. This can lead to a more balanced release of insulin

and glucagon, reducing the necessity for somatostatin's inhibitory action.

4. **Antioxidants and Phytochemicals**: Plant-based foods are rich in antioxidants and phytochemicals, which reduce oxidative stress and inflammation. Lower oxidative stress levels are associated with improved endocrine function and somatostatin activity.
5. **Healthy Fats**: Plant-based sources of fats, such as avocados, nuts, and seeds, provide essential fatty acids that support hormone production and regulation. Omega-3 fatty acids, in particular, have anti-inflammatory properties that can enhance somatostatin activity.

Impact of Plant-Based Diet on Somatostatin-Related Health Outcomes

1. **Diabetes Management**: A plant-based diet can help in managing diabetes by stabilizing blood glucose levels and reducing insulin resistance. The improved glycemic control reduces the need for somatostatin-mediated inhibition of insulin and glucagon, leading to better overall endocrine function.
2. **Digestive Health**: High-fiber and nutrient-rich plant-based diets promote gut health, enhancing the regulation of digestive hormones and processes. This supports the role of somatostatin in modulating gastric acid secretion and digestive enzyme activity.
3. **Weight Management**: Plant-based diets are effective for weight management, reducing body fat and improving metabolic health. Lower body fat reduces the production of somatostatin-inhibiting factors, promoting a healthier hormonal balance.
4. **Anti-Inflammatory Effects**: The anti-inflammatory properties of a plant-based diet help in reducing chronic inflammation, which can positively influence the regulation of somatostatin and other hormones involved in metabolic and digestive health.

Somatostatin plays a crucial role in inhibiting the release of various hormones and regulating digestive processes. Its production and regulation are influenced by complex feedback mechanisms and various physiological factors.

Pancreatic Polypeptide (PP)

Pancreatic Polypeptide (PP) is a peptide hormone produced by the pancreas that plays a crucial role in regulating digestive processes and energy metabolism.

Function of Pancreatic Polypeptide
Pancreatic Polypeptide has several critical functions within the body:

1. **Regulation of Pancreatic Secretions:** PP helps modulate the secretion of pancreatic enzymes and bicarbonate, crucial for digestion. It inhibits the secretion of pancreatic exocrine enzymes, reducing the digestive activity post-meal.
2. **Gastric Emptying:** PP slows down gastric emptying, allowing for a more controlled and efficient digestion process.
3. **Modulation of Appetite:** PP plays a role in appetite regulation by sending satiety signals to the brain, which helps control food intake.
4. **Influence on Hepatic Glycogen Levels:** It impacts liver glycogen storage, aiding in the maintenance of blood glucose levels.
5. **Energy Homeostasis:** PP helps balance energy homeostasis by modulating food intake and energy expenditure.

Production of Pancreatic Polypeptide

PP is produced by PP cells (also known as F cells) in the pancreatic islets of Langerhans. The production process involves several key steps:

1. **Synthesis:** PP is synthesized as a preprohormone and then processed into its active form in the pancreas.
2. **Storage and Release:** It is stored in secretory granules within the PP cells and released in response to various physiological stimuli, including food intake and neural signals.
3. **Stimuli for Secretion:** The primary stimuli for PP release are food ingestion, particularly protein-rich meals, and vagal stimulation, which activates the parasympathetic nervous system.

Regulation of Pancreatic Polypeptide

The regulation of PP is a complex process involving various factors:

1. **Nutrient Intake:** The most significant regulator of PP secretion is food intake. Protein and fat are potent stimulators, while carbohydrates have a lesser effect.
2. **Neural Regulation:** The vagus nerve, which controls many digestive processes, significantly influences PP release. Vagal stimulation during food intake enhances PP secretion.
3. **Hormonal Interactions:** Hormones such as insulin and glucagon, produced by the pancreas, also interact with PP, influencing its secretion and action.
4. **Circadian Rhythms:** PP levels exhibit a circadian pattern, with higher levels during the night, possibly linked to fasting and energy conservation.

Plant-Based Diet and Pancreatic Polypeptide Regulation

A plant-based diet can significantly influence the regulation and function of PP through various mechanisms:

1. **High Fiber Content:** Plant-based diets are rich in dietary fiber, which slows down gastric emptying and promotes satiety, potentially modulating PP levels.
2. **Protein Sources:** Plant-based proteins from legumes, nuts, and seeds can stimulate PP secretion similarly to animal proteins, supporting digestive regulation.
3. **Healthy Fats:** Sources of healthy fats, such as avocados, nuts, and seeds, can enhance PP response, aiding in the modulation of pancreatic secretions.
4. **Low Glycemic Load:** Plant-based diets typically have a lower glycemic load, which can help stabilize blood glucose levels and reduce excessive PP fluctuations.
5. **Antioxidants and Phytochemicals:** The high content of antioxidants and phytochemicals in plant foods can reduce oxidative stress and inflammation, potentially supporting optimal PP function.

Plant-Based Diet on Pancreatic Polypeptide-Related Health Outcomes

1. **Digestive Health:** A plant-based diet, rich in fiber, supports healthy digestion by promoting the controlled release of digestive enzymes and maintaining gut motility.
2. **Weight Management:** The appetite-regulating effects of PP, combined with the satiety provided by fiber-rich plant foods, can aid in weight management and prevent obesity.

3. **Blood Glucose Control:** The stabilizing effect of a low glycemic load plant-based diet on blood glucose levels can help maintain healthy PP levels and improve overall metabolic health.
4. **Reduction in Digestive Disorders:** By modulating pancreatic secretions and promoting efficient digestion, a plant-based diet can help reduce the risk of digestive disorders such as pancreatitis and irritable bowel syndrome (IBS).
5. **Energy Balance:** The regulation of energy homeostasis by PP, supported by a balanced plant-based diet, can improve overall energy levels and prevent metabolic diseases.

6

Gonadal Hormones

Testosterone

Testosterone is a steroid hormone that plays a crucial role in the development and maintenance of male reproductive tissues, secondary sexual characteristics, and overall health.

Function of Testosterone

Testosterone's primary functions are vital to numerous physiological processes, including:

Development and Maintenance of Male Reproductive Tissues:

- **Spermatogenesis**: Testosterone is essential for the production of sperm in the testes. It stimulates the maturation of sperm cells and supports the function of Sertoli cells, which nourish developing sperm.
- **Testicular Function**: Testosterone promotes the development and maintenance of the testes, ensuring their proper function throughout a man's life.

Secondary Sexual Characteristics:

- **Muscle Mass and Strength**: Testosterone increases muscle protein synthesis, leading to greater muscle mass and strength.
- **Bone Density**: It enhances bone density and strength by stimulating the activity of osteoblasts, cells responsible for bone formation.
- **Body Hair**: Testosterone stimulates the growth of facial and body hair during puberty.
- **Voice Deepening**: The hormone causes the larynx to grow and the vocal cords to thicken, resulting in a deeper voice.

Metabolic Effects:

- **Fat Distribution**: Testosterone influences the distribution of body fat, contributing to a leaner body composition with less abdominal fat.
- **Red Blood Cell Production**: It stimulates erythropoiesis, the production of red blood cells, which is crucial for oxygen transport and overall energy levels.

Behavioral and Cognitive Functions:

- **Libido**: Testosterone plays a significant role in regulating sexual desire and arousal.
- **Mood and Cognitive Function**: It is associated with mood regulation, cognitive function, and overall mental well-being. Low testosterone levels have been linked to depression, irritability, and cognitive decline.

Production of Testosterone

Testosterone is produced primarily in the testes in males and in smaller amounts in the ovaries in females and the adrenal glands in both sexes. The production process involves several steps:

Synthesis:

- Testosterone is synthesized from cholesterol through a series of enzymatic reactions. The key enzymes involved in this process include cholesterol side-chain cleavage enzyme (P450scc), 17α-hydroxylase, and 17,20-lyase.
- The Leydig cells in the testes are the primary site of testosterone production in males. In females, the ovaries produce small amounts of testosterone, while the adrenal glands contribute to its production in both sexes.

Regulation by the Hypothalamus and Pituitary Gland:

- The hypothalamus regulates testosterone production through the release of gonadotropin-releasing hormone (GnRH), which stimulates the pituitary gland to secrete luteinizing hormone (LH).
- LH then acts on the Leydig cells in the testes, promoting the synthesis and release of testosterone.

Influencing Factors:

- **Age:** Testosterone levels peak during adolescence and early adulthood and gradually decline with age.
- **Time of Day:** Testosterone levels exhibit a diurnal pattern, peaking in the early morning and declining throughout the day.

- **Health and Lifestyle**: Factors such as diet, exercise, stress, and overall health can influence testosterone production.

Regulation of Testosterone

The regulation of testosterone is a complex process involving feedback mechanisms and external factors:

Feedback Loops:

- High levels of testosterone inhibit the release of GnRH from the hypothalamus and LH from the pituitary gland, reducing testosterone production in a negative feedback loop.

Health and Lifestyle:

- **Exercise**: Regular physical activity, particularly resistance training and high-intensity interval training can boost testosterone levels. Exercise-induced increases in testosterone are thought to be mediated by reduced cortisol levels and increased LH secretion.
- **Sleep**: Adequate sleep is crucial for maintaining healthy testosterone levels. Sleep deprivation can lead to significant reductions in testosterone production.
- **Stress Management**: Chronic stress can elevate cortisol levels, which can suppress testosterone production. Effective stress management techniques are essential for hormonal balance.

Nutritional Status:

- **Caloric Intake**: Both undernutrition and overnutrition can negatively impact testosterone levels. A balanced diet that meets caloric needs is essential for optimal hormone production.

- **Micronutrients**: Certain vitamins and minerals, such as vitamin D, zinc, and magnesium, play crucial roles in testosterone production and regulation. Deficiencies in these nutrients can lead to lower testosterone levels.

Plant-Based Diet and Testosterone Regulation

A plant-based diet, rich in fruits, vegetables, whole grains, nuts, and seeds, can have a profound impact on testosterone regulation through various mechanisms:

Nutrient Density:

- **Vitamin D**: Found in fortified plant milks, mushrooms, and exposure to sunlight, vitamin D is crucial for testosterone production. Studies have shown that vitamin D supplementation can increase testosterone levels in deficient individuals.
- **Zinc and Magnesium**: Nuts, seeds, legumes, and whole grains are excellent sources of zinc and magnesium, both of which are essential for testosterone synthesis.

Healthy Fats:

- **Omega-3 Fatty Acids**: Plant-based sources of omega-3s, such as flaxseeds, chia seeds, and walnuts, have anti-inflammatory properties that support overall hormonal health. These fats help maintain cell membrane integrity and can positively influence testosterone levels.
- **Monounsaturated and Polyunsaturated Fats**: Avocados, nuts, and seeds provide healthy fats that are essential for

hormone production. These fats support the synthesis of cholesterol, the precursor for testosterone.

Antioxidants:

- **Fruits and Vegetables**: Rich in antioxidants, plant-based foods help reduce oxidative stress, which can negatively impact testosterone production. Lower oxidative stress levels are associated with improved hormonal balance.

Fiber:

- High-fiber diets, common in plant-based eating, support gut health and hormone regulation. A healthy gut microbiome can influence testosterone levels through the production of short-chain fatty acids and other metabolites.

Caloric Balance:

- Maintaining a healthy weight through a balanced plant-based diet can prevent obesity-related suppression of testosterone. Excess body fat is linked to lower testosterone levels due to increased production of estrogen and inflammatory cytokines.

Glycemic Control:

- Plant-based diets, which are low in refined sugars and high in complex carbohydrates, help maintain stable blood glucose levels. This stability prevents hyperglycemia-induced suppression of testosterone secretion.

Plant-Based Diet on Testosterone-Related Health Outcomes Muscle Mass and Strength:

- Contrary to the misconception that plant-based diets lack sufficient protein for muscle building, numerous studies show that plant-based proteins can support muscle growth and strength when combined with resistance training. Foods like beans, lentils, quinoa, and tofu provide high-quality protein that supports testosterone synthesis and muscle protein synthesis.

Bone Health:

- Plant-based diets rich in calcium, magnesium, and vitamin K support bone health. Leafy greens, fortified plant milk, and nuts are excellent sources of these nutrients, which work synergistically with testosterone to maintain bone density and reduce the risk of osteoporosis.

Weight Management:

- Plant-based diets are effective for weight management, reducing body fat, and improving insulin sensitivity. Lower body fat and better glycemic control enhance testosterone secretion and overall metabolic health.

Anti-Aging Effects:

- The antioxidant-rich nature of plant-based diets helps combat oxidative stress, a key factor in aging. Improved testosterone levels, coupled with reduced oxidative damage, contribute to healthier aging and better maintenance of lean body mass.

Mental Health:

- Emerging evidence suggests that plant-based diets may benefit mental health by reducing inflammation and oxidative stress, which are linked to mood disorders. Improved testosterone levels also support cognitive function and emotional well-being.

Testosterone plays a pivotal role in the development and maintenance of male reproductive tissues, secondary sexual characteristics, metabolism, and overall health. Its production and regulation are influenced by various factors, including age, sleep, exercise, stress, and diet.

Estrogen

Estrogen is a steroid hormone that plays a critical role in various physiological processes, including reproductive function, cardiovascular health, bone density, and brain function.

Function of Estrogen

Estrogen has a wide range of functions in the body, impacting numerous systems and processes:

1. Reproductive Health

- **Regulation of Menstrual Cycle**: Estrogen is crucial for the development and regulation of the female reproductive system and secondary sexual characteristics. It regulates the menstrual cycle by stimulating the growth of the uterine lining during the first part of the cycle.

- **Development of Secondary Sexual Characteristics**: It is responsible for the development of secondary sexual characteristics such as breast development, widening of the hips, and pubic and armpit hair growth.
- **Fertility**: Estrogen levels influence ovulation and are essential for the maintenance of pregnancy.

2. Bone Health

- **Bone Density**: Estrogen helps maintain bone density by inhibiting bone resorption. It stimulates the activity of osteoblasts (cells that form bone) and reduces the activity of osteoclasts (cells that break down bone), thus playing a protective role against osteoporosis.

3. Cardiovascular Health

- **Vasodilation**: Estrogen promotes vasodilation, which improves blood flow and reduces blood pressure. It also helps maintain the elasticity of blood vessels.
- **Lipid Profile**: Estrogen positively influences the lipid profile by increasing high-density lipoprotein (HDL) cholesterol and reducing low-density lipoprotein (LDL) cholesterol, thus protecting against cardiovascular diseases.

4. Brain Function

- **Cognitive Function**: Estrogen has neuroprotective effects and is involved in the regulation of mood, cognition, and memory. It enhances synaptic plasticity and supports the growth and survival of neurons.

5. Skin Health

- **Collagen Production**: Estrogen stimulates collagen production, which helps maintain skin elasticity and hydration. This contributes to a youthful appearance and delays the onset of wrinkles.

Production of Estrogen

Estrogen is produced primarily in the ovaries, but also in smaller amounts by the adrenal glands and adipose tissue. The production process involves several steps and regulatory mechanisms:

1. Synthesis

- **Ovarian Production**: The majority of estrogen is synthesized in the ovaries. The process begins with the conversion of cholesterol to pregnenolone, which is then converted to androstenedione. Androstenedione is subsequently converted to estrone and estradiol, the primary forms of estrogen.
- **Adrenal Glands and Adipose Tissue**: The adrenal glands and adipose tissue also produce small amounts of estrogen through a similar pathway, contributing to the total circulating levels of the hormone.

2. Regulation by Hypothalamus and Pituitary Gland

- **Gonadotropin-Releasing Hormone (GnRH)**: The hypothalamus secretes GnRH, which stimulates the pituitary gland to release luteinizing hormone (LH) and follicle-stimulating hormone (FSH). These hormones regulate the production of estrogen in the ovaries.
- **Feedback Mechanisms**: Estrogen levels are regulated through negative feedback mechanisms. High levels of estrogen inhibit

the release of GnRH, LH, and FSH, while low levels stimulate their release.

3. Menstrual Cycle and Pregnancy

- **Follicular Phase**: During the follicular phase of the menstrual cycle, rising levels of estrogen stimulate the growth and maturation of the ovarian follicles.
- **Luteal Phase**: After ovulation, the corpus luteum produces progesterone and estrogen, which prepare the uterine lining for the potential implantation of an embryo.
- **Pregnancy**: During pregnancy, the placenta becomes a significant source of estrogen, supporting the maintenance of pregnancy and fetal development.

Regulation of Estrogen

The regulation of estrogen involves complex feedback loops and is influenced by various internal and external factors:

1. Feedback Loops

- **Hypothalamic-Pituitary-Gonadal Axis**: Estrogen levels are regulated through the hypothalamic-pituitary-gonadal axis. High levels of estrogen inhibit the release of GnRH, LH, and FSH, reducing further production of estrogen. Conversely, low levels stimulate their release to increase estrogen production.

2. Age and Life Stages

- **Puberty**: Estrogen levels rise significantly during puberty, leading to the development of secondary sexual characteristics.

- **Menopause**: Estrogen levels decline during menopause, resulting in various physiological changes, including reduced bone density and increased cardiovascular risk.

3. Nutritional Status

- **Diet**: Diet plays a crucial role in estrogen regulation. Certain foods can influence estrogen levels by providing phytoestrogens, compounds that mimic the effects of estrogen in the body.
- **Body Fat**: Adipose tissue contributes to estrogen production, particularly in postmenopausal women. Higher body fat levels can lead to higher estrogen levels.

4. Hormones

- **Insulin and Cortisol**: Insulin and cortisol can influence estrogen production. Insulin resistance and high cortisol levels are associated with disruptions in estrogen balance.

Plant-Based Diet and Estrogen Regulation

A plant-based diet, rich in fruits, vegetables, whole grains, nuts, and seeds, can have a profound impact on estrogen regulation through various mechanisms:

1. Phytoestrogens

- **Sources and Benefits**: Phytoestrogens are naturally occurring plant compounds that mimic the effects of estrogen. Foods rich in phytoestrogens include soy products, flaxseeds, sesame seeds, and whole grains. Phytoestrogens can help balance estrogen levels and alleviate symptoms associated with estrogen deficiency, such as hot flashes during menopause.

- **Isoflavones**: Isoflavones, found in soy products, are a type of phytoestrogen that has been extensively studied for their potential health benefits. They can bind to estrogen receptors, exerting weak estrogenic effects that can be beneficial in maintaining hormonal balance.

2. Nutrient Density

- **Vitamins and Minerals**: A plant-based diet is typically high in essential nutrients, vitamins, and minerals that support overall health and hormonal balance. For example, vitamin D, found in fortified plant milks and mushrooms, is crucial for bone health and estrogen activity.

3. Antioxidants

- **Oxidative Stress Reduction**: Fruits and vegetables are rich in antioxidants, which help reduce oxidative stress. Lower oxidative stress levels are associated with improved estrogen secretion and overall endocrine function. Antioxidants like vitamins C and E play a protective role in maintaining estrogen balance.

4. Healthy Fats

- **Essential Fatty Acids**: Plant-based sources of fats, such as avocados, nuts, and seeds, provide essential fatty acids that support hormone production and regulation. Omega-3 fatty acids, in particular, have anti-inflammatory properties that can enhance estrogen activity.

5. Fiber

- **Gut Health**: High-fiber diets, common in plant-based eating, support gut health and hormone regulation. A healthy gut microbiome can influence estrogen levels through the production of short-chain fatty acids and other metabolites. Fiber also helps in the excretion of excess estrogen, preventing its reabsorption in the intestines.

6. Caloric Balance

- **Weight Management**: Maintaining a healthy weight through a balanced plant-based diet can prevent obesity-related suppression of estrogen. Excess body fat, particularly visceral fat, is linked to higher estrogen levels due to increased production by adipose tissue.

7. Glycemic Control

- **Blood Sugar Stability**: Plant-based diets, which are low in refined sugars and high in complex carbohydrates, help maintain stable blood glucose levels. This stability prevents hyperglycemia-induced disruptions in estrogen secretion.

Plant-Based Diet on Estrogen-Related Health Outcomes

1. Menopausal Symptoms

- **Hot Flashes and Night Sweats**: Phytoestrogens from soy products and flaxseeds can help alleviate menopausal symptoms such as hot flashes and night sweats by mimicking the effects of estrogen in the body.

2. Bone Health

- **Bone Density Maintenance**: Plant-based diets rich in calcium, magnesium, and vitamin K support bone health. Leafy greens, fortified plant milk, and nuts are excellent sources of these nutrients, which work synergistically with estrogen to maintain bone density and reduce the risk of osteoporosis.

3. Cardiovascular Health

- **Lipid Profile Improvement**: Plant-based diets positively influence the lipid profile by increasing HDL cholesterol and reducing LDL cholesterol. The anti-inflammatory and antioxidant properties of plant foods also contribute to cardiovascular health, reducing the risk of heart disease.

4. Cancer Prevention

- **Breast and Prostate Cancer**: Phytoestrogens have been studied for their potential protective effects against hormone-related cancers, such as breast and prostate cancer. The weak estrogenic effects of phytoestrogens can help regulate estrogen levels and reduce cancer risk.

5. Weight Management

- **Obesity Prevention**: Plant-based diets are effective for weight management, reducing body fat, and improving insulin sensitivity. Lower body fat and better glycemic control enhance estrogen secretion and overall metabolic health.

6. Skin Health

- **Collagen Production**: The antioxidant-rich nature of plant-based diets helps combat oxidative stress, which is crucial for maintaining skin health. Improved estrogen levels, coupled with reduced oxidative damage, contribute to healthier, more youthful skin.

7. Mental Health

- **Mood and Cognition**: Emerging evidence suggests that plant-based diets may benefit mental health by reducing inflammation and oxidative stress, which are linked to mood disorders. Improved estrogen levels also support cognitive function and emotional well-being.

8. Fertility

- **Hormonal Balance**: A plant-based diet can help balance hormones, improving fertility in both men and women. Nutrients such as folate, found in leafy greens, and zinc, found in nuts and seeds, are essential for reproductive health.

9. Digestive Health

- **Gut Microbiome**: A diverse and healthy gut microbiome, supported by a plant-based diet, can influence estrogen metabolism and excretion. This helps maintain optimal estrogen levels and prevent estrogen dominance.

10. Anti-Aging Effects

- **Healthy Aging**: The combination of nutrient-dense foods, antioxidants, and healthy fats in a plant-based diet supports overall health and longevity. Improved estrogen levels contribute to better maintenance of lean body mass, bone density, and cognitive function as one age.

Progesterone

Progesterone is a crucial hormone involved in various physiological processes, particularly in the female reproductive system. It plays a key role in regulating the menstrual cycle, supporting pregnancy, and maintaining overall reproductive health.

Function of Progesterone

Progesterone's primary functions are intricately linked to the reproductive system, but its influence extends to other bodily systems as well. The main functions of progesterone include:

1. Regulation of the Menstrual Cycle

Progesterone is essential for the regulation of the menstrual cycle. It works in tandem with estrogen to prepare the endometrium (the lining of the uterus) for potential pregnancy. During the luteal phase of the menstrual cycle, progesterone levels rise, leading to:

- **Endometrial Preparation**: Progesterone causes the endometrium to thicken and become more glandular, creating a suitable environment for a fertilized egg to implant.

- **Menstrual Cycle Regulation**: If pregnancy does not occur, progesterone levels drop, triggering the shedding of the endometrial lining and the onset of menstruation.

2. Support of Pregnancy

Progesterone plays a vital role in maintaining pregnancy. Its functions during pregnancy include:

- **Uterine Quiescence**: Progesterone helps maintain a relaxed state in the uterus, preventing contractions that could lead to premature labor.
- **Immune Modulation**: Progesterone modulates the maternal immune response to prevent the rejection of the developing embryo.
- **Placental Function**: Progesterone supports the development and function of the placenta, which is crucial for nutrient and oxygen exchange between the mother and fetus.

3. Breast Development

Progesterone, along with estrogen, promotes the development of mammary glands in preparation for lactation. This hormonal interplay ensures the breasts are ready to produce milk once the baby is born.

4. Neuroprotective Effects

Recent research has highlighted progesterone's neuroprotective effects, including:

- **Cognitive Function**: Progesterone may play a role in cognitive function and mood regulation, potentially influencing mental health.

- **Nervous System Health**: Progesterone has been found to support the myelination of nerves, contributing to overall nervous system health.

5. Bone Health

Progesterone also contributes to bone health by stimulating the activity of osteoblasts (cells responsible for bone formation) and reducing the activity of osteoclasts (cells responsible for bone resorption). This balance is essential for maintaining bone density and reducing the risk of osteoporosis.

Production of Progesterone

Progesterone is primarily produced in the ovaries, but it is also synthesized in smaller amounts by the adrenal glands and, during pregnancy, by the placenta. The production process involves several steps:

1. Ovarian Production

- **Corpus Luteum**: After ovulation, the ruptured follicle transforms into the corpus luteum, which produces significant amounts of progesterone during the luteal phase of the menstrual cycle.
- **Luteal Phase**: Progesterone levels peak during the luteal phase, ensuring the endometrium is prepared for the potential implantation of a fertilized egg.

2. Adrenal Glands

- **Steroidogenesis**: The adrenal glands produce small amounts of progesterone as part of the steroidogenesis pathway, which also produces cortisol and aldosterone.

3. Placental Production

- **Pregnancy**: During pregnancy, the placenta takes over the production of progesterone from the corpus luteum around the 8th to 10th week of gestation. Placental progesterone is essential for maintaining the pregnancy and supporting fetal development.

Regulation of Progesterone

The regulation of progesterone involves a complex interplay of hormonal signals, feedback mechanisms, and external factors:

1. Hypothalamus and Pituitary Gland

- **Gonadotropin-Releasing Hormone (GnRH)**: The hypothalamus releases GnRH, which stimulates the pituitary gland to produce luteinizing hormone (LH) and follicle-stimulating hormone (FSH).
- **LH Surge**: The mid-cycle LH surge triggers ovulation and the subsequent formation of the corpus luteum, leading to increased progesterone production.

2. Feedback Mechanisms

- **Negative Feedback**: High levels of progesterone exert negative feedback on the hypothalamus and pituitary gland, reducing the secretion of GnRH, LH, and FSH, thereby regulating its own production.

3. External Factors

- **Stress**: Chronic stress can disrupt progesterone production by increasing cortisol levels, which may interfere with the hypothalamic-pituitary-ovarian axis.
- **Diet and Nutrition**: Nutritional status, including the intake of essential vitamins and minerals, plays a role in hormone production and regulation.

Plant-Based Diet and Progesterone Regulation

A plant-based diet, rich in fruits, vegetables, whole grains, nuts, and seeds, can have a significant impact on progesterone regulation through various mechanisms:

1. Nutrient Density

Plant-based diets are typically high in essential nutrients that support overall health and hormonal balance. Key nutrients include:

- **Vitamin B6**: Found in bananas, chickpeas, and potatoes, vitamin B6 is crucial for progesterone synthesis and regulation.
- **Magnesium**: Leafy greens, nuts, and seeds are rich in magnesium, which supports the enzymatic activity involved in progesterone production.
- **Zinc**: Legumes, seeds, and nuts provide zinc, an essential mineral for hormone production and immune function.

2. Phytoestrogens

Phytoestrogens, plant compounds with estrogen-like activity, are found in foods like soy, flaxseeds, and lentils. While they primarily mimic estrogen, they can also influence progesterone levels by:

- **Modulating Hormonal Balance**: Phytoestrogens can help balance estrogen and progesterone levels, particularly in cases of estrogen dominance.
- **Supporting Reproductive Health**: The consumption of phytoestrogens has been linked to improved menstrual cycle regularity and reduced symptoms of PMS.

3. Antioxidants

Fruits and vegetables are rich in antioxidants, which help reduce oxidative stress. Lower oxidative stress levels are associated with improved hormone production and regulation:

- **Vitamin C**: Found in citrus fruits, strawberries, and bell peppers, vitamin C supports adrenal gland function and progesterone synthesis.
- **Vitamin E**: Nuts, seeds, and green leafy vegetables provide vitamin E, which has been shown to support reproductive health and hormonal balance.

4. Healthy Fats

Plant-based sources of fats, such as avocados, nuts, and seeds, provide essential fatty acids that support hormone production:

- **Omega-3 Fatty Acids**: Flaxseeds, chia seeds, and walnuts are rich in omega-3 fatty acids, which have anti-inflammatory properties and support overall hormonal health.
- **Monounsaturated Fats**: Avocados and olives provide monounsaturated fats that are beneficial for hormone synthesis and regulation.

5. Fiber

High-fiber diets, common in plant-based eating, support gut health and hormone regulation:

- **Gut Microbiome**: A healthy gut microbiome can influence hormone levels through the production of short-chain fatty acids and other metabolites.
- **Estrogen Excretion**: Fiber aids in the excretion of excess estrogen, helping to maintain a balance between estrogen and progesterone.

6. Caloric Balance

Maintaining a healthy weight through a balanced plant-based diet can prevent obesity-related suppression of progesterone:

- **Body Fat**: Excess body fat, particularly visceral fat, can disrupt hormonal balance and reduce progesterone levels due to increased production of cortisol and estrogen.
- **Insulin Sensitivity**: Improved insulin sensitivity from a plant-based diet can positively impact hormonal regulation and progesterone production.

Plant-Based Diet on Progesterone-Related Health Outcomes

A plant-based diet can positively influence various health outcomes related to progesterone:

1. Reproductive Health

- **Menstrual Cycle Regularity**: Plant-based diets rich in phytoestrogens and essential nutrients can help regulate menstrual cycles and reduce symptoms of PMS.
- **Fertility**: Nutrient-dense plant foods support overall reproductive health, potentially enhancing fertility and pregnancy outcomes.

2. Bone Health

- **Bone Density**: A diet high in calcium, magnesium, and vitamin K from plant sources supports bone health and helps maintain bone density.
- **Osteoporosis Prevention**: By promoting a healthy balance between estrogen and progesterone, a plant-based diet can reduce the risk of osteoporosis and improve bone strength.

3. Mood and Cognitive Function

- **Mental Health**: Emerging evidence suggests that plant-based diets may benefit mental health by reducing inflammation and oxidative stress, which are linked to mood disorders.
- **Cognitive Function**: Improved progesterone levels, supported by a plant-based diet, can enhance cognitive function and emotional well-being.

4. Weight Management

- **Healthy Weight**: Plant-based diets are effective for weight management, reducing body fat, and improving insulin sensitivity.
- **Hormonal Balance**: Maintaining a healthy weight through a plant-based diet can prevent obesity-related disruptions in hormonal balance.

5. Anti-Aging Effects

- **Oxidative Stress Reduction**: The antioxidant-rich nature of plant-based diets helps combat oxidative stress, a key factor in aging.

- **Hormonal Health**: Improved progesterone levels, coupled with reduced oxidative damage, contribute to healthier aging and better maintenance of reproductive health.

Progesterone plays a pivotal role in reproductive health, bone density, cognitive function, and overall well-being. Its production and regulation are influenced by various factors, including age, stress, diet, and lifestyle.

Inhibin

Inhibin is a glycoprotein hormone that plays a crucial role in the regulation of the reproductive system, particularly in the feedback mechanism that controls the production of follicle-stimulating hormone (FSH).

Function of Inhibin

Inhibin's primary function is to inhibit the secretion of FSH from the anterior pituitary gland. This action is vital for the regulation of the reproductive cycle and fertility in both males and females. The key functions of inhibin include:

1. **Regulation of FSH Secretion**: Inhibin negatively regulates the secretion of FSH by binding to receptors on the pituitary gland, thereby inhibiting its release. This feedback mechanism is essential for maintaining the balance of reproductive hormones.
2. **Spermatogenesis**: In males, inhibin plays a role in regulating spermatogenesis by controlling FSH levels, which in turn influences the production of sperm within the testes.

3. **Menstrual Cycle Regulation**: In females, inhibin is involved in the regulation of the menstrual cycle. It helps modulate the development of ovarian follicles and the timing of ovulation by influencing FSH levels.
4. **Ovarian Function**: Inhibin, particularly inhibin B, is involved in the selection and growth of dominant follicles during the menstrual cycle, playing a critical role in ovarian function and fertility.
5. **Role in Pregnancy**: Inhibin levels change during pregnancy, where it may play a role in placental function and fetal development. Elevated levels of inhibin A, for example, are observed during pregnancy and can be used as a marker for certain conditions.

Production of Inhibin

Inhibin is produced in both the male and female reproductive systems, primarily by the gonads.

1. **Synthesis in Males**: Inhibin is produced by the Sertoli cells of the testes. Sertoli cells, located within the seminiferous tubules, support and nourish developing sperm cells and play a crucial role in spermatogenesis.
2. **Synthesis in Females**: In females, inhibin is produced by the granulosa cells of the ovarian follicles. Granulosa cells surround the developing oocytes and are essential for the growth and maturation of ovarian follicles.
3. **Molecular Structure**: Inhibin is a dimeric protein composed of two subunits: alpha (α) and beta (β). There are two forms of inhibin, inhibin A and inhibin B, which differ in their beta subunit (βA or βB).
4. **Regulation by Gonadotropins**: The production of inhibin is stimulated by gonadotropins, particularly FSH. In turn, inhibin

exerts a negative feedback effect on the pituitary gland to modulate FSH secretion.

Regulation of Inhibin

The regulation of inhibin involves a complex interplay of feedback mechanisms and external factors:

1. **Negative Feedback Loop**: Inhibin functions in a negative feedback loop to regulate FSH secretion. High levels of inhibin lead to decreased secretion of FSH, while low levels of inhibin result in increased FSH secretion.
2. **Hormonal Interactions**: Inhibin interacts with other reproductive hormones, such as luteinizing hormone (LH) and estradiol. These hormones collectively regulate the menstrual cycle and reproductive functions.
3. **Influence of Age**: Inhibin levels change with age. In females, inhibin levels decline with advancing age, particularly during perimenopause and menopause, contributing to changes in FSH levels and ovarian function. In males, inhibin levels also decline with age, affecting spermatogenesis and fertility.
4. **Diet and Nutrition**: Nutritional status can influence inhibin levels. For example, adequate intake of essential nutrients is necessary for the proper function of the reproductive system, including the production and regulation of inhibin.

Plant-Based Diet and Inhibin Regulation

A plant-based diet, which emphasizes the consumption of fruits, vegetables, whole grains, nuts, and seeds, can have significant impacts on the regulation of inhibin through various mechanisms:

1. **Nutrient Density**: Plant-based diets are rich in essential nutrients, vitamins, and minerals that support overall reproductive health. Nutrients such as zinc, selenium, and vitamin E, found abundantly in plant foods, are crucial for gonadal function and hormone production.
2. **Phytoestrogens**: Certain plant foods contain phytoestrogens, which are plant-derived compounds that mimic the action of estrogen in the body. These compounds, found in soy products, flaxseeds, and other plant foods, can influence the hormonal balance and may impact inhibin production and regulation.
3. **Antioxidants**: Fruits and vegetables are rich in antioxidants, which help reduce oxidative stress and support overall cellular health. Lower oxidative stress levels are associated with improved hormonal balance, including the regulation of inhibin.
4. **Healthy Fats**: Plant-based sources of fats, such as avocados, nuts, and seeds, provide essential fatty acids that support hormone production and regulation. Omega-3 fatty acids, in particular, have anti-inflammatory properties that can enhance reproductive hormone activity.
5. **Fiber**: High-fiber diets, common in plant-based eating, support gut health and hormone regulation. A healthy gut microbiome can influence reproductive hormones, including inhibin, through the production of short-chain fatty acids and other metabolites.
6. **Caloric Balance**: Maintaining a healthy weight through a balanced plant-based diet can prevent obesity-related hormonal imbalances. Excess body fat can disrupt the production and regulation of reproductive hormones, including inhibin.
7. **Glycemic Control**: Plant-based diets, which are low in refined sugars and high in complex carbohydrates, help maintain stable blood glucose levels. This stability supports overall hormonal balance and prevents disruptions in inhibin production.

Plant-Based Diet on Inhibin-Related Health Outcomes

1. **Fertility and Reproductive Health**: A plant-based diet, rich in essential nutrients and antioxidants, supports reproductive health by promoting the proper function of the gonads and the regulation of reproductive hormones. This can enhance fertility and overall reproductive outcomes.
2. **Spermatogenesis**: In males, a plant-based diet can support spermatogenesis by providing key nutrients necessary for sperm production and reducing oxidative stress, which can damage sperm cells and impair fertility.
3. **Menstrual Health**: In females, a plant-based diet can help regulate the menstrual cycle by supporting the balance of reproductive hormones, including inhibin. This can reduce the risk of menstrual irregularities and support overall ovarian function.
4. **Pregnancy Outcomes**: Adequate nutrition during pregnancy is essential for fetal development and maternal health. A plant-based diet, rich in essential vitamins and minerals, can support the production and regulation of reproductive hormones, including inhibin, which plays a role in pregnancy.
5. **Hormonal Balance**: The antioxidant and anti-inflammatory properties of plant-based diets help maintain hormonal balance and reduce the risk of conditions associated with hormonal imbalances, such as polycystic ovary syndrome (PCOS) and endometriosis.

Inhibin is a vital hormone in the regulation of the reproductive system, influencing FSH secretion, spermatogenesis, and ovarian function. Its production and regulation are intricately linked to overall reproductive health and are influenced by various factors, including age, hormonal interactions, and diet.

7

Gastrointestinal Hormones

Gastrin

Gastrin is a peptide hormone that plays a critical role in the digestive process, particularly in regulating the secretion of gastric acid in the stomach.

Function of Gastrin

Gastrin's primary function is to stimulate the secretion of gastric acid (HCl) by the parietal cells of the stomach. This hormone facilitates various processes essential for digestion and nutrient absorption:

1. **Stimulating Gastric Acid Secretion**: Gastrin binds to the CCK-B receptors on parietal cells in the stomach lining, leading to the secretion of hydrochloric acid. This acid is crucial for breaking down food, activating digestive enzymes, and providing an acidic environment that inhibits harmful bacteria.
2. **Promoting Gastric Motility**: Gastrin increases the motility of the stomach, enhancing the mechanical breakdown of food and ensuring efficient mixing with gastric juices.
3. **Stimulating Pepsinogen Secretion**: Gastrin promotes the secretion of pepsinogen from chief cells in the stomach. Once activated to pepsin by the acidic environment, pepsin aids in protein digestion.

4. **Trophic Effects on Gastric Mucosa**: Gastrin has trophic (growth-promoting) effects on the gastric mucosa, enhancing the maintenance and growth of the stomach lining.
5. **Influencing Other Digestive Processes**: Gastrin also affects the secretion of pancreatic enzymes and bile, indirectly contributing to the overall digestive process.

Production of Gastrin

Gastrin is produced by G cells located primarily in the antrum of the stomach and, to a lesser extent, in the duodenum. The production process involves several key steps:

1. **Synthesis**: Gastrin is synthesized as a preprohormone and undergoes several post-translational modifications to form its active state. The gene responsible for gastrin production is located on chromosome 17 in humans.
2. **Regulation by Ingested Food**: The presence of partially digested proteins, amino acids, and peptides in the stomach lumen stimulates G cells to secrete gastrin. This secretion is a crucial part of the cephalic and gastric phases of digestion.
3. **Influence of Neural Signals**: The vagus nerve, through the release of acetylcholine, also stimulates gastrin secretion. This neural regulation ensures that gastrin levels increase in response to the sight, smell, or thought of food.
4. **Hormonal Regulation**: Other hormones, such as secretin and somatostatin, play regulatory roles. Secretin inhibits gastrin secretion when the stomach contents are too acidic, while somatostatin directly inhibits G cells.

Regulation of Gastrin

The regulation of gastrin involves complex feedback mechanisms and external factors:

1. **Negative Feedback Loop**: High levels of gastric acid (low pH) inhibit further gastrin release. This feedback mechanism prevents excessive acid production, protecting the stomach lining from damage.
2. **Positive Feedback Mechanisms**: The presence of food and the mechanical stretching of the stomach walls stimulate gastrin release, ensuring adequate acid production for digestion.
3. **Neural Control**: The enteric nervous system and the vagus nerve modulate gastrin secretion in response to various stimuli, integrating the digestive processes.
4. **Hormonal Influences**: Hormones such as cholecystokinin (CCK) can modulate gastrin secretion indirectly by influencing the overall digestive process.

Plant-Based Diet and Gastrin Regulation

A plant-based diet, rich in fruits, vegetables, whole grains, nuts, and seeds, can significantly impact the regulation of gastrin through various mechanisms:

1. **Nutrient Composition**: Plant-based diets are typically high in fiber, which can influence gastrin secretion. Dietary fiber helps modulate the rate of gastric emptying and the physical state of stomach contents, impacting gastrin levels.
2. **Amino Acid Profile**: While animal proteins are known stimulants of gastrin release, plant-based proteins also play a role. Foods such as legumes, nuts, and seeds provide essential amino acids

that can influence gastrin secretion, though typically at a different rate and magnitude compared to animal proteins.

3. **Antioxidants and Phytochemicals**: Plant foods are rich in antioxidants and phytochemicals that can reduce oxidative stress in the gastric mucosa, potentially influencing gastrin activity and promoting overall digestive health.
4. **Gut Microbiome**: A plant-based diet supports a diverse and healthy gut microbiome. Short-chain fatty acids (SCFAs) produced by the fermentation of dietary fiber by gut bacteria can modulate the secretion of various gut hormones, including gastrin.
5. **Anti-inflammatory Properties**: The anti-inflammatory properties of plant-based diets can help maintain a healthy gastric mucosa, reducing the risk of conditions such as gastritis, which can dysregulate gastrin production.

Plant-Based Diet on Gastrin-Related Health Outcomes

1. **Gastric Health**: A plant-based diet can help maintain optimal gastric acid levels, preventing both hyperacidity and hypoacidity conditions. By providing a balanced nutrient profile and supporting a healthy gut microbiome, plant-based diets contribute to the efficient regulation of gastrin.
2. **Gastroesophageal Reflux Disease (GERD)**: Plant-based diets, which are typically lower in fat and more fiber-rich, can help manage GERD symptoms. A balanced gastrin secretion helps maintain appropriate acid levels, reducing the risk of acid reflux.
3. **Peptic Ulcer Disease**: A diet rich in fruits and vegetables, which are high in antioxidants and anti-inflammatory compounds, can protect the gastric mucosa. This protection can help prevent peptic ulcers, which are often associated with dysregulated gastrin and excessive acid production.

4. **Cancer Prevention**: Some studies suggest that high gastrin levels may be linked to certain types of gastric cancers. A plant-based diet, with its anti-inflammatory and antioxidant properties, may help regulate gastrin levels and reduce the risk of such cancers.
5. **Digestive Efficiency**: Plant-based diets promote healthy digestive processes, from efficient gastric emptying to balanced acid production. This efficiency supports overall nutrient absorption and digestive health.

Gastrin plays a pivotal role in regulating gastric acid secretion and overall digestive health. Its production and regulation are influenced by various factors, including diet, neural signals, and hormonal feedback mechanisms.

Cholecystokinin (CCK)

Cholecystokinin (CCK) is a peptide hormone that plays a significant role in digestion and appetite regulation.

Function of Cholecystokinin

Cholecystokinin has several critical functions in the body, primarily related to digestion and satiety:

1. **Stimulation of Digestive Enzymes**: CCK stimulates the pancreas to release digestive enzymes such as amylase, lipase, and proteases, which are essential for the breakdown of carbohydrates, fats, and proteins, respectively. This process is vital for the efficient digestion and absorption of nutrients from food.
2. **Gallbladder Contraction**: One of the primary functions of CCK is to stimulate the contraction of the gallbladder. This

action releases stored bile into the small intestine, aiding in the emulsification and absorption of dietary fats.

3. **Regulation of Satiety**: CCK plays a crucial role in signaling satiety to the brain. When food enters the small intestine, CCK is released and interacts with receptors in the brain, particularly in the hypothalamus, to induce feelings of fullness and reduce food intake.
4. **Gastrointestinal Motility**: CCK helps regulate the motility of the stomach and intestines. It slows gastric emptying, allowing for better digestion and nutrient absorption in the small intestine.
5. **Modulation of Insulin Secretion**: CCK influences insulin secretion by modulating the response of pancreatic beta cells to blood glucose levels. This effect is essential for maintaining glucose homeostasis.

Production of Cholecystokinin

CCK is produced primarily in the small intestine but also in the brain. The production process involves several steps:

1. **Synthesis in the Small Intestine**: CCK is synthesized and secreted by I cells located in the mucosa of the small intestine, particularly in the duodenum and jejunum. The production of CCK is stimulated by the presence of partially digested proteins and fats in the small intestine.
2. **Release and Circulation**: Upon stimulation by chyme entering the small intestine, CCK is released into the bloodstream. It then travels to various target organs, including the pancreas and gallbladder, to exert its effects.
3. **Production in the Brain**: In addition to its synthesis in the small intestine, CCK is also produced in the brain, where it acts as a neurotransmitter. Neuronal CCK is involved in regulating anxiety, pain perception, and appetite.

Regulation of Cholecystokinin

The regulation of CCK involves feedback mechanisms and various external factors:

1. **Nutrient Presence**: The presence of fats and proteins in the small intestine is the primary trigger for CCK release. This nutrient-stimulated release ensures that digestive enzymes and bile are available when needed.
2. **Neuronal Signals**: Vagal afferent neurons play a crucial role in the regulation of CCK. These neurons transmit signals from the gut to the brain, indicating the presence of nutrients and triggering the release of CCK.
3. **Hormonal Interactions**: CCK interacts with other hormones, such as secretin and gastrin, to coordinate digestive processes. Secretin, for example, enhances the effects of CCK on the pancreas, promoting the secretion of bicarbonate-rich fluid to neutralize stomach acid.
4. **Feedback Inhibition**: Once the digestive process is underway, feedback mechanisms help regulate CCK levels. For instance, the digestion and absorption of fats and proteins reduce the stimulus for CCK release, preventing excessive hormone levels.

Plant-Based Diet and Cholecystokinin Regulation

A plant-based diet can significantly impact the regulation of CCK through various mechanisms:

1. **High Fiber Content**: Plant-based diets are rich in dietary fiber, which slows gastric emptying and prolongs the presence of food in the small intestine. This extended presence stimulates sustained CCK release, promoting satiety and aiding in weight management.

2. **Healthy Fats**: Plant-based sources of fats, such as avocados, nuts, and seeds, provide healthy fats that stimulate CCK release without the negative effects associated with saturated fats found in animal products. These healthy fats promote efficient digestion and nutrient absorption.
3. **Protein Sources**: Plant-based proteins, such as legumes, tofu, and quinoa, effectively stimulate CCK production. These proteins, combined with high fiber content, contribute to a prolonged feeling of fullness and reduced calorie intake.
4. **Phytonutrients and Antioxidants**: Plant-based diets are abundant in phytonutrients and antioxidants, which have anti-inflammatory properties. Lower inflammation levels can positively influence gut health and hormone regulation, including CCK.
5. **Gut Microbiota**: A diverse and healthy gut microbiota, fostered by a plant-based diet, can enhance CCK production and secretion. The fermentation of dietary fiber by gut bacteria produces short-chain fatty acids that stimulate CCK release.

Plant-Based Diet on Cholecystokinin-Related Health Outcomes

1. **Weight Management**: Plant-based diets are effective for weight management due to the combined effects of high fiber and protein content, which promote prolonged CCK release and increased satiety. Studies have shown that individuals on plant-based diets tend to have lower body mass indexes (BMIs) compared to those on omnivorous diets.
2. **Digestive Health**: The high fiber content in plant-based diets supports healthy digestion and regular bowel movements. By promoting CCK release, plant-based diets aid in efficient digestion and nutrient absorption, reducing the risk of gastrointestinal disorders such as irritable bowel syndrome (IBS).

3. **Cardiovascular Health**: Healthy fats from plant sources, such as nuts and seeds, support cardiovascular health by promoting favorable lipid profiles and reducing inflammation. Enhanced CCK activity contributes to improved digestion and nutrient absorption, further benefiting heart health.
4. **Mental Health**: Emerging evidence suggests that plant-based diets may benefit mental health by reducing inflammation and oxidative stress, which are linked to mood disorders. Improved CCK levels, coupled with the high antioxidant content of plant-based foods, contribute to better mental well-being.
5. **Diabetes Management**: Plant-based diets have been shown to improve glycemic control and insulin sensitivity, essential for diabetes management. By modulating CCK and other digestive hormones, plant-based diets help maintain stable blood glucose levels.

Cholecystokinin plays a pivotal role in digestion, satiety, and overall health. Its production and regulation are influenced by various factors, including nutrient presence, neuronal signals, and hormonal interactions.

Secretin

Secretin is a peptide hormone essential for the regulation of digestive processes and maintaining the acid-base balance in the body.

Function of Secretin

Secretin plays several critical roles in the digestive system:

1. **Regulation of pH**: Secretin is primarily involved in the regulation of the pH of the duodenum by inhibiting gastric acid secretion from the stomach and stimulating the production of bicarbonate from the pancreas. This bicarbonate neutralizes the acid entering the duodenum from the stomach, providing an optimal pH for digestive enzymes to function.
2. **Stimulating Bicarbonate Secretion**: Secretin prompts the pancreas to release bicarbonate-rich fluid, which helps to neutralize stomach acid and create a suitable environment for enzymes from the pancreas to operate effectively.
3. **Inhibiting Gastric Acid Secretion**: It helps regulate gastric acid production by inhibiting the secretion of gastrin, a hormone that stimulates the production of gastric acid.
4. **Enhancing Bile Production**: Secretin increases bile secretion from the liver, aiding in the digestion and absorption of fats.
5. **Supporting Digestive Enzymes**: It enhances the secretion of digestive enzymes from the pancreas, contributing to the breakdown of carbohydrates, proteins, and fats.

Production of Secretin

Secretin is produced by S cells located in the mucosa of the duodenum and jejunum, parts of the small intestine. The production process involves several key steps:

1. **Synthesis**: Secretin is synthesized as a precursor protein, preprosecretin, which is then processed to its active form.
2. **Release Triggered by pH**: The primary trigger for the release of secretin is the acidic chyme (partially digested food) entering the duodenum from the stomach. When the pH of the chyme is lower than 4.5, S cells release secretin.

3. **Transport**: Once secretin is released, it enters the bloodstream and travels to its target organs, including the pancreas, stomach, and liver, to exert its effects.

Regulation of Secretin

The regulation of secretin involves complex feedback mechanisms and is influenced by several factors:

1. **Feedback Loops**: The secretion of secretin is primarily regulated through a negative feedback loop. When the pH in the duodenum rises (becomes less acidic) due to the neutralizing effect of bicarbonate, the secretion of secretin is reduced.
2. **Nutritional Factors**: Certain nutrients, particularly fats, and amino acids, can stimulate the release of secretin. However, a plant-based diet, rich in fiber and phytonutrients, can modulate this response by promoting a healthy digestive environment.
3. **Hormonal Interactions**: Secretin interacts with other hormones, such as cholecystokinin (CCK) and gastrin, to coordinate digestive processes. CCK, released in response to fats and proteins, works synergistically with secretin to enhance digestive enzymes and bicarbonate secretion.
4. **Gut Microbiome**: The gut microbiome can influence the secretion and activity of secretin. A diverse and balanced microbiome, fostered by a plant-based diet, supports healthy digestion and optimal secretin function.

Plant-Based Diet and Secretin Regulation

A plant-based diet can have significant effects on the regulation and activity of secretin through various mechanisms:

1. **High Fiber Intake**: Plant-based diets are rich in dietary fiber, which promotes gut health and regular bowel movements. Fiber helps maintain a healthy pH in the intestine, supporting the optimal release and function of secretin.
2. **Phytonutrients**: Fruits, vegetables, whole grains, nuts, and seeds contain phytonutrients that have anti-inflammatory and antioxidant properties. These compounds can support the integrity of the gut lining and enhance the secretion and action of digestive hormones, including secretin.
3. **Healthy Fats**: Plant-based sources of healthy fats, such as avocados, nuts, and seeds, provide essential fatty acids that support bile production and overall digestive health. These fats also modulate the release of hormones like CCK, which works in conjunction with secretin.
4. **Probiotics and Prebiotics**: Fermented plant foods, such as sauerkraut, kimchi, and yogurt alternatives, contain probiotics that support a healthy gut microbiome. Prebiotics, found in foods like garlic, onions, and bananas, feed beneficial bacteria. A balanced microbiome enhances secretin function and overall digestive health.
5. **Alkaline Foods**: Many plant-based foods, such as leafy greens, cucumbers, and melons, have an alkalizing effect on the body. These foods can help maintain a healthy pH balance in the digestive system, supporting the optimal activity of secretin.

Plant-Based Diet on Secretin-Related Health Outcomes

1. **Improved Digestion**: A plant-based diet rich in fiber, phytonutrients, and healthy fats supports efficient digestion and nutrient absorption. By promoting a healthy gut environment, this diet enhances the production and function of secretin, leading to better digestive health.

2. **Reduced Inflammation**: Chronic inflammation can disrupt digestive processes and hormone regulation. The anti-inflammatory properties of plant-based foods help reduce inflammation, supporting the proper function of secretin and other digestive hormones.
3. **Enhanced Gut Health**: The high fiber content of plant-based diets promotes regular bowel movements and prevents constipation. A healthy gut environment supports the optimal secretion and activity of secretin, ensuring efficient digestion and nutrient absorption.
4. **Weight Management**: Plant-based diets are effective for weight management due to their high fiber and nutrient density. Maintaining a healthy weight supports the balanced secretion of digestive hormones, including secretin, and reduces the risk of digestive disorders.
5. **Lower Risk of Digestive Disorders**: A plant-based diet can reduce the risk of digestive disorders such as acid reflux, gastritis, and irritable bowel syndrome (IBS). By supporting the optimal function of secretin and other digestive hormones, this diet promotes overall digestive health and reduces the incidence of these conditions.

Ghrelin

Ghrelin, often referred to as the "hunger hormone," is a peptide hormone that plays a critical role in regulating appetite, energy balance, and gastrointestinal motility.

Function of Ghrelin

Ghrelin's primary functions are centered around hunger stimulation, energy homeostasis, and various metabolic processes. It achieves these through several mechanisms:

1. **Appetite Regulation**: Ghrelin is best known for its role in stimulating hunger. It is released primarily by the stomach and acts on the hypothalamus, the brain region responsible for appetite control, to increase food intake. This hormone signals the brain that the body needs energy, promoting eating behavior.
2. **Energy Homeostasis**: Beyond its role in hunger signaling, ghrelin is involved in energy balance. It promotes fat storage and reduces the utilization of fat for energy. This action helps the body prepare for periods of energy scarcity by conserving energy stores.
3. **Gastrointestinal Motility**: Ghrelin also plays a role in gastrointestinal functions, including promoting gastric emptying and enhancing intestinal motility. These effects ensure efficient digestion and nutrient absorption.
4. **Growth Hormone Release**: Ghrelin stimulates the release of growth hormone (GH) from the pituitary gland. GH, in turn, influences growth, cell reproduction, and regeneration, making ghrelin an indirect player in these vital processes.
5. **Cardiovascular Effects**: Emerging research suggests that ghrelin has cardioprotective properties. It can improve cardiac output and reduce vascular resistance, potentially benefiting heart health.
6. **Mood and Cognitive Function**: Ghrelin has been implicated in mood regulation and cognitive functions. It interacts with brain regions involved in reward and motivation, potentially influencing emotional states and mental health.

Production of Ghrelin

Ghrelin is produced in various tissues, with the stomach being the primary source. The production process involves several steps:

1. **Synthesis**: Ghrelin is synthesized predominantly by the gastric mucosa, specifically the oxyntic glands in the stomach lining. Smaller amounts are produced in other tissues, including the small intestine, pancreas, and hypothalamus.
2. **Secretion**: Ghrelin is secreted into the bloodstream in response to fasting and low energy states. Its levels rise before meals, stimulating hunger, and fall after food intake, contributing to satiety.
3. **Activation**: Ghrelin undergoes post-translational modification to become active. The enzyme ghrelin O-acyltransferase (GOAT) adds an acyl group to ghrelin, enabling it to bind to its receptor, the growth hormone secretagogue receptor (GHS-R1a).
4. **Regulation by Nutritional Status**: Ghrelin secretion is tightly regulated by nutritional status. Fasting increases ghrelin levels while feeding suppresses its release. The macronutrient composition of the diet also influences ghrelin secretion, with carbohydrates and proteins having different effects on its levels.

Regulation of Ghrelin

The regulation of ghrelin involves complex feedback mechanisms and interactions with other hormones and nutrients:

1. **Nutrient Intake**: The presence of food in the stomach suppresses ghrelin secretion. Different macronutrients have varying impacts on ghrelin levels; carbohydrates and proteins tend to reduce ghrelin more effectively than fats.
2. **Hormonal Interactions**: Ghrelin interacts with several other hormones involved in energy balance, including leptin, insulin,

and glucagon-like peptide-1 (GLP-1). Leptin, produced by adipose tissue, suppresses ghrelin levels, creating a feedback loop that regulates hunger and energy storage.

3. **Sleep**: Sleep patterns significantly influence ghrelin levels. Sleep deprivation increases ghrelin production, which can lead to increased appetite and weight gain. Conversely, adequate sleep helps maintain balanced ghrelin levels, supporting healthy eating patterns.
4. **Exercise**: Physical activity impacts ghrelin levels, although the effects can vary depending on the type and intensity of exercise. Some studies suggest that high-intensity exercise can reduce ghrelin levels, while moderate exercise may have a neutral or increasing effect.
5. **Body Composition**: Obesity and body fat distribution influence ghrelin secretion. Individuals with higher body fat percentages tend to have lower ghrelin levels, while weight loss can increase ghrelin production, complicating long-term weight maintenance.

Plant-Based Diet and Ghrelin Regulation

A plant-based diet, rich in fruits, vegetables, whole grains, nuts, and seeds, can significantly impact ghrelin regulation through various mechanisms:

1. **Nutrient Density**: Plant-based diets are typically high in essential nutrients, vitamins, and minerals that support overall health and hormonal balance. These nutrients can influence ghrelin secretion and its effects on appetite and metabolism.
2. **Fiber**: High-fiber diets, common in plant-based eating, contribute to satiety and stable ghrelin levels. Dietary fiber slows gastric emptying and prolongs the feeling of fullness, reducing the need for frequent food intake and moderating ghrelin spikes.

3. **Low Energy Density**: Plant-based foods generally have a lower energy density, meaning they provide fewer calories per gram. Consuming low-energy-dense foods helps maintain energy balance and prevents excessive ghrelin-induced hunger.
4. **Healthy Fats**: Plant-based sources of fats, such as avocados, nuts, and seeds, provide essential fatty acids that support hormone production and regulation. Healthy fats also contribute to satiety and may help stabilize ghrelin levels.
5. **Phytochemicals**: Fruits and vegetables are rich in phytochemicals, which have anti-inflammatory and antioxidant properties. These compounds can influence ghrelin secretion and action, promoting a balanced appetite and metabolic health.
6. **Glycemic Control**: Plant-based diets, which are low in refined sugars and high in complex carbohydrates, help maintain stable blood glucose levels. Stable blood glucose prevents hyperglycemia-induced suppression of ghrelin secretion, supporting healthy appetite regulation.

Plant-Based Diet on Ghrelin-Related Health Outcomes

1. **Weight Management**: Plant-based diets are effective for weight management, reducing body fat, and improving insulin sensitivity. Lower body fat and better glycemic control enhance ghrelin regulation, supporting healthy weight maintenance and preventing obesity.
2. **Appetite Control**: The high fiber content and nutrient density of plant-based diets contribute to better appetite control. This dietary pattern helps reduce overeating and supports balanced ghrelin levels, preventing excessive hunger and promoting satiety.
3. **Cardiovascular Health**: Plant-based diets, rich in antioxidants and healthy fats, support cardiovascular health. Balanced ghrelin

levels contribute to improved heart function and reduced risk of cardiovascular diseases.

4. **Metabolic Health**: Improved ghrelin regulation through plant-based eating supports overall metabolic health. This diet helps maintain healthy blood glucose levels, reduces inflammation, and supports efficient energy utilization.
5. **Mental Health**: Emerging evidence suggests that plant-based diets may benefit mental health by reducing inflammation and oxidative stress, which are linked to mood disorders. Balanced ghrelin levels also support cognitive function and emotional well-being.

Research and Evidence

Research on ghrelin and its interaction with diet, particularly plant-based diets, is ongoing. Several studies highlight the beneficial effects of plant-based eating on ghrelin regulation and related health outcomes:

1. **Fiber and Satiety**: A study published in the *American Journal of Clinical Nutrition* found that dietary fiber intake is inversely related to ghrelin levels. Higher fiber intake was associated with reduced hunger and lower ghrelin concentrations.
2. **Nutrient-Dense Foods**: Research in the *Journal of Nutrition* indicates that diets rich in fruits, vegetables, and whole grains support better ghrelin regulation and appetite control. These nutrient-dense foods provide essential vitamins and minerals that influence hormonal balance.
3. **Glycemic Control**: A study in the *Diabetes Care* journal found that plant-based diets improve glycemic control, which in turn supports stable ghrelin levels. The low glycemic index of plant-based foods helps maintain balanced blood sugar and prevents hyperglycemia-induced ghrelin suppression.

4. **Weight Management**: Research published in the *Journal of the Academy of Nutrition and Dietetics* shows that plant-based diets are effective for weight loss and maintenance. These diets reduce body fat and improve insulin sensitivity, supporting healthy ghrelin regulation.
5. **Cardiovascular Health**: A study in the *American Heart Journal* highlights the cardioprotective effects of plant-based diets. Improved ghrelin regulation through plant-based eating contributes to better heart function and reduced risk of cardiovascular diseases.
6. **Mental Health**: Research in the *Frontiers in Psychology* journal suggests that plant-based diets may benefit mental health by reducing inflammation and oxidative stress. Balanced ghrelin levels play a role in supporting cognitive function and emotional well-being.

Ghrelin, the "hunger hormone," plays a pivotal role in appetite regulation, energy balance, and various metabolic processes. Its production and regulation are influenced by multiple factors, including nutrient intake, hormonal interactions, sleep, exercise, and body composition.

Peptide YY (PYY)

Peptide YY (PYY) is a hormone that plays a crucial role in regulating appetite, digestion, and energy balance.

Function of Peptide YY

Peptide YY is primarily known for its role in appetite regulation and digestive processes. It achieves this by:

1. **Appetite Suppression:** PYY is released in response to food intake, particularly meals rich in protein and fiber. It acts on the Y2 receptors in the hypothalamus to reduce appetite and promote a feeling of satiety. This helps to prevent overeating and aids in weight management.
2. **Slowing Gastric Emptying:** PYY slows down the movement of food through the gastrointestinal tract, which prolongs the digestion process and enhances nutrient absorption. This also contributes to a prolonged feeling of fullness.
3. **Reducing Pancreatic Secretion:** PYY inhibits the secretion of digestive enzymes and hormones from the pancreas, thereby modulating the digestive process and improving nutrient utilization.
4. **Enhancing Insulin Sensitivity:** PYY has been shown to improve insulin sensitivity, which helps in better glucose uptake by cells and maintains blood sugar levels within a healthy range.
5. **Modulating Energy Balance:** By regulating appetite and food intake, PYY plays a significant role in maintaining energy balance and preventing obesity-related metabolic disorders.

Production of Peptide YY

Peptide YY is produced by the L-cells in the mucosa of the ileum and colon. The production process involves several steps:

1. **Synthesis:** PYY is synthesized as a precursor protein, prepro-PYY, which is then processed into mature PYY. This process occurs in the L-cells of the ileum and colon.
2. **Release:** PYY is released into the bloodstream in response to food intake, particularly meals high in protein and fiber. The release of PYY is biphasic, with an initial rapid phase followed by a slower, sustained phase.

3. **Transport:** Once released, PYY travels through the bloodstream to reach its target organs, primarily the hypothalamus in the brain, where it exerts its appetite-suppressing effects.
4. **Degradation:** PYY is eventually degraded by enzymes, such as dipeptidyl peptidase IV (DPP-IV), which inactivates the hormone and regulates its levels in the bloodstream.

Regulation of Peptide YY

The regulation of PYY is a complex process involving various factors:

1. **Nutrient Intake:** The composition of the diet significantly influences PYY levels. Meals rich in protein and fiber are potent stimulators of PYY release. Plant-based foods, which are high in fiber, can enhance PYY secretion and promote satiety.
2. **Gastrointestinal Hormones:** Other hormones released during digestion, such as glucagon-like peptide-1 (GLP-1) and cholecystokinin (CCK), also modulate PYY secretion. These hormones work synergistically to regulate appetite and digestive processes.
3. **Gut Microbiota:** The gut microbiota plays a crucial role in the regulation of PYY. Certain bacterial species can influence the release of PYY by fermenting dietary fibers into short-chain fatty acids (SCFAs), which stimulate the L-cells to produce PYY.
4. **Physical Activity:** Regular physical activity has been shown to increase PYY levels, which can help in regulating appetite and maintain energy balance.
5. **Circadian Rhythms:** PYY levels exhibit a circadian rhythm, with higher levels observed during the day and lower levels at night. Disruptions in sleep patterns can affect PYY levels and appetite regulation.

Plant-Based Diet and Peptide YY Regulation

A plant-based diet, rich in fruits, vegetables, whole grains, nuts, and seeds, can have a profound impact on PYY regulation through various mechanisms:

1. **Fiber-Rich Foods:** Plant-based diets are typically high in dietary fiber, which is a key stimulator of PYY release. Soluble fibers, found in foods like oats, beans, and fruits, form a gel-like substance in the gut, slowing digestion and promoting PYY release.
2. **Protein Sources:** Plant-based protein sources, such as legumes, nuts, and seeds, can also stimulate PYY release. These foods provide essential amino acids that are important for overall health and hormone production.
3. **Gut Health:** A diverse and balanced gut microbiota, promoted by a plant-based diet, enhances the production of SCFAs through the fermentation of dietary fibers. SCFAs stimulate PYY release, improving appetite regulation and metabolic health.
4. **Antioxidants and Phytochemicals:** Plant-based foods are rich in antioxidants and phytochemicals, which reduce inflammation and oxidative stress. Lower inflammation levels are associated with improved PYY secretion and overall endocrine function.
5. **Low Glycemic Index:** Plant-based diets typically have a low glycemic index, which helps maintain stable blood glucose levels. Stable glucose levels prevent the suppression of PYY secretion, promoting better appetite control and energy balance.
6. **Healthy Fats:** Plant-based sources of fats, such as avocados, nuts, and seeds, provide essential fatty acids that support hormone production and regulation. Omega-3 fatty acids, in particular, have anti-inflammatory properties that can enhance PYY activity.

Plant-Based Diet on PYY-Related Health Outcomes

1. **Weight Management:** A plant-based diet, rich in fiber and protein, promotes satiety through enhanced PYY secretion, aiding in weight management and preventing obesity-related disorders.
2. **Metabolic Health:** Improved PYY levels contribute to better insulin sensitivity and glucose regulation, reducing the risk of type 2 diabetes and metabolic syndrome.
3. **Digestive Health:** The fiber content in plant-based diets supports gut health by promoting healthy bowel movements and a balanced gut microbiota. This leads to improved digestive processes and nutrient absorption.
4. **Cardiovascular Health:** A plant-based diet, rich in antioxidants and healthy fats, supports cardiovascular health by reducing inflammation and promoting healthy cholesterol levels. Enhanced PYY levels also contribute to weight management, reducing the risk of heart disease.
5. **Mental Health:** Emerging evidence suggests that a plant-based diet may benefit mental health by reducing inflammation and oxidative stress. Improved PYY levels support cognitive function and emotional well-being.

8

Other Endocrine Hormones

Leptin

Leptin is a peptide hormone that plays a crucial role in regulating energy balance, hunger, and metabolism. Discovered in 1994, leptin is primarily produced by adipose (fat) tissue and informs the brain about the state of the body's energy stores.

Function of Leptin

Leptin's primary function is to regulate energy balance by inhibiting hunger, which in turn diminishes fat storage in adipocytes. This hormone achieves this by:

1. **Regulating Appetite**: Leptin acts on receptors in the hypothalamus of the brain, where it inhibits appetite by counteracting the effects of neuropeptide Y (NPY) and anandamide, two hunger-promoting signals, and stimulating the production of alpha-MSH, an appetite suppressant.
2. **Energy Expenditure**: Leptin increases energy expenditure by stimulating the sympathetic nervous system. This leads to increased thermogenesis and higher metabolic rates, thus promoting the utilization of stored fat.
3. **Reproduction**: Leptin plays a role in regulating reproductive function. Adequate levels of leptin signal that the body has

sufficient energy stores for reproduction, affecting fertility and the menstrual cycle in women.

4. **Immune Function**: Leptin modulates the immune response, enhancing the activation and proliferation of T lymphocytes and influencing the production of pro-inflammatory cytokines.
5. **Regulation of Insulin Sensitivity**: Leptin influences glucose metabolism and insulin sensitivity. It helps maintain proper glucose homeostasis and prevents excessive fat accumulation, which can lead to insulin resistance.

Production of Leptin

Leptin is produced by adipocytes, or fat cells, with its levels directly correlated to the amount of body fat. The production process involves several steps:

1. **Synthesis**: The leptin gene (ob gene) located on chromosome 7 in humans is responsible for leptin production. Adipocytes synthesize leptin, which is then secreted into the bloodstream.
2. **Regulation by Nutrient Status**: Leptin production is influenced by the body's energy balance. During periods of energy surplus, adipocytes increase leptin secretion. Conversely, during fasting or weight loss, leptin levels decrease.
3. **Pulsatile Secretion**: Leptin is secreted in a pulsatile manner, with levels peaking during the night. This diurnal rhythm is believed to align with feeding and fasting cycles.
4. **Influencing Factors**: Several factors influence leptin production, including:
    - **Body Fat**: Higher body fat percentage results in increased leptin levels.
    - **Insulin**: Insulin stimulates leptin production, linking it to meal-induced insulin spikes.

- **Cytokines**: Pro-inflammatory cytokines like TNF-α can increase leptin production.

Regulation of Leptin

The regulation of leptin is a complex process involving feedback mechanisms and external factors:

1. **Feedback Loops**: Leptin levels are regulated through feedback mechanisms that involve the brain and other tissues. High leptin levels signal sufficient energy stores, leading to reduced food intake and increased energy expenditure. Low leptin levels trigger hunger and reduce energy expenditure to conserve energy.
2. **Sleep**: Sleep is a critical regulator of leptin production. Disrupted sleep patterns can lead to altered leptin levels and, consequently, impaired energy balance and metabolism.
3. **Exercise**: Physical activity can influence leptin levels. Acute exercise may temporarily reduce leptin levels, while regular physical activity is associated with improved leptin sensitivity.
4. **Nutritional Status**: Nutritional status significantly impacts leptin levels. Fasting decreases leptin levels while refeeding or consuming a meal increases leptin production. Macronutrient composition also plays a role; carbohydrates and proteins, in particular, can stimulate leptin secretion.
5. **Hormones**: Other hormones, such as insulin and cortisol, interact with leptin. Insulin enhances leptin production, while cortisol may impair leptin signaling, contributing to stress-induced weight gain.

Plant-Based Diet and Leptin Regulation

A plant-based diet, rich in fruits, vegetables, whole grains, nuts, and seeds, can profoundly impact leptin regulation through various mechanisms:

1. **Nutrient Density**: Plant-based diets are typically high in essential nutrients, vitamins, and minerals that support overall health and hormonal balance. For example, antioxidants found in fruits and vegetables help reduce oxidative stress, supporting leptin signaling.
2. **Fiber**: High-fiber diets, common in plant-based eating, support gut health and hormone regulation. Dietary fiber can enhance satiety and improve leptin sensitivity, promoting better energy balance and weight management.
3. **Healthy Fats**: Plant-based sources of fats, such as avocados, nuts, and seeds, provide essential fatty acids that support hormone production and regulation. Omega-3 fatty acids, in particular, have anti-inflammatory properties that can enhance leptin activity.
4. **Glycemic Control**: Plant-based diets, which are low in refined sugars and high in complex carbohydrates, help maintain stable blood glucose levels. This stability prevents insulin resistance, which is associated with impaired leptin signaling.
5. **Caloric Balance**: Maintaining a healthy weight through a balanced plant-based diet can prevent obesity-related leptin resistance. Excess body fat is linked to lower leptin sensitivity due to chronic low-grade inflammation and disrupted signaling pathways.
6. **Phytonutrients**: Plant foods are rich in phytonutrients, which have various health benefits, including anti-inflammatory and antioxidant effects. These compounds can improve leptin sensitivity and overall metabolic health.

Plant-Based Diet on Leptin-Related Health Outcomes

1. **Weight Management**: Plant-based diets are effective for weight management, reducing body fat, and improving insulin sensitivity. Lower body fat and better glycemic control enhance leptin sensitivity and overall metabolic health.
2. **Metabolic Health**: Improved leptin sensitivity through a plant-based diet can help regulate energy balance, glucose metabolism, and insulin sensitivity, reducing the risk of metabolic disorders such as type 2 diabetes.
3. **Cardiovascular Health**: Plant-based diets, rich in fiber, antioxidants, and healthy fats, support cardiovascular health by improving lipid profiles, reducing inflammation, and promoting healthy blood pressure levels. Enhanced leptin sensitivity contributes to these benefits by regulating fat storage and energy expenditure.
4. **Inflammation Reduction**: The anti-inflammatory properties of plant-based diets help mitigate chronic inflammation, which is often associated with obesity and leptin resistance. Reduced inflammation enhances leptin signaling and overall hormonal balance.
5. **Reproductive Health**: Improved leptin sensitivity through a plant-based diet can positively impact reproductive health by maintaining proper energy balance and supporting hormonal regulation, which is crucial for fertility and menstrual cycle regularity.

Adiponectin

Adiponectin is a hormone primarily produced by adipocytes (fat cells) and plays a crucial role in regulating glucose levels and fatty acid breakdown.

Function of Adiponectin

Adiponectin is a key player in metabolic processes and has several important functions:

- **Regulation of Glucose Levels**: Adiponectin enhances insulin sensitivity by promoting glucose uptake and utilization in skeletal muscle and adipose tissue. It also inhibits glucose production in the liver, helping to maintain stable blood glucose levels.
- **Fatty Acid Oxidation**: Adiponectin promotes the breakdown of fatty acids, primarily in muscle and liver tissues. This process, known as fatty acid oxidation, is crucial for energy production and maintaining lipid homeostasis.
- **Anti-Inflammatory Effects**: Adiponectin exhibits anti-inflammatory properties by inhibiting the expression of pro-inflammatory cytokines and promoting the production of anti-inflammatory cytokines. This function is particularly important in the context of obesity and metabolic syndrome, where chronic low-grade inflammation is prevalent.
- **Cardioprotective Effects**: Adiponectin has beneficial effects on the cardiovascular system. It enhances endothelial function, reduces atherosclerotic plaque formation, and lowers blood pressure, thereby protecting against cardiovascular diseases.
- **Regulation of Appetite and Weight**: Adiponectin influences appetite regulation and body weight. Higher levels of adiponectin are associated with reduced appetite and lower body weight, while lower levels are linked to increased appetite and obesity.

Production of Adiponectin

Adiponectin is primarily produced by white adipose tissue, but it is also expressed in smaller amounts in other tissues such as brown adipose tissue, muscle, and liver. The production process involves several steps:

- **Synthesis**: Adiponectin is synthesized and secreted by adipocytes. The gene responsible for adiponectin production is located on chromosome 3 in humans.
- **Post-Translational Modifications**: After synthesis, adiponectin undergoes several post-translational modifications, including hydroxylation and glycosylation, which are essential for its proper folding and function.
- **Secretion**: Mature adiponectin is secreted into the bloodstream, where it circulates in three main forms: low-molecular-weight (LMW), middle-molecular-weight (MMW), and high-molecular-weight (HMW) complexes. The HMW form is considered the most biologically active.
- **Influencing Factors**: Several factors influence adiponectin production, including:
    - **Body Weight**: Obesity is associated with lower adiponectin levels, while weight loss increases its levels.
    - **Insulin Sensitivity**: Higher insulin sensitivity is correlated with increased adiponectin production.
    - **Physical Activity**: Regular exercise enhances adiponectin levels.
    - **Diet**: Dietary composition, particularly fat and carbohydrate intake, influences adiponectin production.

Regulation of Adiponectin

The regulation of adiponectin is a complex process involving various factors:

- **Hormonal Regulation**: Several hormones influence adiponectin levels, including:
    - **Insulin**: Insulin increases adiponectin secretion.
    - **Glucocorticoids**: These hormones decrease adiponectin levels.

    - **Thyroid Hormones**: Thyroid hormones positively regulate adiponectin production.
- **Nutritional Regulation**: Dietary factors play a significant role in adiponectin regulation:
    - **Dietary Fats**: Saturated fats decrease adiponectin levels, while unsaturated fats increase them.
    - **Carbohydrates**: High-glycemic-index foods reduce adiponectin levels, whereas low-glycemic-index foods enhance them.
    - **Protein**: Certain amino acids, such as leucine, positively influence adiponectin production.
- **Genetic Factors**: Genetic variations in the adiponectin gene (ADIPOQ) and its regulatory elements affect adiponectin levels and function.
- **Inflammation**: Chronic inflammation, common in obesity and metabolic syndrome, suppresses adiponectin production.
- **Oxidative Stress**: Oxidative stress negatively impacts adiponectin levels. Antioxidant-rich diets can mitigate this effect and promote adiponectin production.

Plant-Based Diet and Adiponectin Regulation

A plant-based diet, rich in fruits, vegetables, whole grains, nuts, and seeds, can significantly influence adiponectin levels through various mechanisms:

- **Nutrient Density**: Plant-based diets are high in essential nutrients, vitamins, and minerals that support overall health and hormonal balance. For example, vitamin E, found in nuts and seeds, has antioxidant properties that can reduce oxidative stress and support adiponectin production.
- **Healthy Fats**: Plant-based sources of fats, such as avocados, nuts, and seeds, provide essential fatty acids that support hormone

production and regulation. Omega-3 fatty acids, found in flax-seeds and walnuts, have anti-inflammatory properties that can enhance adiponectin activity.

- **Fiber**: High-fiber diets, common in plant-based eating, support gut health and hormone regulation. A healthy gut microbiome can influence adiponectin levels through the production of short-chain fatty acids and other metabolites.
- **Phytonutrients**: Fruits and vegetables are rich in phytonutrients, which have antioxidant and anti-inflammatory properties. These compounds help reduce oxidative stress and inflammation, thereby supporting adiponectin production and function.
- **Low Glycemic Index**: Plant-based diets, which are low in refined sugars and high in complex carbohydrates, help maintain stable blood glucose levels. This stability prevents hyperglycemia-induced suppression of adiponectin secretion.

Plant-Based Diet on Adiponectin-Related Health Outcomes

- **Insulin Sensitivity and Diabetes**: Plant-based diets improve insulin sensitivity and reduce the risk of type 2 diabetes. Higher adiponectin levels, promoted by a plant-based diet, enhance glucose uptake and utilization, thereby improving glycemic control.
- **Weight Management and Obesity**: Plant-based diets are effective for weight management, reducing body fat, and improving insulin sensitivity. Lower body fat and better glycemic control enhance adiponectin secretion and overall metabolic health.
- **Cardiovascular Health**: Plant-based diets reduce the risk of cardiovascular diseases by improving lipid profiles, reducing blood pressure, and enhancing endothelial function. Higher adiponectin levels contribute to these cardioprotective effects.
- **Anti-Inflammatory Effects**: The anti-inflammatory properties of plant-based diets help reduce chronic low-grade inflammation,

which is common in obesity and metabolic syndrome. Higher adiponectin levels, supported by a plant-based diet, further mitigate inflammation.

- **Lipid Metabolism**: Plant-based diets promote healthy lipid metabolism, reducing triglycerides and LDL cholesterol levels. Adiponectin plays a crucial role in lipid metabolism by promoting fatty acid oxidation and reducing lipid accumulation in tissues.
- **Oxidative Stress**: The antioxidant-rich nature of plant-based diets helps combat oxidative stress, a key factor in metabolic dysfunction and chronic diseases. Improved adiponectin levels, coupled with reduced oxidative damage, contribute to better metabolic health.

Adiponectin and Specific Plant-Based Foods

- **Nuts and Seeds**: Nuts and seeds are rich in healthy fats, fiber, and phytonutrients that support adiponectin production. Almonds, walnuts, flaxseeds, and chia seeds are particularly beneficial for enhancing adiponectin levels.
- **Fruits**: Berries, apples, and citrus fruits are high in antioxidants and fiber, which help reduce oxidative stress and support adiponectin function. Blueberries and strawberries, in particular, have been shown to increase adiponectin levels.
- **Vegetables**: Leafy greens, cruciferous vegetables, and colorful vegetables provide essential nutrients and phytonutrients that promote adiponectin production. Spinach, kale, broccoli, and bell peppers are excellent choices.
- **Whole Grains**: Whole grains like oats, quinoa, and brown rice are high in fiber and have a low glycemic index, helping to maintain stable blood glucose levels and support adiponectin secretion.

- **Legumes**: Beans, lentils, and chickpeas are rich in protein, fiber, and phytonutrients that enhance adiponectin levels. These foods also support overall metabolic health and insulin sensitivity.

Scientific Evidence on Plant-Based Diets and Adiponectin

Several studies have highlighted the positive impact of plant-based diets on adiponectin levels:

- **Barnard et al. (2009)**: This study found that a low-fat vegan diet increased adiponectin levels and improved insulin sensitivity in overweight women. The diet was rich in fruits, vegetables, whole grains, and legumes, emphasizing the role of plant-based foods in hormonal regulation.
- **Esposito et al. (2004)**: This research demonstrated that a Mediterranean diet, which includes a high intake of plant-based foods, significantly increased adiponectin levels and reduced markers of inflammation in individuals with metabolic syndrome.
- **Madianos et al. (2005)**: This study showed that adherence to a traditional Mediterranean diet, characterized by high consumption of plant-based foods, was associated with higher adiponectin levels and improved cardiovascular health.
- **Pischon et al. (2005)**: This research indicated that a diet rich in fruits, vegetables, and whole grains positively influenced adiponectin levels and reduced the risk of type 2 diabetes.

Adiponectin is a crucial hormone that regulates glucose levels, fatty acid breakdown, inflammation, and cardiovascular health. Its production and regulation are influenced by various factors, including diet, body weight, physical activity, and hormonal balance.

Resistin

Resistin, a relatively recent discovery in the realm of endocrinology, is a hormone primarily known for its role in insulin resistance and inflammation.

Function of Resistin

Resistin is a polypeptide hormone produced by adipose tissue, with significant implications for metabolic processes, particularly concerning insulin resistance and inflammation. Its primary functions include:

1. **Insulin Resistance**: Resistin plays a crucial role in modulating insulin sensitivity. It impairs glucose uptake by cells, leading to higher blood glucose levels and contributing to the development of type 2 diabetes. Resistin interferes with insulin signaling pathways, thereby reducing the effectiveness of insulin in lowering blood sugar levels.
2. **Inflammation**: Resistin is a pro-inflammatory cytokine, meaning it can induce and sustain inflammatory responses. It promotes the production of other inflammatory cytokines, such as TNF-α and IL-6, which are implicated in chronic inflammatory conditions.
3. **Energy Homeostasis**: Resistin influences energy balance by affecting the storage and mobilization of fats. It is involved in adipogenesis (formation of fat cells) and lipolysis (breakdown of fats), impacting overall body fat composition.
4. **Cardiovascular Health**: Elevated resistin levels have been linked to various cardiovascular diseases. It contributes to endothelial dysfunction, a precursor to atherosclerosis, and can exacerbate hypertension by promoting arterial stiffness.
5. **Immune Response**: Resistin also affects the immune system. It modulates the activity of immune cells, including macrophages, and can influence the body's response to infections and other immune challenges.

Production of Resistin

Resistin is primarily produced by adipocytes (fat cells) in humans, although it is also expressed in smaller amounts by other tissues, including immune cells. The production process involves several key steps:

1. **Gene Expression**: The resistin gene (RETN) is located on chromosome 19 in humans. Its expression is regulated by various factors, including hormonal signals, nutritional status, and inflammatory stimuli.
2. **Synthesis**: Once the resistin gene is expressed, the hormone is synthesized as a precursor polypeptide. This precursor undergoes post-translational modifications, including glycosylation, to become the mature, biologically active form of resistin.
3. **Secretion**: Mature resistin is secreted into the bloodstream by adipocytes. The secretion process is influenced by several factors, such as cytokines, free fatty acids, and hormonal signals like insulin and glucocorticoids.
4. **Distribution**: After secretion, resistin circulates in the bloodstream, where it can exert its effects on various tissues, including the liver, muscle, and endothelial cells.

Regulation of Resistin

The regulation of resistin is complex and involves multiple feedback mechanisms and external factors. Key regulatory aspects include:

1. **Hormonal Regulation**: Several hormones influence resistin levels. Insulin and glucocorticoids can upregulate resistin production, while adiponectin, another adipokine, tends to have an inverse relationship with resistin.
2. **Nutritional Status**: Diet plays a crucial role in resistin regulation. High-fat diets and excessive calorie intake can increase

resistin levels, whereas calorie restriction and a balanced diet can help reduce its expression.

3. **Inflammatory Signals**: Inflammatory cytokines like TNF-α and IL-6 can stimulate resistin production. This creates a feedback loop where resistin promotes inflammation, which in turn further increases resistin levels.
4. **Genetic Factors**: Genetic variations can influence resistin production and activity. Polymorphisms in the RETN gene can affect the expression levels and functional properties of resistin.
5. **Physical Activity**: Exercise has been shown to influence resistin levels. Regular physical activity can reduce resistin concentrations, contributing to improved insulin sensitivity and reduced inflammation.

Plant-Based Diet and Resistin Regulation

A plant-based diet, rich in fruits, vegetables, whole grains, nuts, and seeds, can significantly impact resistin regulation through various mechanisms:

1. **Nutrient Density**: Plant-based diets are high in essential nutrients, vitamins, and minerals that support overall health and hormonal balance. For example, magnesium, found in leafy greens and nuts, is crucial for insulin sensitivity and may help modulate resistin levels.
2. **Anti-Inflammatory Properties**: Many plant-based foods possess anti-inflammatory properties. Phytochemicals, such as flavonoids and polyphenols, found in fruits, vegetables, and teas, can reduce inflammation and thereby lower resistin levels.
3. **Fiber Content**: High-fiber diets, common in plant-based eating, support gut health and hormone regulation. A healthy gut microbiome can influence resistin levels through the production of short-chain fatty acids and other metabolites.

4. **Healthy Fats**: Plant-based sources of fats, such as avocados, nuts, and seeds, provide essential fatty acids that support hormone production and regulation. Omega-3 fatty acids, in particular, have anti-inflammatory properties that can help reduce resistin levels.
5. **Glycemic Control**: Plant-based diets, which are low in refined sugars and high in complex carbohydrates, help maintain stable blood glucose levels. This stability prevents hyperglycemia-induced increases in resistin secretion.
6. **Caloric Balance**: Maintaining a healthy weight through a balanced plant-based diet can prevent obesity-related increases in resistin. Excess body fat, particularly visceral fat, is linked to higher resistin levels.

Plant-Based Diet on Resistin-Related Health Outcomes

1. **Insulin Sensitivity**: Numerous studies have shown that plant-based diets can improve insulin sensitivity. By reducing resistin levels and other inflammatory markers, plant-based eating helps enhance the body's response to insulin, lowering the risk of type 2 diabetes.
2. **Inflammation**: The anti-inflammatory properties of plant-based diets contribute to lower resistin levels and reduced systemic inflammation. This can help manage and prevent chronic inflammatory diseases such as rheumatoid arthritis and inflammatory bowel disease.
3. **Cardiovascular Health**: Plant-based diets are associated with better cardiovascular health. By lowering resistin levels and reducing inflammation, these diets help protect against atherosclerosis, hypertension, and other cardiovascular conditions.
4. **Weight Management**: Plant-based diets are effective for weight management, reducing body fat, and improving metabolic health.

Lower body fat and better glycemic control enhance resistin regulation and overall health outcomes.

5. **Gut Health**: The high fiber content of plant-based diets supports a healthy gut microbiome, which plays a role in hormone regulation, including resistin. Improved gut health can lead to better metabolic and inflammatory profiles.

Resistin is a key hormone involved in insulin resistance and inflammation, with significant implications for metabolic health and chronic disease risk. Its production and regulation are influenced by various factors, including diet, hormonal signals, and inflammatory states.

9

Hormones of the Kidneys

Erythropoietin (EPO)

Erythropoietin (EPO) is a glycoprotein hormone that plays a crucial role in the regulation of erythropoiesis, the process of red blood cell production.

Function of Erythropoietin

Erythropoietin's primary function is to regulate red blood cell production to ensure adequate oxygen transport throughout the body. It achieves this through several mechanisms:

1. **Stimulation of Erythropoiesis**: EPO stimulates the differentiation and proliferation of erythroid progenitor cells in the bone marrow. It binds to erythropoietin receptors on these progenitor cells, promoting their survival and maturation into erythrocytes (red blood cells).
2. **Response to Hypoxia**: EPO production is primarily regulated by oxygen levels in the blood. In response to hypoxia (low oxygen levels), EPO synthesis increases, leading to an enhanced production of red blood cells to improve oxygen delivery to tissues.
3. **Regulation of Iron Metabolism**: EPO indirectly influences iron metabolism by increasing the demand for iron needed for

hemoglobin synthesis in red blood cells. This regulation ensures that sufficient iron is available for effective erythropoiesis.

4. **Role in Angiogenesis**: Emerging research suggests that EPO may also play a role in angiogenesis (formation of new blood vessels) and tissue protection, contributing to its functions beyond erythropoiesis.

Production of Erythropoietin

Erythropoietin is produced primarily by the kidneys, with a small amount being produced by the liver. The production process involves several steps:

1. **Synthesis in the Kidneys**: In adults, the kidneys are the main site of EPO production. Specialized cells in the renal cortex, known as interstitial fibroblasts, produce EPO in response to hypoxic conditions.
2. **Liver Production**: In fetuses and to a lesser extent in adults, the liver also produces EPO. Hepatocytes (liver cells) contribute to EPO synthesis, particularly during embryonic development.
3. **Regulation by Hypoxia-Inducible Factors (HIFs)**: The primary regulator of EPO production is the hypoxia-inducible factor (HIF) pathway. Under low oxygen conditions, HIFs stabilize and activate the transcription of the EPO gene, leading to increased EPO synthesis.
4. **Influence of Other Factors**: Various factors, including hormones like androgens, inflammatory cytokines, and nutritional status, can influence EPO production. For instance, androgens (male sex hormones) are known to enhance EPO synthesis.

Regulation of Erythropoietin

The regulation of EPO is a complex process involving feedback mechanisms and external factors:

1. **Hypoxia and Oxygen Sensing**: The primary stimulus for EPO production is hypoxia. Specialized oxygen-sensing cells in the kidneys detect low oxygen levels and trigger the HIF pathway, leading to increased EPO synthesis.
2. **Feedback Loops**: EPO levels are regulated through feedback mechanisms. High levels of circulating EPO and red blood cells can inhibit further EPO production, maintaining homeostasis in red blood cell count.
3. **Iron Availability**: Iron is essential for hemoglobin synthesis in red blood cells. Low iron levels can impair erythropoiesis despite adequate EPO levels. Conversely, sufficient iron availability enhances the effectiveness of EPO.
4. **Nutritional Factors**: Nutritional status, particularly the availability of essential nutrients like iron, vitamin B12, and folate, plays a significant role in EPO regulation and erythropoiesis.
5. **Inflammatory Cytokines**: Chronic inflammation can suppress EPO production and impair erythropoiesis. Inflammatory cytokines such as interleukin-6 (IL-6) and tumor necrosis factor-alpha (TNF-α) can inhibit EPO synthesis and contribute to anemia of chronic disease.

Plant-Based Diet and Erythropoietin Regulation

A plant-based diet, rich in fruits, vegetables, whole grains, nuts, and seeds, can have a profound impact on EPO regulation through various mechanisms:

1. **Iron-Rich Plant Foods**: While heme iron from animal sources is more readily absorbed, non-heme iron from plant sources can

also support healthy erythropoiesis when consumed in sufficient quantities. Foods like lentils, spinach, tofu, and quinoa are rich in iron and can contribute to maintaining adequate iron levels.

2. **Vitamin C for Iron Absorption**: Vitamin C, abundant in fruits and vegetables, enhances the absorption of non-heme iron from plant foods. Consuming vitamin C-rich foods such as citrus fruits, bell peppers, and broccoli with iron-rich plant foods can improve iron status and support EPO function.
3. **Folate and Vitamin B12**: Folate and vitamin B12 are essential for red blood cell production. Leafy greens, legumes, and fortified plant-based foods provide folate, while vitamin B12 can be obtained from fortified plant-based foods and supplements.
4. **Anti-Inflammatory Properties**: Plant-based diets are rich in anti-inflammatory compounds such as polyphenols and antioxidants. These compounds can reduce chronic inflammation and its inhibitory effect on EPO production and erythropoiesis.
5. **Hydration and Kidney Health**: Proper hydration is crucial for kidney function and EPO production. A diet rich in water-dense fruits and vegetables supports kidney health and optimal EPO synthesis.
6. **Fiber and Gut Health**: High-fiber diets support gut health and nutrient absorption, including iron. A healthy gut microbiome can enhance iron bioavailability and support erythropoiesis.

Plant-Based Diet on Erythropoietin-Related Health Outcomes

1. **Anemia Prevention**: A well-planned plant-based diet can prevent and manage anemia by providing sufficient iron, vitamin B12, and folate. Incorporating a variety of iron-rich and vitamin C-rich foods helps maintain healthy hemoglobin levels and supports EPO function.

2. **Cardiovascular Health**: EPO has been linked to cardiovascular health, and a plant-based diet is associated with a lower risk of cardiovascular diseases. By reducing inflammation and supporting optimal blood viscosity, plant-based diets can enhance the cardioprotective effects of EPO.
3. **Enhanced Athletic Performance**: Athletes on plant-based diets can benefit from improved EPO function and red blood cell production, enhancing oxygen delivery and endurance. Proper nutrition and hydration are key to maximizing EPO's benefits for athletic performance.
4. **Kidney Health**: Since the kidneys are the primary site of EPO production, maintaining kidney health is crucial. A plant-based diet can reduce the risk of chronic kidney disease and support overall kidney function, ensuring adequate EPO synthesis.
5. **Reduced Risk of Chronic Diseases**: Plant-based diets are associated with a lower risk of chronic diseases such as diabetes and hypertension, which can impair EPO production and erythropoiesis. By promoting overall health, plant-based diets indirectly support EPO function and red blood cell production.

Erythropoietin plays a pivotal role in red blood cell production and overall oxygen transport throughout the body. Its production and regulation are influenced by various factors, including oxygen levels, iron availability, and nutritional status.

Renin

Renin, a crucial hormone in the regulation of blood pressure and fluid balance, has a significant impact on overall health.

Function of Renin

Renin plays a pivotal role in the renin-angiotensin-aldosterone system (RAAS), which is essential for maintaining blood pressure and electrolyte balance. The primary functions of renin include:

1. **Regulation of Blood Pressure**: Renin catalyzes the conversion of angiotensinogen, a plasma protein produced by the liver, into angiotensin I. Angiotensin I is then converted into angiotensin II by the angiotensin-converting enzyme (ACE) in the lungs. Angiotensin II is a potent vasoconstrictor, which increases blood pressure by narrowing blood vessels.
2. **Sodium and Water Balance**: Angiotensin II stimulates the adrenal cortex to secrete aldosterone, a hormone that promotes sodium retention and potassium excretion by the kidneys. This sodium retention leads to water retention, which increases blood volume and, consequently, blood pressure.
3. **Fluid Homeostasis**: By regulating the reabsorption of sodium and water in the kidneys, renin helps maintain fluid balance in the body. This is crucial for maintaining blood volume and pressure, especially during dehydration or blood loss.

Production of Renin

Renin is produced by the juxtaglomerular cells, which are specialized cells located in the walls of the afferent arterioles of the kidneys. The production process involves several steps:

1. **Synthesis**: Renin is synthesized as an inactive precursor called prorenin. Prorenin is produced and stored in the juxtaglomerular cells of the kidneys.
2. **Activation**: When the body needs to increase blood pressure or when there is a decrease in sodium concentration in the renal tubules, prorenin is cleaved to form active renin. This process

is triggered by signals from the macula densa cells, which sense changes in sodium concentration.

3. **Release**: Active renin is then released into the bloodstream, where it begins the process of converting angiotensinogen to angiotensin I.

Regulation of Renin

The regulation of renin involves a complex interplay of feedback mechanisms and external factors:

1. **Renal Baroreceptors**: These receptors in the kidneys detect changes in blood pressure. When blood pressure decreases, renin release is stimulated. Conversely, when blood pressure increases, renin release is inhibited.
2. **Macula Densa Cells**: Located in the distal convoluted tubule of the nephron, these cells monitor sodium concentration in the filtrate. Low sodium levels trigger the release of renin, while high sodium levels inhibit it.
3. **Sympathetic Nervous System**: Activation of the sympathetic nervous system, often in response to stress or low blood volume, stimulates the release of renin through the β1-adrenergic receptors on juxtaglomerular cells.
4. **Negative Feedback Loop**: Angiotensin II, the product of renin activity, provides negative feedback by inhibiting the further release of renin. This helps maintain balance and prevents excessive increases in blood pressure.

Plant-Based Diet and Renin Regulation

A plant-based diet, rich in fruits, vegetables, whole grains, nuts, and seeds, can have a profound impact on renin regulation through various mechanisms:

1. **Antioxidant Properties**: Plant-based diets are high in antioxidants, which help reduce oxidative stress. Oxidative stress can impair endothelial function and lead to hypertension. Reducing oxidative stress supports better vascular function and renin regulation.
2. **Potassium-Rich Foods**: Many plant-based foods, such as bananas, potatoes, and leafy greens, are high in potassium. Potassium helps balance sodium levels in the body and can reduce the activity of the RAAS, leading to lower renin levels and blood pressure.
3. **Fiber Content**: High-fiber diets, common in plant-based eating, support gut health and can improve the body's response to insulin. Better insulin sensitivity is associated with lower renin activity and improved blood pressure regulation.
4. **Healthy Fats**: Plant-based sources of fats, such as avocados, nuts, and seeds, provide essential fatty acids that support overall health. Omega-3 fatty acids, in particular, have anti-inflammatory properties that can enhance vascular function and reduce renin activity.
5. **Nitric Oxide Production**: Plant-based diets, especially those high in leafy greens, enhance the production of nitric oxide, a vasodilator that improves blood flow and reduces blood pressure. This can lead to decreased renin activity as the body does not need to compensate for low blood flow.

Plant-Based Diet on Renin-Related Health Outcomes

1. **Hypertension Management**: A plant-based diet has been shown to be effective in managing hypertension. Studies indicate that such diets can reduce blood pressure, likely due to their high potassium, low sodium, and antioxidant content. Reduced blood pressure alleviates the need for elevated renin levels, promoting better overall cardiovascular health.
2. **Kidney Health**: Plant-based diets are beneficial for kidney health as they reduce the burden on the kidneys. A lower intake of animal proteins and a higher intake of plant proteins can decrease kidney workload and improve renal function, which in turn can lead to better regulation of renin.
3. **Cardiovascular Health**: By reducing blood pressure and improving lipid profiles, a plant-based diet can significantly reduce the risk of cardiovascular diseases. Lower renin levels, as a result of better blood pressure management, contribute to this improved cardiovascular health.
4. **Weight Management**: Plant-based diets are often associated with lower body weight and reduced obesity rates. Since obesity is a risk factor for increased renin activity and hypertension, maintaining a healthy weight through a plant-based diet supports better renin regulation and overall health.

Renin plays a crucial role in the regulation of blood pressure and fluid balance through its involvement in the RAAS. Its production and regulation are influenced by various physiological mechanisms and external factors.

10

Cardiovascular Hormones

Atrial Natriuretic Peptide (ANP)

Atrial natriuretic peptide (ANP) is a crucial hormone involved in the regulation of blood pressure, electrolyte balance, and fluid homeostasis. Its role extends to influencing cardiovascular health, renal function, and vascular tone.

Function of Atrial Natriuretic Peptide

ANP, produced by the atria of the heart, performs several vital functions in maintaining cardiovascular and renal health:

1. **Regulation of Blood Pressure**: ANP lowers blood pressure by promoting vasodilation, which reduces vascular resistance. It achieves this by relaxing the smooth muscle cells in blood vessel walls, leading to expanded vessels and decreased blood pressure.
2. **Diuresis and Natriuresis**: ANP increases the excretion of sodium (natriuresis) and water (diuresis) by the kidneys. This process helps reduce blood volume and pressure by decreasing the reabsorption of sodium in the renal tubules, leading to increased urine output.
3. **Inhibition of Renin-Angiotensin-Aldosterone System (RAAS)**: ANP inhibits the release of renin from the kidneys, reducing the production of angiotensin II and aldosterone. This

inhibition further promotes sodium and water excretion, contributing to lower blood pressure.

4. **Anti-Proliferative Effects**: ANP has anti-proliferative properties that help prevent the abnormal growth of vascular smooth muscle cells, reducing the risk of atherosclerosis and other cardiovascular diseases.
5. **Modulation of Sympathetic Nervous System**: ANP modulates the activity of the sympathetic nervous system by inhibiting the release of norepinephrine, leading to decreased heart rate and blood pressure.
6. **Promotion of Lipolysis**: ANP stimulates the breakdown of fats (lipolysis), which can contribute to improved lipid profiles and overall cardiovascular health.

Production of Atrial Natriuretic Peptide

ANP is synthesized and secreted by the atrial myocytes (heart muscle cells) in response to various physiological stimuli:

1. **Synthesis**: ANP is synthesized as a preprohormone (preproANP) in the atrial myocytes. It is then cleaved to form proANP, which is stored in granules within the atrial cells. Upon stimulation, proANP is further cleaved to release the active hormone ANP.
2. **Stimuli for Release**: The primary stimulus for ANP release is atrial distension, which occurs when there is increased blood volume or pressure in the atria. Other stimuli include:
    - **Sympathetic Nervous System Activation**: Increased sympathetic activity can enhance ANP release.
    - **Endothelin**: A peptide produced by the endothelial cells lining the blood vessels that can stimulate ANP secretion.
    - **Angiotensin II**: Although ANP inhibits RAAS, angiotensin II can paradoxically stimulate ANP release to counterbalance its effects.

4. **Pulsatile Secretion**: ANP is released in a pulsatile manner, with levels fluctuating throughout the day in response to changes in blood volume and pressure.

Regulation of Atrial Natriuretic Peptide

The regulation of ANP involves a complex interplay of feedback mechanisms and external factors:

1. **Feedback Loops**: ANP levels are regulated through negative feedback loops. High levels of ANP lead to increased diuresis and natriuresis, reducing blood volume and pressure, which in turn decreases atrial distension and ANP release.
2. **Vascular Endothelial Growth Factor (VEGF)**: VEGF can enhance ANP production and release by promoting the proliferation and activity of atrial myocytes.
3. **Exercise**: Physical activity, especially aerobic exercise, can increase ANP levels by enhancing blood flow and atrial distension.
4. **Dietary Sodium Intake**: High sodium intake can stimulate ANP release to promote sodium excretion and maintain fluid balance. Conversely, low sodium intake can reduce ANP levels.
5. **Hormones**: Other hormones, such as aldosterone and vasopressin, can influence ANP levels. Aldosterone promotes sodium retention, which can counteract the effects of ANP, while vasopressin can stimulate ANP release.

Plant-Based Diet and Atrial Natriuretic Peptide Regulation

A plant-based diet, rich in fruits, vegetables, whole grains, nuts, and seeds, can significantly influence the regulation of ANP through various mechanisms:

1. **Nutrient Density**: Plant-based diets are typically high in essential nutrients, vitamins, and minerals that support overall

cardiovascular health. For example, potassium, found in abundance in plant foods like bananas, sweet potatoes, and leafy greens, helps regulate blood pressure and ANP activity.

2. **Antioxidants**: Fruits and vegetables are rich in antioxidants, which help reduce oxidative stress. Lower oxidative stress levels are associated with improved endothelial function and ANP secretion.
3. **Healthy Fats**: Plant-based sources of fats, such as avocados, nuts, and seeds, provide essential fatty acids that support cardiovascular health and hormone production. Omega-3 fatty acids, in particular, have anti-inflammatory properties that can enhance ANP activity.
4. **Fiber**: High-fiber diets, common in plant-based eating, support gut health and hormone regulation. A healthy gut microbiome can influence ANP levels through the production of short-chain fatty acids and other metabolites.
5. **Caloric Balance**: Maintaining a healthy weight through a balanced plant-based diet can prevent obesity-related suppression of ANP. Excess body fat, particularly visceral fat, is linked to lower ANP levels due to increased production of inflammatory cytokines.
6. **Glycemic Control**: Plant-based diets, which are low in refined sugars and high in complex carbohydrates, help maintain stable blood glucose levels. This stability prevents hyperglycemia-induced suppression of ANP secretion.
7. **Phytochemicals**: Plant foods contain various bioactive compounds, such as flavonoids and polyphenols, that can modulate ANP levels and cardiovascular health. These compounds have been shown to enhance endothelial function and reduce inflammation.

Plant-Based Diet on Atrial Natriuretic Peptide-Related Health Outcomes

1. **Cardiovascular Health**: A plant-based diet can improve cardiovascular health by supporting healthy blood pressure levels and reducing the risk of hypertension. The high potassium and low sodium content of plant-based foods, along with their anti-inflammatory and antioxidant properties, enhance ANP activity and overall cardiovascular function.
2. **Weight Management**: Plant-based diets are effective for weight management, reducing body fat, and improving insulin sensitivity. Lower body fat and better glycemic control enhance ANP secretion and overall metabolic health.
3. **Renal Function**: The diuretic and natriuretic effects of ANP are crucial for maintaining renal function and preventing fluid overload. A plant-based diet, rich in hydration and kidney-supportive nutrients, can promote optimal ANP activity and kidney health.
4. **Anti-Aging Effects**: The antioxidant-rich nature of plant-based diets helps combat oxidative stress, a key factor in aging. Improved ANP levels, coupled with reduced oxidative damage, contribute to healthier aging and better maintenance of cardiovascular function.
5. **Mental Health**: Emerging evidence suggests that plant-based diets may benefit mental health by reducing inflammation and oxidative stress, which are linked to mood disorders. Improved ANP levels also support cognitive function and emotional well-being.

Atrial natriuretic peptide plays a pivotal role in regulating blood pressure, fluid balance, and overall cardiovascular health. Its production and regulation are influenced by various factors, including blood volume, exercise, diet, and hormonal interactions.

11

Bone Hormones

Osteocalcin

Osteocalcin, also known as bone gamma-carboxyglutamic acid-containing protein (BGLAP), is a non-collagenous protein hormone found in bone and dentin. It plays a critical role in the regulation of bone metabolism and has been increasingly recognized for its endocrine functions, particularly in energy metabolism and glucose regulation.

Function of Osteocalcin

Osteocalcin is a multi-functional hormone with diverse roles in the body:

- **Bone Formation and Mineralization**: Osteocalcin is produced by osteoblasts, the cells responsible for bone formation. It is involved in the regulation of bone mineralization and turnover. Osteocalcin binds calcium ions and integrates them into the bone matrix, thereby contributing to bone strength and density.
- **Regulation of Energy Metabolism**: Recent studies have shown that osteocalcin plays a significant role in energy metabolism. It influences insulin secretion and sensitivity, adiponectin production, and energy expenditure. Osteocalcin enhances insulin

secretion from pancreatic beta cells and increases insulin sensitivity in peripheral tissues, helping to regulate blood glucose levels.

- **Fertility**: Osteocalcin has been implicated in male fertility. It acts on the Leydig cells in the testes to promote the production of testosterone, which is essential for spermatogenesis and overall male reproductive health.
- **Brain Function**: Emerging research suggests that osteocalcin can cross the blood-brain barrier and influence brain function. It has been associated with cognitive functions, including learning and memory. Osteocalcin deficiency has been linked to cognitive decline and neurodegenerative diseases.

Production of Osteocalcin

Osteocalcin production is a complex process primarily occurring in osteoblasts:

- **Synthesis**: Osteocalcin is synthesized by osteoblasts in the bone. The gene responsible for osteocalcin production is located on chromosome 1 in humans.
- **Vitamin K-Dependent Carboxylation**: For osteocalcin to become biologically active, it undergoes a process known as gamma-carboxylation, which is vitamin K-dependent. This modification allows osteocalcin to bind calcium and be incorporated into the bone matrix.
- **Secretion**: Once synthesized and carboxylated, osteocalcin is secreted into the bone matrix. Some osteocalcin remains in the bone, while a portion is released into the bloodstream, where it can exert its endocrine effects.

Regulation of Osteocalcin

The regulation of osteocalcin involves multiple factors, including hormonal control, nutritional status, and physical activity:

Hormonal Regulation:

- **Parathyroid Hormone (PTH)**: PTH stimulates osteocalcin production by promoting osteoblast activity.
- **Insulin**: Insulin signaling enhances osteocalcin activation by influencing its carboxylation process.
- **Glucocorticoids**: These hormones inhibit osteocalcin production by reducing osteoblast activity, which can lead to decreased bone formation and density.

Nutritional Influences:

- **Vitamin K**: Adequate intake of vitamin K is crucial for the gamma-carboxylation and activation of osteocalcin.
- **Calcium and Phosphorus**: These minerals are vital for bone health and the incorporation of osteocalcin into the bone matrix.

Physical Activity: Weight-bearing exercises stimulate osteoblast activity and osteocalcin production, contributing to stronger bones and improved metabolic health.

Plant-Based Diet and Osteocalcin Regulation

A plant-based diet, which is rich in fruits, vegetables, whole grains, nuts, and seeds, can have a profound impact on osteocalcin regulation through various mechanisms:

Nutrient Density:

- **Vitamin K:** Leafy green vegetables such as kale, spinach, and broccoli are excellent sources of vitamin K, which is essential for osteocalcin activation. Studies have shown that higher dietary intake of vitamin K is associated with improved bone health and increased osteocalcin levels.
- **Calcium:** Plant-based sources of calcium, such as fortified plant milk, tofu, and almonds, contribute to bone mineralization and osteocalcin function.

Magnesium and Phosphorus: These minerals, found in nuts, seeds, and whole grains, are crucial for bone health and support the function of osteocalcin.

Amino Acids: Plant-based proteins, such as those found in legumes, quinoa, and nuts, provide essential amino acids necessary for osteocalcin synthesis. Arginine and lysine, in particular, play a role in collagen production and bone health.

Antioxidants: Fruits and vegetables are rich in antioxidants, which help reduce oxidative stress. Lower oxidative stress levels are associated with better bone health and higher osteocalcin activity.

Healthy Fats: Plant-based sources of fats, such as avocados, nuts, and seeds, provide essential fatty acids that support overall health. Omega-3 fatty acids, in particular, have anti-inflammatory properties that can enhance bone health and osteocalcin function.

Fiber: High-fiber diets, common in plant-based eating, support gut health and nutrient absorption, which are important for bone health and osteocalcin regulation.

Caloric Balance: Maintaining a healthy weight through a balanced plant-based diet can prevent obesity-related suppression of osteocalcin. Excess body fat, particularly visceral fat, is linked to lower osteocalcin levels and impaired bone health.

Plant-Based Diet on Osteocalcin-Related Health Outcomes
Bone Health:

- **Density and Strength**: Plant-based diets rich in calcium, vitamin K, and magnesium support bone health. Studies have shown that individuals following a plant-based diet have higher bone mineral density and stronger bones compared to those consuming a typical Western diet.
- **Fracture Risk**: Adequate intake of nutrients found in plant-based diets can reduce the risk of fractures. Leafy greens, nuts, and fortified plant milk are particularly beneficial in providing essential nutrients for bone health.

Metabolic Health:

- **Glucose Regulation**: Osteocalcin plays a role in glucose metabolism, and a plant-based diet can enhance its effects. Diets high in fiber and low in refined sugars help maintain stable blood glucose levels, preventing hyperglycemia-induced suppression of osteocalcin secretion.
- **Insulin Sensitivity**: The nutrient profile of a plant-based diet, including antioxidants and healthy fats, can improve insulin sensitivity and support osteocalcin's role in glucose regulation.

Weight Management:

- **Body Fat Reduction**: Plant-based diets are effective for weight management, reducing body fat, and improving insulin sensitivity. Lower body fat enhances osteocalcin secretion and overall metabolic health.

Cognitive Function:

- **Brain Health**: The anti-inflammatory and antioxidant properties of plant-based diets can support cognitive function and protect against neurodegenerative diseases. Improved osteocalcin levels also contribute to better cognitive health and reduced risk of cognitive decline.

Osteocalcin is a critical hormone involved in bone formation, energy metabolism, fertility, and brain function. Its production and regulation are influenced by various factors, including hormonal control, nutritional status, and physical activity.

12

Neurohormones

Dopamine

Dopamine is a neurotransmitter that plays a pivotal role in various physiological functions, including mood regulation, reward processing, and motor control.

Function of Dopamine
Dopamine's primary functions include:

1. **Mood Regulation**: Dopamine is crucial for regulating mood and emotional responses. It is often referred to as the "feel-good" neurotransmitter because it contributes to feelings of pleasure and satisfaction.
2. **Reward Processing**: Dopamine is essential in the brain's reward system, influencing motivation and the pursuit of rewarding stimuli. It plays a role in reinforcing behaviors by providing a sense of pleasure or accomplishment.
3. **Motor Control**: Dopamine is involved in coordinating smooth and controlled movements. A deficit in dopamine levels is linked to motor disorders such as Parkinson's disease, characterized by tremors and difficulty in movement.

4. **Cognitive Function**: Dopamine influences cognitive processes such as attention, memory, and problem-solving. It helps in maintaining focus and organizing thoughts.
5. **Endocrine Regulation**: Dopamine inhibits the release of prolactin from the pituitary gland, playing a role in reproductive health and lactation.

Production of Dopamine

Dopamine is produced through a multi-step biochemical pathway:

Synthesis: Dopamine is synthesized from the amino acid tyrosine, which is derived from dietary sources or synthesized from phenylalanine. The process involves two key enzymatic reactions:

- **Tyrosine Hydroxylation**: Tyrosine is converted to L-DOPA (L-3,4-dihydroxyphenylalanine) by the enzyme tyrosine hydroxylase, which is the rate-limiting step in dopamine synthesis.
- **Decarboxylation**: L-DOPA is then converted to dopamine by the enzyme aromatic L-amino acid decarboxylase.

Storage: Dopamine is stored in vesicles within nerve terminals, where it is ready for release into the synaptic cleft in response to neuronal signals.

Release and Reuptake: Dopamine is released into the synaptic cleft and binds to dopamine receptors on the postsynaptic neuron. The action of dopamine is terminated by reuptake into the presynaptic neuron via dopamine transporters or by enzymatic degradation.

Regulation of Dopamine

The regulation of dopamine involves multiple feedback mechanisms and external factors:

1. **Feedback Loops**: Dopamine levels are regulated by feedback loops involving dopamine receptors and transporters. High levels of dopamine inhibit further release, while low levels stimulate production and release.
2. **Sleep**: Sleep patterns significantly affect dopamine levels. Adequate sleep supports optimal dopamine function, while sleep deprivation can lead to reduced dopamine sensitivity and impaired mood regulation.
3. **Exercise**: Physical activity, especially aerobic exercise, boosts dopamine levels and receptor sensitivity. Exercise-induced dopamine release contributes to improved mood and cognitive function.
4. **Nutrition**: Diet plays a crucial role in dopamine production. Nutrients such as tyrosine, found in protein-rich foods, are essential for dopamine synthesis. Conversely, diets high in saturated fats and refined sugars can impair dopamine signaling.
5. **Hormones**: Other hormones, such as cortisol (the stress hormone), influence dopamine levels. Chronic stress can deplete dopamine stores, leading to mood disorders and cognitive impairments.

Plant-Based Diet and Dopamine Regulation

A plant-based diet, rich in fruits, vegetables, whole grains, nuts, and seeds, can significantly impact dopamine regulation through various mechanisms:

Nutrient Density: Plant-based diets are typically high in essential nutrients, vitamins, and minerals that support overall brain health and dopamine synthesis. For example:

- **Tyrosine and Phenylalanine**: Found in legumes, nuts, seeds, and soy products, these amino acids are precursors for dopamine production.

- ◦ **Vitamin B6**: Crucial for the conversion of L-DOPA to dopamine, vitamin B6 is abundant in bananas, chickpeas, and fortified cereals.
- ◦ **Folate**: Important for the methylation process involved in neurotransmitter synthesis, folate is found in leafy greens, beans, and lentils.

Antioxidants: Fruits and vegetables are rich in antioxidants, such as flavonoids and polyphenols, which protect dopamine neurons from oxidative stress and inflammation. Berries, citrus fruits, and green tea are particularly beneficial.

Healthy Fats: Omega-3 fatty acids, found in flaxseeds, chia seeds, and walnuts, support brain health and enhance dopamine receptor function. These fatty acids also have anti-inflammatory properties that protect neural pathways.

Fiber: High-fiber diets, common in plant-based eating, support gut health and the production of short-chain fatty acids, which can influence brain function and dopamine regulation.

Caloric Balance: Maintaining a healthy weight through a balanced plant-based diet can prevent obesity-related impairments in dopamine signaling. Excess body fat is linked to decreased dopamine receptor sensitivity.

Glycemic Control: Plant-based diets, low in refined sugars and high in complex carbohydrates, help maintain stable blood glucose levels. Stable blood sugar prevents hyperglycemia-induced dopamine dysregulation.

Plant-Based Diet on Dopamine-Related Health Outcomes

1. **Mood and Mental Health**: Plant-based diets have been associated with lower rates of depression and anxiety. The high nutrient density, antioxidant content, and anti-inflammatory effects contribute to better mood regulation and mental well-being.

2. **Cognitive Function**: Improved dopamine signaling from a plant-based diet can enhance cognitive performance, including memory, attention, and problem-solving skills. Foods rich in antioxidants and omega-3 fatty acids are particularly beneficial for cognitive health.
3. **Neuroprotection**: Plant-based diets can provide neuroprotective benefits, reducing the risk of neurodegenerative diseases such as Parkinson's disease. The anti-inflammatory and antioxidant properties of plant foods help protect dopamine neurons from damage.
4. **Weight Management**: A plant-based diet is effective for weight management, which is crucial for maintaining dopamine receptor sensitivity. Lower body fat and better glycemic control enhance dopamine function and overall metabolic health.
5. **Energy and Motivation**: Enhanced dopamine signaling from a nutrient-rich plant-based diet can improve energy levels and motivation, contributing to better physical performance and overall quality of life.

Dopamine plays a critical role in regulating mood, reward processing, motor control, cognitive function, and endocrine health. Its production and regulation are influenced by various factors, including diet, sleep, exercise, and stress.

Serotonin

Serotonin, also known as 5-hydroxytryptamine (5-HT), is a key neurotransmitter that significantly influences mood, cognition, and various physiological processes.

Function of Serotonin

Serotonin's primary functions span a wide range of physiological and psychological processes:

1. **Mood Regulation**: Serotonin is well-known for its role in mood stabilization. It is often referred to as the "feel-good" neurotransmitter due to its association with feelings of well-being and happiness. Low levels of serotonin are linked to depression and anxiety disorders.
2. **Cognition and Memory**: Serotonin influences cognitive functions such as memory, learning, and concentration. It modulates synaptic plasticity, which is essential for learning and memory formation.
3. **Sleep Regulation**: Serotonin is a precursor to melatonin, a hormone that regulates sleep-wake cycles. It helps promote healthy sleep patterns and circadian rhythms.
4. **Appetite and Digestion**: Serotonin impacts appetite, satiety, and digestion. Approximately 90% of the body's serotonin is found in the gastrointestinal tract, where it regulates bowel movements and function.
5. **Cardiovascular Health**: Serotonin contributes to the regulation of heart rate and blood vessel constriction. It plays a role in maintaining cardiovascular health and blood pressure.
6. **Bone Health**: Emerging research suggests that serotonin may influence bone density and health. It affects bone formation and resorption, thus playing a role in maintaining bone strength.
7. **Social Behavior**: Serotonin impacts social behavior, including aggression and social dominance. Altered serotonin levels are associated with social anxiety and other social disorders.

Production of Serotonin

Serotonin production involves several steps and key components:

- **Synthesis**: Serotonin is synthesized from the amino acid tryptophan. The conversion process involves two main enzymes:
    - **Tryptophan hydroxylase (TPH)**: This enzyme converts tryptophan to 5-hydroxytryptophan (5-HTP).
    - **Aromatic L-amino acid decarboxylase (AAAD)**: This enzyme converts 5-HTP to serotonin (5-HT).
- **Storage and Release**: Once synthesized, serotonin is stored in vesicles within neurons. It is released into the synaptic cleft in response to nerve impulses, where it binds to specific serotonin receptors on the post-synaptic neuron.
- **Reuptake and Degradation**: After exerting its effects, serotonin is reabsorbed by the pre-synaptic neuron through the serotonin transporter (SERT). It can then be reused or broken down by the enzyme monoamine oxidase (MAO) into inactive metabolites.
- **Location**: While serotonin is primarily found in the gastrointestinal tract, a significant amount is also present in the central nervous system (CNS). The pineal gland, part of the brain, also uses serotonin to produce melatonin.

Regulation of Serotonin

The regulation of serotonin involves various feedback mechanisms and external factors:

1. **Genetic Factors**: Genetic variations can affect serotonin production, transport, and receptor function. Polymorphisms in the serotonin transporter gene (SLC6A4) are linked to mood disorders and altered serotonin levels.

2. **Diet**: Dietary intake of tryptophan, the precursor of serotonin, plays a crucial role in its production. Foods rich in tryptophan, such as nuts, seeds, tofu, and bananas, can boost serotonin synthesis.
3. **Exercise**: Physical activity enhances serotonin production and release. Exercise increases tryptophan availability in the brain, promoting serotonin synthesis.
4. **Light Exposure**: Sunlight exposure stimulates serotonin production in the brain. Lack of sunlight, particularly during winter months, can lead to reduced serotonin levels and seasonal affective disorder (SAD).
5. **Gut Health**: The gut microbiome influences serotonin production. Certain gut bacteria synthesize serotonin and other metabolites that impact its levels. A healthy, diverse gut microbiome supports optimal serotonin regulation.
6. **Sleep**: Quality sleep is essential for maintaining balanced serotonin levels. Sleep deprivation or irregular sleep patterns can disrupt serotonin production and function.

Plant-Based Diet and Serotonin Regulation

A plant-based diet, rich in fruits, vegetables, whole grains, nuts, and seeds, can profoundly impact serotonin regulation through various mechanisms:

1. **Tryptophan-Rich Foods**: Plant-based sources of tryptophan include nuts, seeds, soy products, and bananas. These foods provide the necessary precursor for serotonin synthesis.
2. **Carbohydrate Intake**: Carbohydrates stimulate the release of insulin, which helps increase the uptake of amino acids by muscles, leaving more tryptophan available for serotonin production

in the brain. Whole grains, legumes, and starchy vegetables are excellent plant-based carbohydrate sources.

3. **Antioxidants**: Fruits and vegetables are rich in antioxidants, which help reduce oxidative stress. Lower oxidative stress levels are associated with improved serotonin function and overall mental health.
4. **Healthy Fats**: Omega-3 fatty acids, found in flaxseeds, chia seeds, walnuts, and algae, support brain health and serotonin regulation. Omega-3s have anti-inflammatory properties that enhance neurotransmitter function.
5. **Gut Health**: A plant-based diet high in fiber supports a healthy gut microbiome. Fermented foods like sauerkraut, kimchi, and tempeh promote gut health, which in turn positively affects serotonin production.
6. **B Vitamins**: B vitamins, particularly B6, B12, and folate, are essential for neurotransmitter synthesis, including serotonin. Plant-based sources include leafy greens, legumes, nutritional yeast, and fortified foods.

Plant-Based Diet on Serotonin-Related Health Outcomes

- **Mood and Mental Health**: Numerous studies have shown that plant-based diets can improve mood and reduce symptoms of depression and anxiety. The anti-inflammatory and antioxidant properties of plant foods support brain health and serotonin function.
    - A study published in the journal *Nutrients* found that higher consumption of fruits and vegetables was associated with lower levels of depressive symptoms.
    - Another study in *Psychiatry Research* reported that a plant-based diet was linked to better mental health outcomes, including reduced anxiety and depression.

- **Sleep Quality**: Plant-based diets, rich in magnesium and tryptophan, support better sleep quality. Magnesium, found in leafy greens, nuts, and seeds, helps regulate neurotransmitters and melatonin production.
    - Research published in *Sleep Medicine Reviews* suggests that dietary magnesium intake is associated with improved sleep quality.
- **Gut Health**: The high fiber content in plant-based diets promotes a healthy gut microbiome, which is essential for serotonin production. A diverse gut microbiome supports the production of short-chain fatty acids and other metabolites that influence serotonin levels.
    - A study in the journal *Cell Host & Microbe* highlights the connection between gut bacteria and serotonin synthesis in the gut.
- **Cardiovascular Health**: Serotonin plays a role in cardiovascular function, and a plant-based diet supports heart health by reducing inflammation, lowering cholesterol levels, and improving blood pressure.
    - The *Journal of the American College of Cardiology* reports that plant-based diets are associated with a lower risk of cardiovascular disease.
- **Bone Health**: Although more research is needed, the potential link between serotonin and bone health suggests that a plant-based diet, rich in calcium, magnesium, and vitamin K, may support bone density and reduce the risk of osteoporosis.
    - According to a study in the journal *Nutrients*, plant-based diets can provide adequate nutrients for bone health, potentially benefiting bone density.

Serotonin is a multifaceted neurotransmitter with critical roles in mood regulation, cognition, sleep, appetite, cardiovascular health, bone health, and social behavior. Its production and regulation are influenced by genetic, dietary, environmental, and lifestyle factors.

Melatonin

Melatonin, a hormone produced primarily by the pineal gland in the brain, plays a critical role in regulating sleep-wake cycles, also known as circadian rhythms. Its influence extends to various physiological processes, including immune function, antioxidant activity, and reproductive health.

Function of Melatonin

Melatonin's primary function is to regulate the sleep-wake cycle, but it also influences other critical bodily functions:

1. **Regulating Sleep-Wake Cycles**: Melatonin levels rise in the evening, signaling the body that it is time to prepare for sleep. This hormone promotes the onset and maintenance of sleep, helping to synchronize the circadian rhythms with the external environment.
2. **Antioxidant Activity**: Melatonin is a potent antioxidant, scavenging free radicals and protecting cells from oxidative damage. This function is particularly important in protecting neural tissue and other sensitive organs from oxidative stress.
3. **Immune System Support**: Melatonin modulates immune responses, enhancing the activity of various immune cells such as T lymphocytes and natural killer cells. It helps to regulate the balance between pro-inflammatory and anti-inflammatory cytokines, supporting overall immune health.
4. **Regulation of Reproductive Hormones**: Melatonin influences reproductive hormones by modulating the release of

gonadotropin-releasing hormone (GnRH). This regulation can affect the timing of puberty and reproductive cycles.

5. **Mood and Cognitive Function**: Melatonin has been implicated in mood regulation and cognitive functions. Its ability to regulate sleep patterns indirectly affects mental health, reducing the risk of mood disorders and cognitive decline associated with sleep disturbances.

Production of Melatonin

Melatonin is produced primarily in the pineal gland, with smaller amounts produced in other tissues such as the retina, gastrointestinal tract, and immune cells. The production process involves several steps:

- **Synthesis**: Melatonin is synthesized from the amino acid tryptophan through a multi-step process:
- **Tryptophan Hydroxylation**: Tryptophan is first hydroxylated to 5-hydroxytryptophan by the enzyme tryptophan hydroxylase.
- **Decarboxylation**: 5-hydroxytryptophan is then decarboxylated to serotonin by the enzyme aromatic L-amino acid decarboxylase.
- **Acetylation**: Serotonin is acetylated to N-acetylserotonin by the enzyme arylalkylamine N-acetyltransferase (AANAT).
- **Methylation**: Finally, N-acetylserotonin is methylated to melatonin by the enzyme hydroxyindole-O-methyltransferase (HIOMT).
- **Regulation by Light**: The production of melatonin is highly sensitive to light exposure. During the day, light exposure inhibits melatonin synthesis, while darkness stimulates its production. The suprachiasmatic nucleus (SCN) in the hypothalamus serves as the central regulator, relaying information about light exposure to the pineal gland.
- **Circadian Rhythm**: Melatonin production follows a circadian rhythm, with levels rising in the evening, peaking during the

night, and falling in the early morning. This rhythm helps regulate sleep-wake cycles and aligns them with the day-night cycle.

- **Influencing Factors**: Several factors influence melatonin production, including age, light exposure, and certain lifestyle factors:
- **Age**: Melatonin levels decline with age, contributing to sleep disturbances in older adults.
- **Light Exposure**: Light exposure, particularly blue light from screens, can suppress melatonin production and disrupt sleep patterns.
- **Lifestyle**: Shift work, travel across time zones, and irregular sleep schedules can affect melatonin synthesis and circadian rhythms.

Regulation of Melatonin

The regulation of melatonin is a complex process involving feedback mechanisms and external factors:

1. **Feedback Loops**: Melatonin production is regulated through feedback loops involving the SCN and pineal gland. The SCN receives light information from the retina and adjusts melatonin synthesis accordingly. High melatonin levels during the night signal the SCN to reduce melatonin production as morning approaches.
2. **Light Exposure**: Light is the most significant regulator of melatonin production. Exposure to light, especially blue light, inhibits melatonin synthesis. This regulation is crucial for aligning sleep-wake cycles with the external environment. Minimizing exposure to artificial light in the evening can help maintain healthy melatonin levels.
3. **Diet and Nutrients**: Diet plays a role in melatonin regulation, with certain nutrients and dietary patterns influencing its production:

    - **Tryptophan-Rich Foods**: Foods rich in tryptophan, such as nuts, seeds, soy products, and whole grains, provide the precursor needed for melatonin synthesis.
    - **Vitamin B6**: This vitamin, found in bananas, chickpeas, and potatoes, is essential for converting tryptophan to serotonin, a precursor of melatonin.
    - **Magnesium**: Magnesium, found in leafy greens, nuts, and seeds, supports overall sleep health and melatonin synthesis.
4. **Lifestyle Factors**: Regular sleep schedules, managing stress, and maintaining a healthy lifestyle support melatonin regulation. Practices such as maintaining a consistent bedtime, reducing screen time before bed, and incorporating relaxation techniques can enhance melatonin production.

Plant-Based Diet and Melatonin Regulation

A plant-based diet can significantly impact melatonin regulation through various mechanisms:

1. **Nutrient Density**: Plant-based diets are typically rich in essential nutrients, vitamins, and minerals that support overall health and hormonal balance. For example, foods high in antioxidants, such as berries, leafy greens, and nuts, can protect the pineal gland from oxidative damage, supporting melatonin production.
2. **Tryptophan-Rich Foods**: Plant-based sources of tryptophan, such as nuts, seeds, soy products, and whole grains, provide the necessary precursor for melatonin synthesis. Incorporating these foods into the diet can enhance melatonin levels and improve sleep quality.
3. **Antioxidants**: Fruits and vegetables are rich in antioxidants, which help reduce oxidative stress. Lower oxidative stress levels

are associated with improved melatonin secretion and overall endocrine function.

4. **Healthy Fats**: Plant-based sources of fats, such as avocados, nuts, and seeds, provide essential fatty acids that support hormone production and regulation. Omega-3 fatty acids, in particular, have anti-inflammatory properties that can enhance melatonin activity.
5. **Fiber**: High-fiber diets, common in plant-based eating, support gut health and hormone regulation. A healthy gut microbiome can influence melatonin levels through the production of short-chain fatty acids and other metabolites.
6. **Caloric Balance**: Maintaining a healthy weight through a balanced plant-based diet can prevent obesity-related suppression of melatonin. Excess body fat, particularly visceral fat, is linked to lower melatonin levels due to increased production of pro-inflammatory cytokines.
7. **Glycemic Control**: Plant-based diets, which are low in refined sugars and high in complex carbohydrates, help maintain stable blood glucose levels. This stability prevents hyperglycemia-induced suppression of melatonin secretion.

Plant-Based Diet on Melatonin-Related Health Outcomes

1. **Sleep Quality**: A plant-based diet can improve sleep quality by enhancing melatonin production. The high levels of tryptophan and other nutrients in plant-based foods support the synthesis and regulation of melatonin, leading to better sleep patterns.
2. **Mood and Mental Health**: Improved melatonin levels, supported by a plant-based diet, can positively affect mood and mental health. Better sleep quality and antioxidant intake reduce the risk of mood disorders and cognitive decline.

3. **Immune Function**: The immune-modulating effects of melatonin are enhanced by a plant-based diet rich in antioxidants and anti-inflammatory compounds. This can lead to improved immune responses and reduced risk of infections.
4. **Chronic Disease Prevention**: Melatonin's antioxidant and anti-inflammatory properties, combined with the health benefits of a plant-based diet, can reduce the risk of chronic diseases such as cardiovascular disease, diabetes, and certain cancers.
5. **Longevity and Aging**: A plant-based diet can support healthy aging by maintaining optimal melatonin levels. The antioxidants and nutrients in plant foods help protect against oxidative stress and inflammation, promoting longevity and overall health.

Melatonin plays a pivotal role in regulating sleep-wake cycles and supporting various physiological processes, including immune function, antioxidant activity, and mood regulation. Its production and regulation are influenced by factors such as light exposure, diet, and lifestyle.

13

Thymus Hormones

Thymosin

Thymosin is a peptide hormone that plays a crucial role in the development and function of the immune system. It is involved in the maturation of T-cells, which are essential for adaptive immunity.

Function of Thymosin

Thymosin's primary functions are related to the immune system, including:

1. **T-Cell Maturation**: Thymosin is vital for the differentiation and maturation of T-cells in the thymus gland. These cells are crucial for the adaptive immune response, recognizing and attacking pathogens and infected cells.
2. **Immune Modulation**: Thymosin modulates the immune response by influencing the activity and proliferation of various immune cells, including macrophages and natural killer cells. This helps in maintaining immune homeostasis.
3. **Wound Healing**: Thymosin beta-4, a specific form of thymosin, promotes wound healing by accelerating the migration of cells to the wound site, reducing inflammation, and enhancing tissue regeneration.

4. **Anti-Inflammatory Effects**: Thymosin exhibits anti-inflammatory properties, helping to control excessive inflammatory responses that can lead to tissue damage.

Production of Thymosin

Thymosin is produced in the thymus gland, with its production involving several key steps:

1. **Synthesis**: Thymosin is synthesized in the thymus gland from a precursor protein. The gene responsible for thymosin production is located on chromosome 22 in humans.
2. **Processing**: The precursor protein undergoes post-translational modifications to form active thymosin peptides, including thymosin alpha-1 and thymosin beta-4.
3. **Secretion**: Thymosin peptides are secreted by thymic epithelial cells into the bloodstream, where they exert their immunomodulatory effects.

Regulation of Thymosin

The regulation of thymosin involves complex mechanisms influenced by various internal and external factors:

1. **Thymic Hormones**: The production of thymosin is regulated by other thymic hormones, such as thymopoietin and thymulin, which coordinate the maturation and differentiation of immune cells.
2. **Age**: Thymosin production declines with age, corresponding with the gradual involution of the thymus gland. This reduction in thymosin levels contributes to the decreased immune function observed in elderly individuals.

3. **Stress and Infections**: Physical and psychological stress, as well as infections, can influence thymosin levels. Chronic stress and persistent infections tend to suppress thymosin production, impairing immune function.
4. **Nutritional Status**: Nutritional factors, particularly those derived from diet, play a significant role in regulating thymosin production. Deficiencies in essential nutrients can impair thymic function and thymosin synthesis.

Plant-Based Diet and Thymosin Regulation

A plant-based diet, rich in fruits, vegetables, whole grains, nuts, and seeds, can have a profound impact on thymosin regulation through various mechanisms:

1. **Nutrient Density**: Plant-based diets are typically high in essential nutrients, vitamins, and minerals that support overall health and hormonal balance. For example, vitamin D, found in fortified plant milks and mushrooms, is crucial for immune function and thymosin activity.
2. **Antioxidants**: Fruits and vegetables are rich in antioxidants, which help reduce oxidative stress. Lower oxidative stress levels are associated with improved thymosin secretion and overall immune function.
3. **Healthy Fats**: Plant-based sources of fats, such as avocados, nuts, and seeds, provide essential fatty acids that support hormone production and regulation. Omega-3 fatty acids, in particular, have anti-inflammatory properties that can enhance thymosin activity.
4. **Fiber**: High-fiber diets, common in plant-based eating, support gut health and immune regulation. A healthy gut microbiome can influence thymosin levels through the production of short-chain fatty acids and other metabolites.

5. **Phytochemicals**: Plant-based foods contain various phytochemicals, such as flavonoids and polyphenols, which possess anti-inflammatory and immunomodulatory properties. These compounds can positively impact thymosin production and immune function.

Plant-Based Diet on Thymosin-Related Health Outcomes

1. **Immune Function**: A plant-based diet supports robust immune function by providing essential nutrients, antioxidants, and phytochemicals that enhance thymosin activity and T-cell function. This leads to better protection against infections and improved immune surveillance.
2. **Wound Healing**: Nutrient-rich plant-based foods promote wound healing through the anti-inflammatory and cell-regenerative properties of compounds like vitamin C and beta-carotene. Thymosin beta-4, in particular, benefits from the nutrient support provided by such diets.
3. **Anti-Aging Effects**: The antioxidant-rich nature of plant-based diets helps combat oxidative stress, a key factor in aging. Improved thymosin levels, coupled with reduced oxidative damage, contribute to healthier aging and better maintenance of immune function.
4. **Inflammatory Diseases**: A plant-based diet can help manage chronic inflammatory diseases by reducing systemic inflammation. The anti-inflammatory effects of plant-derived nutrients and phytochemicals support thymosin's role in controlling excessive immune responses.

Nutrient-Specific Influences on Thymosin

1. **Vitamin D**: Vitamin D is crucial for immune function and thymosin activity. Plant-based sources of vitamin D include fortified plant milks, mushrooms exposed to UV light, and supplements. Adequate vitamin D levels support thymic health and thymosin production.
2. **Vitamin C**: Vitamin C, abundant in fruits and vegetables, supports immune function by promoting the production and function of immune cells. It also helps in the synthesis and function of thymosin beta-4, enhancing wound healing and reducing inflammation.
3. **Zinc**: Zinc is essential for immune function and thymic hormone activity. Plant-based sources of zinc include nuts, seeds, legumes, and whole grains. Adequate zinc intake is necessary for thymosin synthesis and T-cell function.
4. **Selenium**: Selenium, found in nuts (especially Brazil nuts), seeds, and whole grains, is a critical nutrient for immune function and antioxidant defense. Selenium supports thymosin production and protects thymic cells from oxidative damage.
5. **Iron**: Iron is vital for immune cell proliferation and function. Plant-based sources of iron include legumes, tofu, spinach, and fortified cereals. Consuming vitamin C-rich foods alongside iron-rich foods enhances iron absorption, supporting thymic health and thymosin production.

Thymosin in Plant-Based Research

Recent research highlights the benefits of plant-based diets on immune function and thymosin activity:

1. **Antioxidant Impact**: Studies have shown that diets rich in antioxidants from fruits and vegetables enhance immune function

by reducing oxidative stress. This reduction in oxidative stress supports thymosin production and overall thymic health.

2. **Anti-Inflammatory Effects**: Research indicates that plant-based diets reduce systemic inflammation, which positively impacts thymosin levels and immune function. Phytochemicals in plant foods have been shown to modulate immune responses and enhance thymosin activity.
3. **Gut Health and Immunity**: A healthy gut microbiome, supported by a high-fiber plant-based diet, plays a critical role in immune regulation. Short-chain fatty acids produced by gut bacteria influence thymosin production and T-cell function, highlighting the importance of dietary fiber.

Optimizing Thymosin Levels through a Plant-Based Diet

1. **Diverse Diet**: Consume a diverse range of fruits, vegetables, whole grains, nuts, and seeds to ensure a broad spectrum of nutrients and phytochemicals that support thymosin production and immune function.
2. **Fortified Foods**: Include fortified plant-based foods, such as plant milk and cereals, to ensure adequate intake of essential nutrients like vitamin D and vitamin B12.
3. **Supplementation**: Consider supplements for nutrients that are challenging to obtain in sufficient amounts from a plant-based diet alone, such as vitamin D, vitamin B12, and possibly zinc, after consulting with a healthcare provider.
4. **Hydration**: Maintain proper hydration to support overall health and nutrient transport, which indirectly supports thymosin production and immune function.
5. **Balanced Meals**: Ensure balanced meals that include sources of protein, healthy fats, and complex carbohydrates. This balance

helps in maintaining steady blood glucose levels and provides essential nutrients for thymosin synthesis.

6. **Regular Exercise**: Engage in regular physical activity to enhance immune function and thymosin production. Exercise promotes healthy circulation and reduces inflammation, which benefits thymic health.

Thymosin plays a pivotal role in the immune system, particularly in the maturation and function of T-cells. Its production and regulation are influenced by various factors, including age, stress, infections, and nutrition.

14

Other Important Hormones

Calcitonin

Calcitonin, a peptide hormone, plays a crucial role in regulating calcium homeostasis and bone metabolism.

Function of Calcitonin

Calcitonin's primary function is to regulate calcium levels in the blood and bone metabolism. It achieves this by:

1. **Lowering Blood Calcium Levels**: Calcitonin helps to reduce the concentration of calcium in the blood. When blood calcium levels rise above normal, calcitonin is released to counteract this increase by inhibiting the activity of osteoclasts, the cells responsible for bone resorption.
2. **Inhibiting Bone Resorption**: Calcitonin directly inhibits osteoclast activity, which slows down the breakdown of bone tissue. This action helps maintain bone density and strength, particularly during periods of high bone turnover, such as growth and remodeling.
3. **Enhancing Bone Formation**: By reducing bone resorption, calcitonin indirectly supports bone formation. Osteoblasts, the cells responsible for bone formation, are more active when bone resorption is minimized, leading to increased bone mass.

4. **Renal Calcium Excretion**: Calcitonin promotes the excretion of calcium through the kidneys, further contributing to the reduction of blood calcium levels. This process helps prevent hypercalcemia, a condition characterized by excessively high calcium levels in the blood.
5. **Protecting Against Postprandial Hypercalcemia**: After a meal, calcitonin prevents a significant rise in blood calcium levels by promoting calcium uptake in bones and its excretion via urine. This regulation is crucial for maintaining stable calcium levels throughout the day.

Production of Calcitonin

Calcitonin is produced by the parafollicular cells (also known as C cells) in the thyroid gland. The production process involves several steps:

1. **Synthesis:** Calcitonin is synthesized as a precursor molecule called preprocalcitonin. This precursor undergoes proteolytic cleavage to form procalcitonin, which is further processed to produce mature calcitonin.
2. **Regulation by Calcium Levels**: The primary regulator of calcitonin secretion is the calcium concentration in the blood. High blood calcium levels stimulate the release of calcitonin, while low calcium levels inhibit its secretion.
3. **Pulsatile Secretion**: Calcitonin is secreted in a pulsatile manner, with variations throughout the day. This secretion pattern is influenced by factors such as dietary calcium intake and bone metabolism rates.
4. **Influencing Factors**: Several factors influence calcitonin production, including:

- **Age**: Calcitonin levels are higher in children and adolescents, reflecting the increased bone growth and turnover during these stages. Levels decline with age.
- **Gender**: Women may have slightly higher baseline calcitonin levels than men, which could be related to differences in bone metabolism and hormonal regulation.
- **Diet**: Dietary calcium intake directly impacts calcitonin secretion. High calcium diets stimulate calcitonin production to help regulate blood calcium levels.

Regulation of Calcitonin

The regulation of calcitonin involves complex feedback mechanisms and external factors:

1. **Feedback Loops**: Blood calcium levels regulate calcitonin secretion through negative feedback mechanisms. Elevated calcium levels stimulate calcitonin release, which then acts to lower blood calcium levels. Once calcium levels are reduced, calcitonin secretion decreases.
2. **Dietary Calcium Intake**: A diet high in calcium can increase calcitonin production. This relationship helps to prevent hypercalcemia by promoting the storage of excess calcium in bones and its excretion via the kidneys.
3. **Vitamin D**: Vitamin D plays a crucial role in calcium metabolism and influences calcitonin activity. Adequate levels of vitamin D enhance calcium absorption in the intestines and its deposition in bones, thereby supporting calcitonin's role in maintaining calcium balance.
4. **Physical Activity**: Regular physical activity, particularly weight-bearing exercises, positively affects bone health and calcitonin levels. Exercise stimulates bone formation and reduces the risk of osteoporosis, partly through its impact on calcitonin secretion.

5. **Hormones**: Other hormones, such as parathyroid hormone (PTH) and estrogen, interact with calcitonin to regulate calcium and bone metabolism. PTH and calcitonin have opposing effects on calcium levels, creating a balanced regulatory system.

Plant-Based Diet and Calcitonin Regulation

A plant-based diet, rich in fruits, vegetables, whole grains, nuts, and seeds, can profoundly impact calcitonin regulation through various mechanisms:

1. **Calcium-Rich Plant Foods**: Plant-based sources of calcium, such as leafy greens (kale, bok choy, and collard greens), fortified plant milk, and tofu, provide adequate calcium to support bone health and calcitonin function. These foods help maintain optimal calcium levels without the risks associated with high animal-based calcium sources.
2. **Magnesium**: Magnesium, found in abundance in nuts, seeds, whole grains, and leafy greens, is essential for bone health and the proper functioning of calcitonin. Magnesium helps regulate calcium transport and supports bone mineralization.
3. **Vitamin K**: Vitamin K, present in green leafy vegetables, plays a vital role in bone metabolism and calcitonin activity. It helps in the carboxylation of osteocalcin, a protein necessary for bone mineralization, indirectly supporting calcitonin's function in bone health.
4. **Antioxidants**: Fruits and vegetables are rich in antioxidants, which help reduce oxidative stress. Lower oxidative stress levels are associated with improved overall endocrine function, including calcitonin secretion and activity.
5. **Healthy Fats**: Plant-based sources of fats, such as avocados, nuts, and seeds, provide essential fatty acids that support hormone production and regulation. Omega-3 fatty acids, in particular,

have anti-inflammatory properties that can enhance calcitonin activity.

6. **Fiber**: High-fiber diets, common in plant-based eating, support gut health and hormone regulation. A healthy gut microbiome can influence calcitonin levels through the production of short-chain fatty acids and other metabolites.
7. **Glycemic Control**: Plant-based diets, which are low in refined sugars and high in complex carbohydrates, help maintain stable blood glucose levels. This stability prevents metabolic stress that could affect calcitonin regulation.

Plant-Based Diet on Calcitonin-Related Health Outcomes

1. **Bone Health**: Plant-based diets rich in calcium, magnesium, and vitamin K support bone health. Leafy greens, fortified plant milk, and nuts are excellent sources of these nutrients, which work synergistically with calcitonin to maintain bone density and reduce the risk of osteoporosis.
2. **Calcium Balance**: A plant-based diet helps maintain optimal calcium levels in the body, reducing the risk of both hypercalcemia and hypocalcemia. By providing a steady supply of bioavailable calcium, plant-based foods support calcitonin's role in calcium homeostasis.
3. **Weight Management**: Plant-based diets are effective for weight management, reducing body fat, and improving metabolic health. Lower body fat reduces the risk of conditions like hyperparathyroidism, which can negatively impact calcitonin regulation and bone health.
4. **Anti-Aging Effects**: The antioxidant-rich nature of plant-based diets helps combat oxidative stress, a key factor in aging. Improved calcitonin levels, coupled with reduced oxidative damage,

contribute to healthier aging and better maintenance of bone mass.

5. **Mental Health**: Emerging evidence suggests that plant-based diets may benefit mental health by reducing inflammation and oxidative stress, which are linked to mood disorders. Improved overall hormonal balance, including calcitonin, supports cognitive function and emotional well-being.

Calcitonin plays a pivotal role in regulating calcium homeostasis and bone metabolism throughout life. Its production and regulation are influenced by various factors, including age, dietary intake, physical activity, and overall hormonal balance.

Prostaglandins (PGs)

Prostaglandins (PGs) are a group of physiologically active lipid compounds derived from fatty acids. They play a critical role in various bodily functions, including inflammation, pain, fever, and the regulation of blood flow, among others.

Function of Prostaglandins

Prostaglandins perform a variety of functions in the body, which are essential for maintaining homeostasis and responding to injury and infection. These functions can be broadly categorized into several key areas:

1. Inflammation and Immune Response

Prostaglandins are central mediators of inflammation. They are produced at sites of tissue damage or infection and contribute to the development of the inflammatory response. Specific functions include:

- **Vasodilation**: Prostaglandins cause the dilation of blood vessels, increasing blood flow to the affected area, which brings in immune cells to fight infection and clear debris.
- **Pain Sensation**: Prostaglandins sensitize nerve endings to pain, leading to the sensation of pain at the site of inflammation or injury.
- **Fever Induction**: Certain prostaglandins, particularly PGE2, act on the hypothalamus to raise the body temperature, resulting in fever, which is a common response to infection.

2. Reproductive Health

Prostaglandins play a vital role in reproductive health, including:

- **Ovulation**: They are involved in the process of ovulation, facilitating the release of the egg from the ovary.
- **Menstrual Cycle**: Prostaglandins are responsible for the contraction of the uterus during menstruation, which helps shed the uterine lining.
- **Labor and Delivery**: During childbirth, prostaglandins help induce labor by stimulating uterine contractions.

3. Cardiovascular System

In the cardiovascular system, prostaglandins help regulate blood pressure and maintain blood flow. Functions include:

- **Vasodilation and Vasoconstriction**: Prostaglandins can either dilate or constrict blood vessels, thus playing a role in the regulation of blood pressure.
- **Platelet Aggregation**: Some prostaglandins inhibit platelet aggregation (e.g., prostacyclin), preventing blood clots, while others promote aggregation (e.g., thromboxane), which is essential for stopping bleeding.

4. Gastrointestinal System

Prostaglandins protect the gastrointestinal tract by:

- **Mucus Production**: They stimulate the production of mucus in the stomach lining, which helps protect against the corrosive effects of stomach acid.
- **Regulation of Acid Secretion**: They modulate the secretion of gastric acid, contributing to the balance and protection of the stomach lining.

5. Renal System

In the kidneys, prostaglandins regulate various functions, including:

- **Renal Blood Flow**: They help maintain adequate blood flow to the kidneys, ensuring proper filtration and urine formation.
- **Salt and Water Balance**: Prostaglandins influence the reabsorption of sodium and water, affecting fluid balance and blood pressure.

Production of Prostaglandins

Prostaglandins are synthesized from arachidonic acid, a polyunsaturated fatty acid found in the phospholipids of cell membranes. The production process involves several steps:

1. Release of Arachidonic Acid

When a cell is stimulated by physical, chemical, or biological signals (e.g., injury or infection), enzymes called phospholipases release arachidonic acid from the cell membrane.

2. Cyclooxygenase Pathway

Arachidonic acid is then converted into prostaglandin H2 (PGH2) by the enzyme cyclooxygenase (COX). There are two main isoforms of COX:

- **COX-1**: This isoform is constitutively expressed in most tissues and is involved in maintaining physiological functions, such as protecting the stomach lining and regulating blood flow.
- **COX-2**: This isoform is inducible and primarily involved in the inflammatory response. It is upregulated in response to inflammatory stimuli, leading to the production of pro-inflammatory prostaglandins.

3. Specific Prostaglandin Formation

PGH2 is a precursor that is further converted into various specific prostaglandins by different enzymes. These include:

- **Prostaglandin E2 (PGE2)**: Involved in inflammation, fever, and pain.
- **Prostaglandin I2 (PGI2 or Prostacyclin)**: Acts as a vasodilator and inhibits platelet aggregation.
- **Prostaglandin D2 (PGD2)**: Involved in sleep regulation and allergic responses.
- **Prostaglandin F2α (PGF2α)**: Induces uterine contractions and is involved in reproductive processes.
- **Thromboxane A2 (TXA2)**: Promotes platelet aggregation and vasoconstriction.

Regulation of Prostaglandins

The regulation of prostaglandin production is a complex process involving various feedback mechanisms and external factors:

1. Enzyme Expression

The expression of COX-1 and COX-2 enzymes is tightly regulated:

- **COX-1**: As it is constitutively expressed, its activity is relatively stable and contributes to baseline prostaglandin levels involved in homeostatic functions.

- **COX-2**: Its expression is highly inducible by inflammatory cytokines, growth factors, and other stimuli. This regulation ensures that prostaglandins are produced in response to injury or infection, contributing to the inflammatory response.

2. Feedback Inhibition

Prostaglandins themselves can regulate their production through feedback mechanisms:

- **PGE2**: High levels of PGE2 can inhibit further production of prostaglandins by downregulating COX-2 expression.
- **PGI2 and TXA2**: The balance between prostacyclin (PGI2) and thromboxane (TXA2) is crucial for maintaining vascular homeostasis and preventing excessive clotting or bleeding.

3. Nutritional Factors

Diet and nutrition significantly influence prostaglandin production and activity. Key factors include:

- **Fatty Acid Composition**: The types of fats consumed in the diet affect the availability of substrates for prostaglandin synthesis. Diets high in omega-6 fatty acids (e.g., from animal products and certain vegetable oils) can lead to increased production of pro-inflammatory prostaglandins. Conversely, omega-3 fatty acids (e.g., from flaxseeds, chia seeds, and walnuts) can compete with arachidonic acid for COX enzymes, leading to the production of anti-inflammatory eicosanoids.
- **Antioxidants**: Antioxidants found in plant-based foods (e.g., fruits, vegetables, and whole grains) can reduce oxidative stress and inflammation, potentially influencing prostaglandin production and activity.

- **Phytonutrients**: Certain plant compounds, such as flavonoids and polyphenols, can modulate the activity of COX enzymes and influence prostaglandin synthesis.

Plant-Based Diet and Prostaglandin Regulation

A plant-based diet can have profound effects on the regulation of prostaglandins through various mechanisms:

1. Omega-3 Fatty Acids

Plant-based sources of omega-3 fatty acids, such as flaxseeds, chia seeds, and walnuts, provide alpha-linolenic acid (ALA), which can be converted into eicosapentaenoic acid (EPA) and docosahexaenoic acid (DHA) in the body. These fatty acids compete with arachidonic acid for COX enzymes, leading to the production of less inflammatory eicosanoids, such as prostaglandin E3 (PGE3) and prostacyclin I3 (PGI3).

2. Antioxidants and Anti-Inflammatory Compounds

Plant-based diets are rich in antioxidants and anti-inflammatory compounds, which can reduce oxidative stress and inflammation. For example, polyphenols found in fruits, vegetables, and whole grains have been shown to inhibit COX-2 activity, thereby reducing the production of pro-inflammatory prostaglandins.

3. Phytochemicals

Various phytochemicals found in plant foods can modulate prostaglandin synthesis. For instance, curcumin (from turmeric) and resveratrol (from grapes) have been shown to inhibit COX-2 activity and reduce inflammation.

4. Fiber

High-fiber diets support a healthy gut microbiome, which can influence inflammation and prostaglandin production. Short-chain fatty acids (SCFAs) produced by the fermentation of dietary fiber in the gut have anti-inflammatory effects and can modulate the production of prostaglandins.

5. Overall Dietary Patterns

Adopting a plant-based diet, which emphasizes whole, unprocessed foods, can help maintain a balanced production of prostaglandins. By reducing the intake of pro-inflammatory foods (e.g., refined sugars, and processed meats) and increasing the consumption of anti-inflammatory foods (e.g., fruits, vegetables, nuts, and seeds), a plant-based diet supports overall health and reduces the risk of chronic inflammatory conditions.

Plant-Based Diet on Prostaglandin-Related Health Outcomes

1. Inflammation and Pain Management

Plant-based diets have been shown to reduce inflammation and pain, partly due to their impact on prostaglandin production. By increasing the intake of anti-inflammatory omega-3 fatty acids and antioxidants, plant-based diets can help manage conditions like arthritis and other inflammatory disorders.

2. Cardiovascular Health

The balance between prostacyclin and thromboxane is crucial for cardiovascular health. Plant-based diets, rich in omega-3 fatty acids and antioxidants, can promote the production of prostacyclin, which inhibits platelet aggregation and supports vasodilation, thereby reducing the risk of cardiovascular diseases.

3. Reproductive Health

Dietary factors influence prostaglandin production involved in reproductive health. Plant-based diets can help regulate menstrual cycles and reduce the severity of menstrual cramps by modulating the production of prostaglandins involved in uterine contractions.

4. Gastrointestinal Health

By promoting the production of protective prostaglandins and reducing inflammation, plant-based diets support gastrointestinal health. The high fiber content of plant-based diets also supports gut health and reduces the risk of conditions like gastritis and peptic ulcers.

5. Chronic Disease Prevention
Chronic diseases, such as diabetes and cancer, are often associated with chronic inflammation. Plant-based diets, which reduce the production of pro-inflammatory prostaglandins and promote anti-inflammatory pathways, can help prevent and manage these diseases.

Prostaglandins are vital lipid compounds with diverse roles in inflammation, pain, fever, reproductive health, cardiovascular function, and gastrointestinal protection. Their production and regulation are influenced by various factors, including enzyme expression, feedback mechanisms, and nutritional factors.

Histamine

Histamine is a biogenic amine involved in local immune responses, regulating physiological functions in the gut, and acting as a neurotransmitter for the brain, spinal cord, and uterus.

Function of Histamine
Histamine plays several crucial roles in the body, including:

1. **Immune Response:** Histamine is stored in mast cells and basophils and is released during immune responses, such as allergic reactions. It contributes to inflammation by causing vasodilation, increasing the permeability of blood vessels, and attracting other immune cells to the site of infection or injury.
2. **Gastrointestinal Function:** In the gut, histamine stimulates the secretion of gastric acid by parietal cells, which is essential for digestion and maintaining the acidic environment of the stomach.

3. **Neurotransmission:** Histamine functions as a neurotransmitter in the brain, where it is involved in regulating the sleep-wake cycle, appetite, and cognitive functions.
4. **Vascular Regulation:** Histamine plays a role in regulating blood pressure and heart rate through its effects on blood vessels and cardiac tissue.
5. **Smooth Muscle Contraction:** Histamine causes the contraction of smooth muscles, such as those in the bronchi, which can lead to symptoms like bronchoconstriction in asthma.

Production of Histamine

Histamine is produced through the decarboxylation of the amino acid histidine by the enzyme histidine decarboxylase. This process occurs in various tissues, including the brain, stomach, and immune cells.

1. **Synthesis:** The enzyme histidine decarboxylase converts histidine into histamine. This enzyme is widely distributed in the body, with high concentrations in the brain, gastric mucosa, and immune cells.
2. **Storage and Release:** Histamine is stored in granules within mast cells and basophils in the immune system. Upon activation by allergens, physical injury, or other triggers, these cells release histamine into the surrounding tissues.
3. **Degradation:** After its release, histamine is rapidly broken down by two main enzymes: histamine-N-methyltransferase (HMT) and diamine oxidase (DAO). HMT methylates histamine in the central nervous system, while DAO oxidatively deaminates histamine primarily in the digestive tract.

Regulation of Histamine

The regulation of histamine involves complex feedback mechanisms and external factors:

1. **Feedback Loops:** The release of histamine is regulated through feedback mechanisms involving histamine receptors (H1, H2, H3, and H4). These receptors modulate histamine release and action, ensuring balanced physiological responses.
2. **Immune Signals:** Cytokines and other immune signals can induce the synthesis and release of histamine from immune cells during inflammatory and allergic responses.
3. **Gastrointestinal Regulation:** In the stomach, histamine release is regulated by neural and hormonal signals, such as gastrin and acetylcholine, which stimulate histamine-producing cells (enterochromaffin-like cells) to enhance gastric acid secretion.
4. **Neurotransmission:** In the brain, histamine levels are modulated by neuronal activity and interactions with other neurotransmitter systems, including acetylcholine, dopamine, and serotonin.

Plant-Based Diet and Histamine Regulation

A plant-based diet, rich in fruits, vegetables, whole grains, nuts, and seeds, can influence histamine regulation through various mechanisms:

1. **Antioxidants:** Plant-based foods are rich in antioxidants, which help reduce oxidative stress. Lower oxidative stress levels can prevent excessive histamine release and reduce inflammation.
2. **Anti-inflammatory Compounds:** Many plant-based foods contain anti-inflammatory compounds, such as flavonoids and polyphenols, which can inhibit the release of histamine from immune cells and reduce allergic reactions.

3. **Probiotics and Prebiotics:** Fermented foods and dietary fibers from plant-based sources support gut health by promoting a healthy microbiome. A balanced gut microbiome can modulate immune responses and histamine metabolism, reducing symptoms of histamine intolerance.
4. **Nutrient Density:** Plant-based diets provide essential nutrients, such as vitamin C and vitamin B6, which are co-factors for DAO, the enzyme responsible for degrading histamine. Adequate intake of these vitamins can enhance histamine degradation and reduce histamine-related symptoms.
5. **Low Histamine Foods:** Some plant-based foods naturally contain low levels of histamine, making them suitable for individuals with histamine intolerance. Examples include fresh fruits and vegetables (excluding tomatoes, spinach, and eggplant), grains, and certain nuts.

Plant-Based Diet on Histamine-Related Health Outcomes

1. **Allergy Management:** A diet rich in anti-inflammatory and antioxidant-rich plant foods can help manage allergic conditions by reducing histamine release and activity. Foods such as berries, apples, and green tea contain quercetin, a natural antihistamine that can alleviate allergy symptoms.
2. **Gut Health:** Consuming a variety of plant-based fibers supports a healthy gut microbiome, which plays a crucial role in regulating histamine production and degradation. Fermented foods like sauerkraut and kimchi, although typically avoided in a low-histamine diet, can be beneficial in moderation for gut health.
3. **Mental Health:** Histamine's role as a neurotransmitter implies that its balanced levels are important for mental health. Plant-based diets that support brain health through nutrients like

omega-3 fatty acids (found in flaxseeds and walnuts) and antioxidants can help maintain optimal histamine function in the brain.

4. **Cardiovascular Health:** By reducing oxidative stress and inflammation, plant-based diets can support cardiovascular health, indirectly influencing histamine's role in vascular regulation and blood pressure management.
5. **Asthma and Respiratory Health:** Anti-inflammatory foods and natural antihistamines found in a plant-based diet can help manage asthma and other respiratory conditions by reducing bronchoconstriction and histamine-related inflammation.

Plant-Based Foods and Their Impact on Histamine Levels

1. **Quercetin:** Found in onions, apples, and capers, quercetin is a flavonoid with potent antihistamine and anti-inflammatory properties. It stabilizes mast cells, preventing them from releasing histamine and reducing allergy symptoms.
2. **Vitamin C:** Citrus fruits, bell peppers, and strawberries are rich in vitamin C, which acts as a natural antihistamine. Vitamin C can reduce histamine levels in the blood, alleviating symptoms of histamine intolerance and allergies.
3. **Vitamin B6:** Bananas, chickpeas, and potatoes provide vitamin B6, a co-factor for DAO. Adequate vitamin B6 levels support the efficient breakdown of histamine, reducing the risk of histamine accumulation and intolerance.
4. **Polyphenols:** Green tea, berries, and grapes are high in polyphenols, which have anti-inflammatory and antihistamine effects. These compounds can modulate immune responses and decrease histamine release from mast cells.
5. **Probiotic Foods:** Non-dairy probiotic sources like coconut yogurt, tempeh, and miso can support gut health and enhance the breakdown of histamine by promoting a healthy gut microbiome.

Probiotics help balance immune responses and reduce histamine-related symptoms.

Managing Histamine Intolerance with a Plant-Based Diet

Histamine intolerance occurs when there is an imbalance between histamine intake or production and the body's ability to degrade it. A plant-based diet can be tailored to manage histamine intolerance effectively:

1. **Low-Histamine Foods:** Focus on fresh, minimally processed plant-based foods that are naturally low in histamine. Examples include most fresh vegetables (excluding tomatoes, spinach, and eggplant), fresh fruits (excluding citrus and bananas), rice, quinoa, and certain nuts.
2. **Avoiding High-Histamine Foods:** Certain plant-based foods are high in histamine or can trigger its release. These include fermented foods (like sauerkraut and soy sauce), aged foods, and certain vegetables (like tomatoes, spinach, and eggplant).
3. **Supporting Histamine Degradation:** Ensure adequate intake of vitamins and minerals that support DAO activity, such as vitamin C, vitamin B6, copper, and zinc. Foods like bell peppers, chickpeas, sunflower seeds, and leafy greens can help maintain these nutrient levels.
4. **Anti-Inflammatory Diet:** Incorporate anti-inflammatory foods like berries, turmeric, and leafy greens to reduce overall inflammation and histamine release. These foods contain bioactive compounds that can modulate immune responses and decrease histamine levels.
5. **Hydration:** Drinking plenty of water helps dilute histamine levels in the body and supports overall detoxification processes. Proper hydration is essential for maintaining histamine balance and reducing symptoms of histamine intolerance.

Histamine plays a vital role in immune response, gastrointestinal function, neurotransmission, vascular regulation, and smooth muscle contraction. Its production and regulation involve complex mechanisms influenced by immune signals, neurotransmitter interactions, and dietary factors.

Bradykinin

Bradykinin is a peptide hormone that plays a critical role in numerous physiological processes, including vasodilation, inflammation, pain, and blood pressure regulation.

Function of Bradykinin

Bradykinin's primary functions involve various aspects of cardiovascular and inflammatory responses:

1. **Vasodilation**: Bradykinin is a potent vasodilator, meaning it causes blood vessels to widen. This process is crucial for regulating blood pressure and ensuring adequate blood flow to various tissues. Bradykinin achieves this by stimulating the production of nitric oxide and prostacyclin, both of which are key vasodilatory agents.
2. **Inflammation**: Bradykinin plays a significant role in the inflammatory response. It increases the permeability of blood vessels, allowing immune cells and proteins to enter tissues where they can combat infection or injury. This increased permeability can also lead to edema, or swelling, a common feature of inflammation.
3. **Pain Sensation**: Bradykinin contributes to the sensation of pain. It directly stimulates pain receptors (nociceptors) and increases the sensitivity of these receptors to other pain-inducing

substances. This makes bradykinin an important mediator of pain in conditions like arthritis and other inflammatory diseases.

4. **Blood Pressure Regulation**: By promoting vasodilation and influencing the release of other vasoactive substances, bradykinin helps regulate blood pressure. Its actions counterbalance the effects of vasoconstrictors, such as angiotensin II, thereby contributing to cardiovascular homeostasis.

Production of Bradykinin

The production of bradykinin involves a complex biochemical pathway known as the kallikrein-kinin system:

1. **Kallikrein Activation**: Bradykinin is produced from its precursor, kininogen, through the action of enzymes called kallikreins. There are two main types of kallikreins involved in this process: plasma kallikrein and tissue kallikrein. Plasma kallikrein is activated in the bloodstream, while tissue kallikrein acts within tissues.
2. **Kininogen Cleavage**: Kallikreins cleave kininogen to release bradykinin. High-molecular-weight kininogen (HMWK) is cleaved by plasma kallikrein to produce bradykinin, while low-molecular-weight kininogen (LMWK) is cleaved by tissue kallikrein to produce kallidin, which is subsequently converted to bradykinin by aminopeptidases.
3. **Degradation**: Bradykinin is rapidly degraded by enzymes such as angiotensin-converting enzyme (ACE), neprilysin, and aminopeptidases. These enzymes ensure that bradykinin's effects are short-lived, preventing excessive vasodilation and inflammation.

Regulation of Bradykinin

The regulation of bradykinin levels and activity is a finely tuned process involving several factors:

1. **Feedback Mechanisms**: The kallikrein-kinin system is regulated through feedback mechanisms that control the activation of kallikreins and the degradation of bradykinin. For instance, increased levels of bradykinin can inhibit further kallikrein activation.
2. **Enzyme Inhibitors**: Specific inhibitors of kallikrein, such as C1-inhibitor, regulate bradykinin production by preventing the activation of kallikrein. Similarly, ACE inhibitors, commonly used to treat hypertension, can increase bradykinin levels by reducing its degradation.
3. **Inflammatory Signals**: Inflammatory mediators, such as cytokines and other immune signals, can upregulate the production of bradykinin during inflammation. This ensures an adequate response to injury or infection but can also lead to excessive inflammation if not properly controlled.
4. **Genetic Factors**: Genetic variations in the genes encoding kallikreins, kininogens, and bradykinin receptors can affect bradykinin production and activity. These genetic factors can influence an individual's susceptibility to conditions such as hereditary angioedema, where bradykinin levels are abnormally high.

Plant-Based Diet and Bradykinin Regulation

A plant-based diet, rich in fruits, vegetables, whole grains, nuts, and seeds, can influence bradykinin regulation through various mechanisms:

1. **Antioxidants**: Plant-based diets are rich in antioxidants, such as flavonoids, vitamin C, and vitamin E, which can modulate the inflammatory response. Antioxidants reduce oxidative stress, which is a key factor in the activation of the kallikrein-kinin system. For example, quercetin, a flavonoid found in many fruits and vegetables, has been shown to inhibit bradykinin-induced inflammation.
2. **Omega-3 Fatty Acids**: Plant-based sources of omega-3 fatty acids, such as flaxseeds, chia seeds, and walnuts, have anti-inflammatory properties. Omega-3 fatty acids can inhibit the production of pro-inflammatory cytokines and reduce bradykinin-mediated inflammation.
3. **Fiber**: High-fiber diets, common in plant-based eating, support gut health and the production of short-chain fatty acids (SCFAs) by the gut microbiota. SCFAs, such as butyrate, have anti-inflammatory effects and can downregulate the production of bradykinin during inflammatory responses.
4. **Polyphenols**: Polyphenols, found in a variety of plant foods, have been shown to modulate the activity of the kallikrein-kinin system. For example, resveratrol, a polyphenol in grapes and berries, can inhibit kallikrein activity and reduce bradykinin levels.
5. **Magnesium**: Magnesium, abundant in leafy greens, nuts, and seeds, is essential for numerous enzymatic reactions, including those involved in the regulation of bradykinin. Adequate magnesium intake supports cardiovascular health and helps maintain balanced bradykinin levels.

Plant-Based Diet on Bradykinin-Related Health Outcomes

1. **Cardiovascular Health**: Bradykinin's vasodilatory effects are beneficial for cardiovascular health. A plant-based diet, with its emphasis on whole, unprocessed foods, supports endothelial

function and reduces the risk of hypertension. By promoting nitric oxide production and reducing inflammation, plant-based diets help maintain healthy blood pressure levels.

2. **Anti-Inflammatory Benefits**: The anti-inflammatory properties of plant-based diets are well-documented. By modulating bradykinin levels and activity, a plant-based diet can reduce chronic inflammation and the risk of inflammatory diseases such as arthritis, inflammatory bowel disease, and asthma.
3. **Pain Management**: Bradykinin-induced pain can be mitigated by a plant-based diet. The anti-inflammatory and analgesic properties of certain plant compounds, such as curcumin from turmeric and gingerol from ginger, can help alleviate pain associated with bradykinin-mediated conditions.
4. **Allergic Reactions**: Bradykinin plays a role in allergic reactions, particularly in conditions like angioedema. A plant-based diet, rich in anti-inflammatory nutrients, can help manage allergic symptoms by regulating bradykinin levels and reducing histamine release.
5. **Gut Health**: A healthy gut microbiome is crucial for the regulation of bradykinin and overall inflammatory responses. Plant-based diets promote a diverse and balanced gut microbiota, which in turn produces metabolites that can influence bradykinin activity and reduce inflammation.

Bradykinin plays a pivotal role in cardiovascular, inflammatory, and pain processes. Its production and regulation are influenced by various factors, including genetic predisposition, feedback mechanisms, and inflammatory signals.

Angiotensin II

Angiotensin II is a potent vasoconstrictor hormone that plays a critical role in blood pressure regulation, fluid balance, and cardiovascular health.

Function of Angiotensin II

Angiotensin II exerts its physiological effects through several mechanisms, primarily focusing on blood pressure regulation and fluid homeostasis. Its functions include:

1. **Vasoconstriction**: Angiotensin II causes the constriction of blood vessels, which increases vascular resistance and raises blood pressure. This action is vital in maintaining adequate perfusion to organs during hypotensive states.
2. **Aldosterone Secretion**: It stimulates the adrenal cortex to release aldosterone, a hormone that promotes sodium retention and potassium excretion by the kidneys. This process enhances water reabsorption, contributing to increased blood volume and pressure.
3. **Antidiuretic Hormone (ADH) Release**: Angiotensin II promotes the release of ADH from the posterior pituitary gland. ADH increases water reabsorption in the kidneys, further supporting blood volume and pressure regulation.
4. **Thirst Stimulation**: It triggers the hypothalamus to induce thirst, encouraging water intake to maintain fluid balance.
5. **Sympathetic Nervous System Activation**: Angiotensin II enhances sympathetic nervous system activity, which increases heart rate and contractility, contributing to elevated blood pressure.
6. **Cell Growth and Inflammation**: Angiotensin II promotes the proliferation of vascular smooth muscle cells and has pro-

inflammatory effects, which can contribute to cardiovascular remodeling and pathology if chronically elevated.

Production of Angiotensin II

The production of Angiotensin II involves a multi-step enzymatic process primarily centered in the kidneys, liver, and lungs:

1. **Renin Release**: The juxtaglomerular cells of the kidneys release renin in response to low blood pressure, low sodium concentration, or sympathetic nervous system activation. Renin is an enzyme that catalyzes the conversion of angiotensinogen to angiotensin I.
2. **Angiotensinogen Production**: The liver continuously produces and releases angiotensinogen into the bloodstream. Angiotensinogen is an inactive precursor protein.
3. **Conversion to Angiotensin I**: Renin cleaves angiotensinogen to form angiotensin I, a decapeptide with minimal physiological activity.
4. **Conversion to Angiotensin II**: Angiotensin I is converted to angiotensin II by the angiotensin-converting enzyme (ACE), primarily in the lungs. ACE removes two amino acids from angiotensin I to form the active octapeptide, angiotensin II.

Regulation of Angiotensin II

The regulation of Angiotensin II involves intricate feedback mechanisms and is influenced by various factors:

1. **Renin-Angiotensin-Aldosterone System (RAAS)**: The RAAS is the primary regulator of Angiotensin II production. Low blood pressure, low sodium levels, and increased sympathetic

activity stimulate renin release, initiating the cascade that leads to Angiotensin II formation.

2. **Negative Feedback Mechanism**: Elevated levels of Angiotensin II inhibit further renin release through a negative feedback loop, preventing excessive Angiotensin II production.
3. **Angiotensin-Converting Enzyme 2 (ACE2)**: ACE2 is an enzyme that degrades Angiotensin II to angiotensin-(1-7), which counteracts the effects of Angiotensin II by promoting vasodilation and anti-inflammatory actions. This balance between ACE and ACE2 activity is crucial for maintaining cardiovascular health.
4. **Hormonal Influences**: Hormones such as aldosterone and ADH, stimulated by Angiotensin II, further regulate fluid and electrolyte balance, indirectly affecting Angiotensin II levels.
5. **Dietary Factors**: Nutritional status and dietary composition can influence the RAAS and Angiotensin II activity. High sodium intake, for example, can suppress renin release, while low sodium diets can stimulate the RAAS.

Plant-Based Diet and Angiotensin II Regulation

A plant-based diet, rich in fruits, vegetables, whole grains, nuts, and seeds, can have significant effects on the regulation of Angiotensin II through various mechanisms:

1. **Antioxidant-Rich Foods**: Plant-based diets are abundant in antioxidants, which reduce oxidative stress and inflammation. Oxidative stress can activate the RAAS, leading to increased Angiotensin II levels. Consuming antioxidant-rich foods helps mitigate this effect, promoting cardiovascular health.
2. **Low Sodium Intake**: A plant-based diet naturally tends to be lower in sodium compared to diets high in processed foods. Reduced sodium intake decreases the stimulation of the RAAS,

leading to lower Angiotensin II levels and improved blood pressure control.

3. **High Potassium Intake**: Fruits and vegetables are excellent sources of potassium, which counteracts the effects of sodium and helps regulate blood pressure. Potassium-rich foods support kidney function and reduce RAAS activation.
4. **Magnesium and Calcium**: Plant-based foods provide essential minerals like magnesium and calcium, which have vasodilatory effects and help modulate blood pressure. These minerals can influence RAAS activity and Angiotensin II production.
5. **Omega-3 Fatty Acids**: Nuts, seeds, and certain plant oils contain omega-3 fatty acids, which have anti-inflammatory properties and support cardiovascular health. Omega-3s can reduce RAAS activation and lower Angiotensin II levels.
6. **Fiber**: High-fiber diets, common in plant-based eating, support gut health and reduce systemic inflammation. A healthy gut microbiome can influence RAAS activity and Angiotensin II levels.
7. **Phytochemicals**: Plant-based diets are rich in phytochemicals, such as flavonoids and polyphenols, which have been shown to modulate the RAAS and reduce Angiotensin II activity. These compounds support endothelial function and cardiovascular health.

Plant-Based Diet on Angiotensin II-Related Health Outcomes

1. **Blood Pressure Control**: Numerous studies have demonstrated that plant-based diets are effective in lowering blood pressure. The DASH (Dietary Approaches to Stop Hypertension) diet, which emphasizes plant-based foods, has been shown to reduce blood pressure significantly. Lower Angiotensin II levels contribute to this effect.

2. **Cardiovascular Health**: By reducing Angiotensin II levels, a plant-based diet helps lower the risk of cardiovascular diseases, such as heart attacks and strokes. The anti-inflammatory and antioxidant properties of plant foods protect against vascular damage and improve endothelial function.
3. **Kidney Health**: High Angiotensin II levels can contribute to kidney damage and chronic kidney disease. A plant-based diet, with its beneficial effects on blood pressure and inflammation, supports kidney health and reduces the progression of kidney disease.
4. **Weight Management**: Plant-based diets are effective for weight management, reducing body fat, and improving insulin sensitivity. Lower body fat and better glycemic control help regulate the RAAS and Angiotensin II levels.
5. **Diabetes Management**: Angiotensin II can contribute to insulin resistance and the development of type 2 diabetes. A plant-based diet, rich in fiber and antioxidants, improves insulin sensitivity and glycemic control, reducing the impact of Angiotensin II on metabolic health.

Angiotensin II plays a pivotal role in blood pressure regulation, fluid balance, and cardiovascular health. Its production and regulation are influenced by various factors, including the renin-angiotensin-aldosterone system, dietary composition, and hormonal balance.

Endothelin (ET)

Endothelin (ET) is a peptide hormone with significant physiological and pathological roles in the cardiovascular system and beyond.

Function of Endothelin

Endothelin exerts multiple effects on the body, particularly in vascular homeostasis, where it serves as one of the most potent vasoconstrictors. It also influences other systems, contributing to various physiological and pathological processes.

1. **Vasoconstriction**: Endothelin-1 (ET-1), the most studied isoform, is a powerful vasoconstrictor. It acts on the smooth muscle cells of blood vessels to induce contraction, thereby increasing blood pressure. This function is crucial for maintaining vascular tone and blood flow regulation.
2. **Cardiac Function**: Endothelin contributes to cardiac contractility and growth. It enhances the force of contraction in the heart muscle, supporting cardiac output, especially during stress conditions.
3. **Cell Proliferation and Inflammation**: Endothelin has mitogenic properties, meaning it promotes cell division, particularly in vascular smooth muscle cells and fibroblasts. It is also involved in inflammatory processes, contributing to the pathogenesis of various cardiovascular diseases.
4. **Renal Function**: In the kidneys, endothelin regulates sodium and water excretion, thus influencing fluid balance and blood pressure. It also affects renal blood flow and glomerular filtration rate.
5. **Neurological Effects**: Endothelin influences the central nervous system, affecting neuronal activity and contributing to neurovascular regulation.

Production of Endothelin

Endothelin is produced by various cell types throughout the body, with vascular endothelial cells being the primary source. The production process is tightly regulated and involves several key steps:

1. **Gene Expression**: The gene for endothelin-1 (EDN1) is located on chromosome 6 in humans. Its expression is regulated by multiple factors, including shear stress, hypoxia, and cytokines.
2. **Preproendothelin Synthesis**: The EDN1 gene encodes a precursor protein called preproendothelin, which is further processed into big endothelin (an intermediate form) by the action of endothelin-converting enzymes (ECEs).
3. **Conversion to Active Form**: Big endothelin is cleaved by ECEs to produce the active 21-amino acid peptide, endothelin-1, which can then exert its biological effects by binding to endothelin receptors (ETA and ETB) on target cells.

Regulation of Endothelin

The regulation of endothelin involves complex feedback mechanisms and interactions with various physiological stimuli:

1. **Feedback Inhibition**: High levels of endothelin can inhibit its own production through negative feedback loops involving the ETA and ETB receptors. These receptors mediate different responses, with ETA primarily inducing vasoconstriction and cell proliferation, while ETB can cause vasodilation and clearance of endothelin from circulation.
2. **Shear Stress and Hypoxia**: Increased shear stress, often due to elevated blood flow, upregulates endothelin production. Hypoxia, a condition of low oxygen levels, also stimulates endothelin synthesis, particularly in the lungs and heart.

3. **Hormonal Regulation**: Hormones such as angiotensin II and vasopressin can increase endothelin production. Conversely, nitric oxide (NO) and prostacyclin inhibit endothelin synthesis, creating a balance in vascular tone regulation.
4. **Inflammatory Cytokines**: Pro-inflammatory cytokines, such as interleukin-1 (IL-1) and tumor necrosis factor-alpha (TNF-alpha), can stimulate endothelin production, linking inflammation to vascular dysfunction.

Plant-Based Diet and Endothelin Regulation

A plant-based diet can influence endothelin levels through various mechanisms, potentially contributing to improved cardiovascular health and reduced risk of related diseases.

1. **Antioxidants**: Plant-based diets are rich in antioxidants, such as vitamins C and E, flavonoids, and polyphenols, which can reduce oxidative stress and inflammation. Lower oxidative stress levels are associated with decreased endothelin production.
2. **Nitric Oxide Production**: Many plant foods, especially leafy greens and beets, are high in nitrates, which are converted to nitric oxide in the body. Nitric oxide is a potent vasodilator that inhibits endothelin synthesis, promoting vascular health.
3. **Anti-Inflammatory Properties**: Fruits, vegetables, nuts, and seeds have anti-inflammatory properties due to their high content of phytochemicals and fiber. Reducing inflammation can decrease endothelin levels, mitigating its pathological effects.
4. **Magnesium and Potassium**: Plant-based diets are typically high in magnesium and potassium, minerals that contribute to vascular health. Magnesium acts as a natural calcium channel blocker, reducing vascular resistance and endothelin levels.
5. **Omega-3 Fatty Acids**: Omega-3 fatty acids, found in flaxseeds, chia seeds, and walnuts, have anti-inflammatory effects and

can modulate endothelin production. They enhance endothelial function and reduce the risk of cardiovascular diseases.

Plant-Based Diet on Endothelin-Related Health Outcomes

1. **Cardiovascular Health**: A plant-based diet can improve cardiovascular health by reducing endothelin levels and enhancing endothelial function. This diet lowers blood pressure, decreases arterial stiffness, and reduces the risk of atherosclerosis.
2. **Renal Function**: By reducing inflammation and oxidative stress, a plant-based diet supports kidney health and can mitigate the progression of chronic kidney disease. Lower endothelin levels contribute to improved renal function and reduced proteinuria.
3. **Pulmonary Health**: In conditions like pulmonary hypertension, a plant-based diet's anti-inflammatory and antioxidant properties can help reduce endothelin-mediated vasoconstriction, improving overall lung function and oxygenation.
4. **Neurological Health**: A diet rich in antioxidants and anti-inflammatory compounds can protect against endothelin-related neurovascular disorders. This may include conditions such as stroke and dementia, where endothelin levels are elevated.
5. **Cancer Prevention**: Given endothelin's role in cell proliferation, a plant-based diet's ability to modulate endothelin production may help reduce the risk of certain cancers. High-fiber diets, in particular, have been associated with lower endothelin levels and reduced cancer risk.

Endothelin plays a critical role in vascular homeostasis and various other physiological processes. Its production and regulation are influenced by factors such as oxidative stress, inflammation, hormonal signals, and dietary components.

Neuropeptide Y (NPY)

Neuropeptide Y (NPY) is a 36-amino acid peptide neurotransmitter, one of the most abundant and widely distributed peptides in the central and peripheral nervous systems. NPY plays a crucial role in regulating various physiological processes, including appetite control, energy homeostasis, circadian rhythms, and stress response.

Function of Neuropeptide Y

NPY exerts its effects through interactions with a family of G-protein-coupled receptors (Y1, Y2, Y4, Y5, and Y6 in humans). The functions of NPY are diverse and include:

1. Appetite Regulation

NPY is a potent stimulator of food intake and is involved in the regulation of hunger and satiety. It acts primarily in the hypothalamus, where it stimulates feeding behavior by:

- **Increasing Appetite:** NPY promotes the sensation of hunger by activating NPY receptors in the hypothalamus, leading to increased food intake.
- **Modulating Satiety Signals:** NPY counteracts the effects of anorexigenic (appetite-suppressing) peptides such as leptin and insulin, thereby enhancing feeding behavior.

2. Energy Homeostasis

NPY plays a vital role in maintaining energy balance by influencing metabolic processes:

- **Fat Storage:** NPY promotes the accumulation of fat in adipose tissues by increasing lipogenesis (fat synthesis) and reducing lipolysis (fat breakdown).
- **Energy Expenditure:** NPY decreases energy expenditure by reducing thermogenesis (heat production) in brown adipose tissue.

3. Stress Response

NPY is involved in the body's response to stress:

- **Stress Resilience:** NPY is released during stressful situations and acts to buffer the stress response, reducing anxiety and promoting calmness.
- **Stress-Induced Eating:** NPY levels increase under stress, leading to stress-induced eating behaviors and potentially contributing to obesity.

4. Circadian Rhythms

NPY influences circadian rhythms, which are the body's natural cycles of sleep and wakefulness:

- **Synchronization of Biological Clocks:** NPY helps synchronize the circadian clocks in peripheral tissues with the central circadian pacemaker in the hypothalamus.

5. Cardiovascular Function

NPY has various effects on the cardiovascular system:

- **Blood Pressure Regulation:** NPY can cause vasoconstriction (narrowing of blood vessels), leading to increased blood pressure.
- **Heart Rate Modulation:** NPY can influence heart rate and cardiac output.

Production of Neuropeptide Y

The production of NPY involves multiple steps, primarily occurring in the nervous system:

1. Synthesis

NPY is synthesized in neurons located in the central and peripheral nervous systems. The NPY gene is located on chromosome 7 in humans, and its expression is regulated by various factors, including nutritional status and stress.

2. Regulation by the Hypothalamus

The hypothalamus plays a central role in regulating NPY production:

- **Hypothalamic Neurons:** NPY is produced by neurons in the arcuate nucleus of the hypothalamus, a critical area for appetite and energy balance regulation.
- **Influence of Leptin and Insulin:** Leptin and insulin, hormones involved in energy homeostasis, inhibit NPY production, thereby reducing hunger and food intake.

3. Circadian Influence

The production and release of NPY are influenced by circadian rhythms, with peak levels occurring during the dark phase in nocturnal animals and during the light phase in diurnal animals.

Regulation of Neuropeptide Y

The regulation of NPY involves complex feedback mechanisms and external factors:

1. Feedback Loops

NPY levels are regulated through negative feedback loops:

- **Inhibition by Leptin and Insulin:** High levels of leptin and insulin inhibit NPY production, reducing appetite and food intake.

- **Activation by Ghrelin:** Ghrelin, the "hunger hormone," stimulates NPY production, increasing hunger and food intake.

2. Nutritional Status
Nutritional status has a significant impact on NPY levels:

- **Fasting and Caloric Restriction:** Fasting and caloric restriction increase NPY levels, promoting hunger and food-seeking behavior.
- **Obesity and Overeating:** Obesity and overconsumption of high-calorie foods can lead to dysregulation of NPY, contributing to further weight gain.

3. Stress and Circadian Rhythms
Stress and circadian rhythms also influence NPY regulation:

- **Stress-Induced NPY Release:** Acute and chronic stress increase NPY release, which can lead to stress-induced eating and metabolic changes.
- **Circadian Modulation:** Circadian rhythms regulate the timing of NPY production, influencing feeding behavior and metabolic processes.

Plant-Based Diet and Neuropeptide Y Regulation

A plant-based diet, rich in fruits, vegetables, whole grains, nuts, and seeds, can significantly impact NPY regulation through various mechanisms:

1. Nutrient Density

Plant-based diets are typically high in essential nutrients, vitamins, and minerals that support overall health and hormonal balance:

- **Micronutrients:** Nutrients such as magnesium, found in leafy greens and nuts, are crucial for proper nervous system function and may influence NPY production.

2. Antioxidants

Fruits and vegetables are rich in antioxidants, which help reduce oxidative stress:

- **Oxidative Stress Reduction:** Lower oxidative stress levels are associated with improved NPY regulation and reduced stress-induced NPY release.

3. Fiber

High-fiber diets, common in plant-based eating, support gut health and hormonal regulation:

- **Gut-Brain Axis:** A healthy gut microbiome can influence NPY levels through the production of short-chain fatty acids and other metabolites.

4. Healthy Fats

Plant-based sources of fats, such as avocados, nuts, and seeds, provide essential fatty acids that support hormone production and regulation:

- **Omega-3 Fatty Acids:** Omega-3 fatty acids have anti-inflammatory properties that can enhance NPY activity and reduce stress-induced NPY release.

5. Glycemic Control

Plant-based diets, which are low in refined sugars and high in complex carbohydrates, help maintain stable blood glucose levels:

- **Blood Glucose Stability:** Stable blood glucose levels prevent hyperglycemia-induced suppression of NPY secretion, supporting balanced energy homeostasis.

6. Caloric Balance

Maintaining a healthy weight through a balanced plant-based diet can prevent obesity-related dysregulation of NPY:

- **Weight Management:** Excess body fat is linked to altered NPY levels due to increased production of leptin and insulin resistance.

Plant-Based Diet on Neuropeptide Y-Related Health Outcomes

1. Appetite and Weight Management

A plant-based diet can support healthy appetite regulation and weight management:

- **Satiety:** High-fiber foods increase satiety, reducing overall calorie intake and helping to regulate NPY levels.
- **Healthy Weight:** Maintaining a healthy weight through a plant-based diet reduces the risk of NPY dysregulation associated with obesity.

2. Stress Reduction

Plant-based diets can help reduce stress and its impact on NPY levels:

- **Nutrient-Rich Foods:** Foods rich in vitamins and minerals, such as leafy greens and nuts, support the nervous system and reduce stress-induced NPY release.
- **Antioxidant Intake:** High intake of antioxidants from fruits and vegetables can mitigate the effects of oxidative stress on NPY regulation.

3. Metabolic Health

A plant-based diet can improve metabolic health by influencing NPY and related pathways:

- **Improved Insulin Sensitivity:** Stable blood glucose levels and improved insulin sensitivity reduce the risk of NPY dysregulation.
- **Reduced Inflammation:** Anti-inflammatory properties of plant-based foods support overall metabolic health and NPY regulation.

4. Cardiovascular Health

Plant-based diets can benefit cardiovascular health through the regulation of NPY:

- **Blood Pressure Control:** Reduced intake of saturated fats and increased consumption of heart-healthy nutrients can mitigate the vasoconstrictive effects of NPY on blood vessels.
- **Cholesterol Management:** Plant-based diets are typically lower in cholesterol and can support overall cardiovascular health, reducing the risk of NPY-related cardiovascular issues.

Neuropeptide Y plays a pivotal role in regulating appetite, energy homeostasis, stress response, and circadian rhythms. Its production and regulation are influenced by various factors, including nutritional status, stress, and circadian rhythms.

Substance P (SP)

Substance P (SP) is a neuropeptide that plays a critical role in the transmission of pain, mood regulation, and various physiological functions. Its influence extends from the nervous system to the immune and cardiovascular systems.

Function of Substance P

Substance P serves several key functions within the body, primarily involving the nervous system but also impacting other systems:

1. **Pain Transmission**: Substance P is a key player in the transmission of pain signals from peripheral receptors to the central nervous system. It is released from sensory nerves and contributes to the sensation of pain by binding to the neurokinin-1 (NK1) receptor, facilitating the communication of pain signals.
2. **Inflammation**: Substance P has pro-inflammatory properties, contributing to the inflammatory response by promoting the release of cytokines and other inflammatory mediators. It is involved in the process of neurogenic inflammation, where nerve endings release neuropeptides to mediate inflammation.
3. **Mood Regulation**: Substance P influences mood and emotional regulation. It has been implicated in conditions such as depression and anxiety, where altered levels of SP and its receptor have been observed.
4. **Cardiovascular Effects**: Substance P affects cardiovascular functions, including vasodilation and blood pressure regulation. It can cause the release of nitric oxide (NO) from endothelial cells, leading to vasodilation and improved blood flow.
5. **Gastrointestinal Function**: SP is involved in regulating gastrointestinal motility and secretion. It stimulates smooth muscle contraction and glandular secretion in the gastrointestinal tract.
6. **Immune System**: SP modulates immune responses by influencing the activity of various immune cells, including macrophages,

mast cells, and T cells. It can enhance or suppress immune functions depending on the context.

Production of Substance P

Substance P is produced in several tissues, with a predominant synthesis in the nervous system:

1. **Synthesis**: SP is synthesized from its precursor, preprotachykinin A (PPT-A), which undergoes post-translational modifications to produce the active peptide. The gene encoding PPT-A is located on chromosome 7 in humans.
2. **Neurons**: SP is primarily produced by sensory neurons in the dorsal root ganglia and other parts of the nervous system. It is stored in large dense-core vesicles and released upon stimulation.
3. **Peripheral Tissues**: In addition to the nervous system, SP is also produced in peripheral tissues, including the gastrointestinal tract, respiratory system, and immune cells.
4. **Release Mechanism**: SP is released from nerve endings in response to various stimuli, such as noxious stimuli, stress, and inflammatory signals. The release process involves the influx of calcium ions and the fusion of vesicles with the cell membrane.

Regulation of Substance P

The regulation of SP is a complex process involving multiple factors and feedback mechanisms:

1. **Receptor-Mediated Feedback**: SP exerts its effects through the NK1 receptor. The binding of SP to NK1 can initiate a feedback mechanism that regulates SP release and synthesis. Prolonged stimulation can lead to receptor desensitization and internalization, modulating SP's effects.

2. **Enzymatic Degradation**: SP is degraded by several enzymes, including neutral endopeptidase (NEP) and angiotensin-converting enzyme (ACE). These enzymes cleave SP into inactive fragments, terminating its activity.
3. **Neural Regulation**: Neural pathways and neurotransmitters, such as glutamate and GABA, influence SP release and synthesis. For example, excitatory neurotransmitters like glutamate can enhance SP release, while inhibitory neurotransmitters like GABA can suppress it.
4. **Inflammatory Mediators**: Pro-inflammatory cytokines, such as interleukin-1 (IL-1) and tumor necrosis factor-alpha (TNF-α), can upregulate SP synthesis and release. This regulation is part of the neuro-immune interaction during inflammation.
5. **Hormonal Influence**: Hormones such as cortisol and adrenaline can modulate SP levels. Stress-induced hormonal changes can lead to increased SP release, contributing to stress-related symptoms.

Plant-Based Diet and Substance P Regulation

A plant-based diet, rich in fruits, vegetables, whole grains, nuts, and seeds, can impact the regulation of Substance P through various mechanisms:

1. **Anti-Inflammatory Properties**: Plant-based diets are rich in anti-inflammatory compounds, such as polyphenols and flavonoids, found in fruits and vegetables. These compounds can reduce the levels of pro-inflammatory cytokines that upregulate SP, thereby modulating its inflammatory effects.
2. **Antioxidants**: High antioxidant content in plant-based foods helps reduce oxidative stress, which can otherwise enhance SP release. Lower oxidative stress is associated with better regulation of SP and overall neural health.

3. **Omega-3 Fatty Acids**: Plant sources of omega-3 fatty acids, such as flaxseeds, chia seeds, and walnuts, have anti-inflammatory effects that can modulate SP activity. Omega-3 fatty acids help in maintaining the balance of pro- and anti-inflammatory mediators.
4. **Amino Acids**: Certain amino acids, like tryptophan, found in plant foods like legumes and seeds, can influence SP synthesis. Tryptophan is a precursor to serotonin, which can interact with SP pathways and influence mood and pain perception.
5. **Fiber**: High-fiber diets support gut health and the production of short-chain fatty acids (SCFAs) by the gut microbiota. SCFAs have been shown to have anti-inflammatory properties that can impact SP regulation indirectly.
6. **Phytochemicals**: Various phytochemicals found in plant-based foods can influence SP pathways. For instance, capsaicin, found in chili peppers, can deplete SP from sensory neurons, reducing pain transmission.

Plant-Based Diet on Substance P-Related Health Outcomes

1. **Pain Management**: A plant-based diet can aid in managing chronic pain conditions by reducing inflammation and oxidative stress, both of which are linked to elevated SP levels. Foods rich in anti-inflammatory compounds, such as turmeric, ginger, and berries, can help modulate pain signals mediated by SP.
2. **Mental Health**: By influencing serotonin levels and reducing inflammation, a plant-based diet can improve mental health outcomes. Studies have shown that diets high in fruits, vegetables, and whole grains are associated with lower rates of depression and anxiety, conditions linked to altered SP levels.
3. **Cardiovascular Health**: Plant-based diets support cardiovascular health by promoting vasodilation and reducing inflammation.

The intake of antioxidants and omega-3 fatty acids can help maintain healthy blood vessels and modulate SP's cardiovascular effects.

4. **Gastrointestinal Health**: High-fiber plant-based diets promote gut health and regular bowel movements. The anti-inflammatory properties of plant foods can also reduce gastrointestinal inflammation, potentially influenced by SP.
5. **Immune Function**: Plant-based diets enhance immune function through their high content of vitamins, minerals, and phytochemicals. By modulating inflammatory pathways and supporting a healthy gut microbiome, these diets can influence SP-related immune responses.

Substance P is a multifaceted neuropeptide with significant roles in pain transmission, inflammation, mood regulation, and various physiological functions. Its production and regulation are influenced by a complex interplay of neural, hormonal, and inflammatory signals.

Vasopressin

Vasopressin, also known as antidiuretic hormone (ADH), is a peptide hormone crucial for maintaining water balance, blood pressure, and overall homeostasis.

Function of Vasopressin

Vasopressin's primary functions include regulating water retention in the kidneys, maintaining blood pressure, and managing blood volume. It achieves these functions through the following mechanisms:

1. Water Retention

Vasopressin promotes water reabsorption in the kidneys by acting on the collecting ducts. It binds to V2 receptors on the cells of the collecting ducts, leading to the insertion of aquaporin-2 channels into the cell membranes. This process increases water permeability, allowing more water to be reabsorbed back into the bloodstream, thus concentrating the urine and reducing water excretion.

2. Blood Pressure Regulation

Vasopressin contributes to blood pressure regulation by inducing vasoconstriction, which is the narrowing of blood vessels. It binds to V1 receptors on the smooth muscle cells of blood vessels, causing them to contract. This vasoconstriction increases peripheral resistance, thereby raising blood pressure.

3. Blood Volume Management

By regulating water reabsorption and vascular tone, vasopressin helps maintain adequate blood volume. Proper blood volume is essential for ensuring efficient circulation and oxygen delivery to tissues, as well as for maintaining stable blood pressure levels.

4. Social and Behavioral Functions

Recent research has indicated that vasopressin also plays a role in social behaviors, including bonding, aggression, and social communication. Its effects on the brain's neural circuits influence these complex behaviors, although this aspect is less understood compared to its physiological functions.

Production of Vasopressin

Vasopressin is produced by the hypothalamus, a region of the brain that regulates various physiological processes. The production process involves several steps:

1. Synthesis

Vasopressin is synthesized in the hypothalamus's supraoptic and paraventricular nuclei. The precursor molecule, preprovasopressin, is first synthesized and then processed into the active hormone, vasopressin.

2. Transport

Once synthesized, vasopressin is transported along the axons of the hypothalamic neurons to the posterior pituitary gland. It is stored in the nerve endings of the posterior pituitary until it is needed.

3. Release

Vasopressin is released into the bloodstream in response to specific stimuli, such as increased plasma osmolality (a measure of the concentration of solutes in the blood) and decreased blood volume or pressure. These stimuli are detected by osmoreceptors and baroreceptors, respectively, which signal the hypothalamus to release vasopressin.

4. Regulation by Feedback Mechanisms

The release of vasopressin is tightly regulated by feedback mechanisms to maintain homeostasis. For example, when plasma osmolality decreases (indicating sufficient water intake), vasopressin release is inhibited to prevent excessive water retention.

Regulation of Vasopressin

The regulation of vasopressin involves a complex interplay of various factors, including osmotic and non-osmotic stimuli, feedback loops, and hormonal interactions. Key regulatory mechanisms include:

1. Osmotic Regulation

Plasma osmolality is the primary regulator of vasopressin release. Osmoreceptors in the hypothalamus detect changes in plasma osmolality and signal the release or inhibition of vasopressin accordingly. Increased plasma osmolality (hypertonicity) stimulates vasopressin release to promote water reabsorption and dilute the blood. Conversely, decreased plasma osmolality (hypotonicity) inhibits vasopressin release.

2. Non-Osmotic Regulation

Non-osmotic factors, such as blood volume and pressure, also influence vasopressin release. Baroreceptors in the cardiovascular system detect changes in blood volume and pressure. A decrease in blood volume or pressure stimulates vasopressin release to promote water retention and vasoconstriction, thereby restoring normal blood volume and pressure.

3. Feedback Loops

Vasopressin release is modulated by feedback loops involving other hormones and physiological states. For example, high levels of cortisol (a stress hormone) can inhibit vasopressin release, while angiotensin II (a hormone involved in blood pressure regulation) can stimulate vasopressin release.

4. Circadian Rhythm

Vasopressin secretion follows a circadian rhythm, with higher levels at night to promote water retention and prevent dehydration during sleep. This rhythm is regulated by the body's internal clock, located in the suprachiasmatic nucleus of the hypothalamus.

5. Influence of Diet and Lifestyle

Dietary and lifestyle factors can also affect vasopressin regulation. For instance, a high-salt diet can increase plasma osmolality and stimulate vasopressin release. Conversely, a diet rich in fruits, vegetables, and whole grains (characteristic of a plant-based diet) can help maintain proper fluid balance and support vasopressin regulation.

Plant-Based Diet and Vasopressin Regulation

A plant-based diet, rich in fruits, vegetables, whole grains, nuts, and seeds, can significantly impact vasopressin regulation through various mechanisms:

1. Hydration Status

Plant-based diets typically include a high intake of fruits and vegetables, which have high water content. This natural hydration helps maintain proper plasma osmolality, reducing the need for vasopressin release to retain water. Adequate hydration from these foods supports optimal kidney function and overall fluid balance.

2. Electrolyte Balance

Fruits and vegetables provide essential electrolytes, such as potassium and magnesium, which play crucial roles in maintaining fluid and electrolyte balance. Proper electrolyte balance helps regulate plasma osmolality and supports vasopressin's role in water retention and blood pressure regulation.

3. Antioxidants and Anti-Inflammatory Compounds

Plant-based foods are rich in antioxidants and anti-inflammatory compounds, which can help reduce oxidative stress and inflammation. Lower levels of oxidative stress and inflammation contribute to overall hormonal balance, including the regulation of vasopressin.

4. Fiber and Gut Health

High-fiber diets, common in plant-based eating, support gut health and can influence hormone regulation. A healthy gut microbiome can produce short-chain fatty acids and other metabolites that impact vasopressin levels and fluid balance.

5. Blood Pressure Management

A plant-based diet is effective in managing blood pressure due to its low sodium and high potassium content. Lower blood pressure reduces the need for vasopressin-induced vasoconstriction, promoting a balanced vasopressin release.

6. Weight Management

Maintaining a healthy weight through a balanced plant-based diet can prevent obesity-related disturbances in vasopressin regulation. Excess body fat, particularly visceral fat, can affect hormone levels and increase the risk of hypertension and other metabolic disorders.

7. Glycemic Control

Plant-based diets, which are low in refined sugars and high in complex carbohydrates, help maintain stable blood glucose levels. Stable blood glucose prevents hyperglycemia-induced suppression of vasopressin secretion, supporting its regulatory functions.

Plant-Based Diet on Vasopressin-Related Health Outcomes

1. Kidney Health

A plant-based diet supports kidney health by promoting proper hydration, electrolyte balance, and reduced oxidative stress. By maintaining optimal vasopressin levels, this diet can help prevent conditions like kidney stones and chronic kidney disease.

2. Cardiovascular Health

The vasoconstrictive effects of vasopressin are balanced by the blood pressure-lowering benefits of a plant-based diet. This dietary approach can reduce the risk of hypertension and related cardiovascular diseases, supporting overall cardiovascular health.

3. Hydration and Fluid Balance

Proper hydration from plant-based foods helps regulate plasma osmolality and reduces the need for excessive vasopressin release. This balance supports overall fluid homeostasis and prevents dehydration-related issues.

4. Weight Management

A plant-based diet is effective for weight management, reducing body fat, and improving insulin sensitivity. Lower body fat and better glycemic control enhance vasopressin regulation and overall metabolic health.

5. Mental Health

Emerging evidence suggests that plant-based diets may benefit mental health by reducing inflammation and oxidative stress, which are linked to mood disorders. Improved vasopressin levels also support cognitive function and emotional well-being.

6. Bone Health

While vasopressin primarily regulates water balance, its overall impact on hormonal balance can influence bone health. A plant-based diet rich in calcium, magnesium, and vitamin K supports bone health and can help prevent osteoporosis.

7. Anti-Aging Effects

The antioxidant-rich nature of plant-based diets helps combat oxidative stress, a key factor in aging. Improved vasopressin levels, coupled with reduced oxidative damage, contribute to healthier aging and better maintenance of lean body mass.

8. Gut Health

High-fiber diets, common in plant-based eating, support gut health and hormone regulation. A healthy gut microbiome can influence vasopressin levels through the production of short-chain fatty acids and other metabolites.

9. Metabolic Health

A plant-based diet can improve overall metabolic health by supporting proper hormone regulation, including vasopressin. This dietary approach can help prevent and manage metabolic disorders such as diabetes and obesity.

Vasopressin plays a pivotal role in maintaining water balance, blood pressure, and overall homeostasis throughout life. Its production and regulation are influenced by various factors, including osmotic and non-osmotic stimuli, feedback mechanisms, and dietary influences.

Corticotropin-Releasing Hormone (CRH)

Corticotropin-Releasing Hormone (CRH), also known as corticotropin-releasing factor (CRF), is a critical peptide hormone involved in the stress response. Its impact spans from regulating the hypothalamic-pituitary-adrenal (HPA) axis to influencing various physiological and behavioral processes.

Function of Corticotropin-Releasing Hormone

CRH's primary function is to regulate the stress response by controlling the release of adrenocorticotropic hormone (ACTH) from the pituitary gland. It achieves this by:

1. **Stress Response**: CRH is pivotal in the body's response to stress. When a stressor is perceived, CRH is released from the hypothalamus, triggering a cascade of events that lead to the secretion of glucocorticoids (such as cortisol) from the adrenal glands. These hormones help mobilize energy, suppress the immune system, and prepare the body to cope with stress.
2. **HPA Axis Regulation**: CRH is the central regulator of the HPA axis. It stimulates the synthesis and release of ACTH from the anterior pituitary gland. ACTH then prompts the adrenal cortex to produce cortisol, which helps the body manage stress.
3. **Behavioral Effects**: CRH influences behavior and mood. Elevated CRH levels are associated with anxiety and depression-like behaviors. It affects neurotransmitter systems, including serotonin and norepinephrine, which are crucial for mood regulation.
4. **Immune Modulation**: CRH plays a role in modulating the immune response. It can have pro-inflammatory or anti-inflammatory effects depending on the context and the presence of glucocorticoids. CRH receptors are present in immune cells, influencing their activity.
5. **Autonomic Nervous System Activation**: CRH contributes to the activation of the sympathetic nervous system, leading to increased heart rate, blood pressure, and energy mobilization during stress.

Production of Corticotropin-Releasing Hormone

CRH is produced by the hypothalamus, a small region of the brain responsible for maintaining homeostasis. The production process involves several steps:

1. **Synthesis**: CRH is synthesized in the paraventricular nucleus (PVN) of the hypothalamus. The gene responsible for CRH production is located on chromosome 8 in humans.
2. **Release**: In response to stress, CRH is released from the hypothalamic neurons into the hypophyseal portal system, a network of blood vessels connecting the hypothalamus to the anterior pituitary gland.
3. **ACTH Stimulation**: Upon reaching the anterior pituitary, CRH binds to its receptors on corticotroph cells, stimulating the production and release of ACTH into the bloodstream.
4. **Circadian Rhythm**: The production and release of CRH follow a circadian rhythm, with levels peaking in the early morning and declining throughout the day. This rhythm aligns with the body's natural sleep-wake cycle and cortisol production patterns.

Regulation of Corticotropin-Releasing Hormone

The regulation of CRH is a complex process involving feedback mechanisms and external factors:

1. **Feedback Loops**: CRH is regulated by negative feedback loops involving cortisol. High levels of cortisol inhibit the release of CRH from the hypothalamus and ACTH from the pituitary gland, thus reducing cortisol production.
2. **Stressors**: Physical and psychological stressors, such as injury, infection, or emotional distress, stimulate CRH release. The body's

response to these stressors involves increased CRH production to activate the HPA axis.

3. **Neurotransmitters**: Several neurotransmitters, including norepinephrine and serotonin, influence CRH production. For example, norepinephrine from the locus coeruleus can enhance CRH release, while serotonin may have inhibitory effects.
4. **Cytokines**: Pro-inflammatory cytokines, such as interleukin-1 (IL-1) and tumor necrosis factor-alpha (TNF-α), can stimulate CRH production. This links the immune response to the activation of the HPA axis during inflammation.
5. **Nutrition**: Diet and nutritional status can influence CRH levels. For instance, hypoglycemia (low blood glucose levels) can trigger CRH release to mobilize energy stores.

Plant-Based Diet and Corticotropin-Releasing Hormone Regulation

A plant-based diet, rich in fruits, vegetables, whole grains, nuts, and seeds, can impact CRH regulation through various mechanisms:

1. **Nutrient Density**: Plant-based diets are typically high in essential nutrients, vitamins, and minerals that support overall health and hormonal balance. For example, magnesium, found in leafy greens and nuts, is crucial for regulating stress and CRH levels. Magnesium deficiency is associated with increased stress and CRH release.
2. **Antioxidants**: Fruits and vegetables are rich in antioxidants, which help reduce oxidative stress. Lower oxidative stress levels are associated with a balanced HPA axis and reduced CRH secretion (Packer, 1995). For example, foods high in vitamin C, such as citrus fruits and bell peppers, can help mitigate the effects of stress.

3. **Healthy Fats**: Plant-based sources of fats, such as avocados, nuts, and seeds, provide essential fatty acids that support hormone production and regulation. Omega-3 fatty acids, in particular, have anti-inflammatory properties that can modulate CRH activity.
4. **Fiber**: High-fiber diets, common in plant-based eating, support gut health and hormone regulation. A healthy gut microbiome can influence CRH levels through the gut-brain axis. Short-chain fatty acids produced by gut bacteria have been shown to affect stress responses and HPA axis activity.
5. **Phytochemicals**: Plant-based diets are rich in phytochemicals, such as flavonoids and polyphenols, which have been shown to have anti-stress and anti-inflammatory effects. For example, flavonoids found in berries and green tea can reduce CRH levels and improve stress resilience.
6. **Glycemic Control**: Plant-based diets, which are low in refined sugars and high in complex carbohydrates, help maintain stable blood glucose levels. Stable blood glucose levels prevent hypoglycemia-induced CRH release and reduce overall stress on the body.

Plant-Based Diet on CRH-Related Health Outcomes

1. **Mental Health**: A plant-based diet may benefit mental health by reducing inflammation and oxidative stress, which are linked to mood disorders. Lower CRH levels, resulting from a balanced diet, support better mood regulation and reduce the risk of anxiety and depression.
2. **Immune Function**: By modulating CRH levels and reducing chronic stress, a plant-based diet can support a balanced immune response. This reduces the risk of stress-related immune dysregulation and chronic inflammation.

3. **Sleep Quality**: Improved nutritional status and reduced stress levels from a plant-based diet can enhance sleep quality. Better sleep supports the natural circadian rhythm of CRH production, promoting overall hormonal balance and health.
4. **Weight Management**: Plant-based diets are effective for weight management, reducing body fat, and improving insulin sensitivity. Lower body fat and better glycemic control enhance overall metabolic health and reduce stress-induced CRH release.
5. **Cognitive Function**: The anti-inflammatory and antioxidant properties of plant-based diets support brain health and cognitive function. Lower CRH levels contribute to better cognitive performance and reduced risk of neurodegenerative diseases.

Corticotropin-Releasing Hormone (CRH) plays a pivotal role in the stress response, HPA axis regulation, behavior, immune modulation, and autonomic nervous system activation. Its production and regulation are influenced by various factors, including stressors, neurotransmitters, cytokines, and nutritional status.

15

Digestive Enzymes

Understanding Enzymes in the Human Body

Enzymes are biological catalysts that speed up chemical reactions in the body without being consumed in the process. They are crucial for various physiological processes, including digestion, metabolism, and cellular repair. Understanding enzymes involves exploring their structure, function, and the role they play in maintaining health and homeostasis.

The Nature and Structure of Enzymes

Enzymes are typically proteins, although some RNA molecules can also function as enzymes (ribozymes). The structure of an enzyme is vital for its function and consists of one or more polypeptide chains folded into a unique three-dimensional shape. This structure includes an active site, where substrates bind and undergo a chemical reaction. The specificity of enzymes to their substrates is often described by the "lock and key" model, where the enzyme (lock) is precisely shaped to fit the substrate (key). Alternatively, the "induced fit" model suggests that enzymes are flexible and adjust their shape to fit the substrate upon binding.

Enzyme Function and Mechanism

Enzymes accelerate reactions by lowering the activation energy required for the reaction to proceed. This is achieved through various mechanisms:

1. **Proximity and Orientation:** Enzymes bring substrates close together and in the correct orientation to facilitate the reaction.
2. **Microenvironment:** Enzymes provide an optimal environment, such as the correct pH and temperature, to enhance reaction rates.
3. **Strain Induction:** Enzymes can induce strain in substrate bonds, making them easier to break and thus lowering the activation energy.

Types of Enzymes and Their Functions

Enzymes are classified based on the types of reactions they catalyze. The major classes of enzymes include:

1. **Oxidoreductases:** Catalyze oxidation-reduction reactions. Example: Lactate dehydrogenase, which converts lactate to pyruvate.
2. **Transferases:** Transfer functional groups from one molecule to another. Example: Alanine transaminase, which transfers amino groups.
3. **Hydrolases:** Catalyze the hydrolysis of various bonds. Example: Amylase, which breaks down starch into sugars.
4. **Lyases:** Break bonds by means other than hydrolysis and oxidation. Example: Adenylate cyclase, which forms cyclic AMP.
5. **Isomerases:** Catalyze the rearrangement of atoms within a molecule. Example: Phosphoglucose isomerase, which converts glucose-6-phosphate to fructose-6-phosphate.
6. **Ligases:** Join two molecules together with covalent bonds. Example: DNA ligase, which joins DNA fragments during replication.

Enzyme Regulation

Enzyme activity is tightly regulated to maintain homeostasis and respond to changes in the environment. Regulation can occur through several mechanisms:

1. **Allosteric Regulation:** Enzymes have allosteric sites where regulatory molecules can bind, causing a change in the enzyme's activity. This can either activate or inhibit the enzyme.
2. **Covalent Modification:** Enzymes can be activated or deactivated by the addition or removal of chemical groups, such as phosphorylation.
3. **Feedback Inhibition:** The end product of a metabolic pathway can inhibit an enzyme involved early in the pathway, thus regulating the pathway's activity.
4. **Gene Expression:** The synthesis of enzymes can be regulated at the genetic level, affecting the amount of enzymes available.

Enzymes in Digestion

Digestion relies heavily on enzymes to break down food into absorbable nutrients. Key digestive enzymes include:

1. **Amylases:** Break down carbohydrates into simple sugars. Salivary amylase begins the process in the mouth, while pancreatic amylase continues in the small intestine.
2. **Proteases:** Break down proteins into amino acids. Pepsin in the stomach, and trypsin and chymotrypsin in the small intestine, are critical proteases.
3. **Lipases:** Break down fats into fatty acids and glycerol. Pancreatic lipase is essential for fat digestion in the small intestine.

Enzymes in Metabolism

Metabolic pathways are a series of chemical reactions within a cell, facilitated by enzymes. These pathways can be anabolic (building molecules) or catabolic (breaking down molecules). Enzymes in metabolism include:

1. **Glycolytic Enzymes:** Such as hexokinase and pyruvate kinase, are involved in glycolysis, the breakdown of glucose to pyruvate.
2. **Citric Acid Cycle Enzymes:** Such as citrate synthase and succinate dehydrogenase, facilitate the citric acid cycle (Krebs cycle) in energy production.
3. **Electron Transport Chain Enzymes:** Such as cytochrome c oxidase, which play a role in oxidative phosphorylation and ATP production.

Enzymes in DNA Replication and Repair

Enzymes are essential for the accurate replication and repair of DNA. Key enzymes include:

1. **DNA Polymerase:** Synthesizes new DNA strands by adding nucleotides to a pre-existing strand.
2. **Helicase:** Unwinds the DNA double helix, allowing replication to occur.
3. **Topoisomerase:** Prevents the over-winding of DNA ahead of the replication fork.
4. **DNA Ligase:** Joins Okazaki fragments on the lagging strand during DNA replication.
5. **Nucleases:** Remove damaged or mismatched DNA, allowing for repair.

Enzymes in Cellular Signaling

Enzymes play crucial roles in cellular signaling pathways, which regulate various cellular functions and responses to external stimuli. Important signaling enzymes include:

1. **Kinases:** Such as protein kinase A, adds phosphate groups to proteins, modifying their activity.
2. **Phosphatases:** Such as protein phosphatase 1, which removes phosphate groups from proteins, reversing the action of kinases.
3. **Cyclases:** Such as adenylate cyclase, which converts ATP to cyclic AMP, a second messenger in signal transduction.

Enzymes in Disease and Medicine

Enzyme malfunction can lead to various diseases. For example:

1. **Lysosomal Storage Disorders:** Caused by deficiencies in lysosomal enzymes, leading to the accumulation of undigested molecules. Example: Tay-Sachs disease, caused by a deficiency in hexosaminidase A.
2. **Metabolic Disorders:** Such as phenylketonuria (PKU), is caused by a deficiency in phenylalanine hydroxylase, leading to the accumulation of phenylalanine.
3. **Cancer:** Abnormal enzyme activity can lead to uncontrolled cell growth. For instance, mutations in enzymes involved in DNA repair can result in cancer.

Enzymes are also crucial in medicine, both as therapeutic agents and in diagnostics. For instance:

1. **Enzyme Replacement Therapy:** Used to treat diseases like Gaucher's disease by providing patients with the deficient enzyme.

2. **Enzymes in Diagnostics:** Enzymes like glucose oxidase are used in glucose meters to monitor blood sugar levels in diabetics.

Plant-Based Foods and Enzyme Activity

A plant-based diet can influence enzyme activity positively. Certain foods contain compounds that can enhance or inhibit enzyme activity:

1. **Bromelain:** Found in pineapples, it is a proteolytic enzyme that aids in protein digestion and has anti-inflammatory properties.
2. **Papain:** Found in papayas, it also aids in protein digestion and has been used in wound care.
3. **Quercetin:** A flavonoid found in many fruits and vegetables that can inhibit enzymes involved in inflammation and cancer progression.
4. **Sulforaphane:** Found in cruciferous vegetables, it can activate enzymes involved in detoxification and antioxidant defense.

Enzymes are indispensable to human health, driving the biochemical reactions necessary for life. Understanding their structure, function, and regulation is crucial for advancing medical science and developing therapies for enzyme-related diseases. A plant-based diet can support enzyme function, highlighting the interplay between diet and enzymatic activity. As research continues, the role of enzymes in health and disease will become even clearer, paving the way for novel treatments and preventive strategies.

Amylase

Amylase is a crucial enzyme in the human body, playing a vital role in the digestion of carbohydrates. This enzyme helps break down complex carbohydrates into simpler sugars, facilitating their absorption and utilization by the body. Understanding amylase's function, production, and regulation provides insights into how the human digestive system works and highlights the benefits of a plant-based diet in optimizing amylase activity and overall health.

Function of Amylase

Amylase is a type of hydrolase enzyme that catalyzes the hydrolysis of starch into sugars. There are two main types of amylase in the human body: alpha-amylase and beta-amylase.

Alpha-Amylase

Alpha-amylase (salivary and pancreatic amylase) is the primary form of amylase found in humans. It is secreted by the salivary glands and the pancreas. This enzyme acts on starches in the mouth and the small intestine, breaking them down into maltose and dextrin, which are further digested into glucose.

Salivary Amylase:

- **Function:** Salivary amylase begins the process of starch digestion in the mouth. It breaks down polysaccharides into smaller oligosaccharides.
- **Optimal pH:** The optimal pH for salivary amylase activity is around 6.7 to 7.0, which corresponds to the pH of the oral cavity.

Pancreatic Amylase:

- **Function:** Pancreatic amylase continues the digestion of starches in the small intestine. It breaks down the oligosaccharides into disaccharides like maltose and isomaltose, which are further broken down into glucose by other enzymes.

- **Optimal pH**: The optimal pH for pancreatic amylase activity is around 7.0 to 8.0, matching the slightly alkaline environment of the small intestine.

Beta-Amylase

Beta-amylase is less prevalent in humans but is significant in the plant kingdom. It acts on the non-reducing end of starch chains to produce maltose. Although humans primarily rely on alpha-amylase, beta-amylase is found in certain plant-based foods and supplements.

Production of Amylase

The production of amylase is a well-coordinated process involving the salivary glands and the pancreas.

Salivary Glands

The salivary glands (parotid, submandibular, and sublingual) produce salivary amylase. This process is stimulated by the presence of food in the mouth and the act of chewing, which signals the autonomic nervous system to secrete saliva.

1. **Parotid Glands**: These are the largest salivary glands and produce a significant amount of amylase-rich saliva.
2. **Submandibular and Sublingual Glands**: These glands produce a mixture of serous (watery) and mucous saliva, contributing to the overall enzyme activity in the mouth.

Pancreas

The pancreas is the primary source of digestive enzymes, including pancreatic amylase. The production and secretion of pancreatic amylase are regulated by hormonal and neural mechanisms.

1. **Hormonal Regulation**: The hormone cholecystokinin (CCK) plays a crucial role in stimulating the pancreas to release digestive enzymes, including amylase.

2. **Neural Regulation**: The vagus nerve (cranial nerve X) also stimulates the secretion of pancreatic enzymes during the cephalic phase of digestion, which begins even before food enters the stomach.

Regulation of Amylase

The regulation of amylase involves multiple factors, including genetic, hormonal, and dietary influences.

Genetic Factors

Genetic variations can influence the production and activity of amylase. For example, individuals with more copies of the AMY1 gene, which encodes for salivary amylase, tend to have higher salivary amylase levels. This genetic variability can affect carbohydrate digestion efficiency.

Hormonal Regulation

Hormones such as insulin and glucagon can modulate amylase production and secretion.

1. **Insulin**: Insulin, secreted by the pancreas in response to high blood glucose levels, can enhance the synthesis of pancreatic amylase.
2. **Glucagon**: Glucagon, released during low blood glucose levels, can have a modulatory effect on enzyme production.

Dietary Influences

Dietary habits significantly impact amylase production and activity.

1. **Carbohydrate Intake**: A diet rich in carbohydrates can stimulate increased production of amylase to facilitate efficient digestion. Conversely, low carbohydrate intake might reduce amylase levels.
2. **Plant-Based Diet**: A plant-based diet, which typically includes high amounts of complex carbohydrates, can promote optimal

amylase activity. Foods such as whole grains, fruits, and vegetables provide substrates that amylase can act upon, enhancing its production and efficiency.

Plant-Based Foods that Enhance Amylase Activity

Several plant-based foods have been shown to enhance amylase activity and overall digestive health.

Whole Grains

Whole grains like oats, barley, and brown rice are excellent sources of complex carbohydrates. These foods provide a steady supply of starch, stimulating amylase production and activity.

Fruits

Fruits such as apples, bananas, and mangoes contain natural sugars and fibers that support amylase activity. Bananas, in particular, have been shown to increase salivary amylase levels due to their high carbohydrate content.

Vegetables

Starchy vegetables like sweet potatoes, corn, and peas are rich in carbohydrates, promoting the production of amylase. These vegetables also provide essential nutrients that support overall digestive health.

The Role of Fiber in Amylase Regulation

Dietary fiber, found abundantly in plant-based foods, plays a crucial role in regulating amylase activity and promoting digestive health.

Soluble Fiber

Soluble fiber, found in foods like oats, legumes, and fruits, can slow down the digestion of carbohydrates, providing a sustained release of glucose. This steady supply of carbohydrates ensures continuous amylase activity.

Insoluble Fiber

Insoluble fiber, present in whole grains, vegetables, and seeds, adds bulk to the stool and promotes regular bowel movements. While it does not directly affect amylase, it supports overall digestive health, indirectly aiding enzyme function.

Benefits of a Plant-Based Diet on Amylase Activity and Digestive Health

A plant-based diet offers numerous benefits for amylase activity and overall digestive health.

Enhanced Enzyme Production

Plant-based diets are typically rich in complex carbohydrates, which stimulate the production and activity of amylase. This enhanced enzyme activity leads to more efficient digestion and absorption of nutrients.

Improved Gut Health

A diet high in fiber supports a healthy gut microbiome, which is essential for optimal digestive enzyme activity. A balanced gut microbiome can enhance the efficiency of amylase and other digestive enzymes.

Regulation of Blood Glucose Levels

Efficient carbohydrate digestion by amylase ensures a steady release of glucose into the bloodstream, preventing spikes and crashes in blood sugar levels. This regulation is particularly beneficial for individuals with diabetes or insulin resistance.

Amylase is a critical enzyme in the human digestive system, essential for breaking down complex carbohydrates into simple sugars. Its production and activity are influenced by genetic, hormonal, and dietary factors. A plant-based diet, rich in whole grains, fruits, and vegetables, supports optimal amylase activity and overall digestive health.

Pepsin

Pepsin is a vital enzyme in the human body, playing a critical role in the digestion of proteins. This enzyme helps break down proteins into smaller peptides, facilitating their absorption and utilization by the body.

Function of Pepsin

Pepsin is a proteolytic enzyme, meaning it breaks down proteins into peptides. It is one of the main digestive enzymes in the stomach and is particularly effective in the acidic environment of the stomach.

Mechanism of Action

Pepsin catalyzes the hydrolysis of peptide bonds in proteins. It preferentially cleaves bonds involving aromatic amino acids such as phenylalanine, tryptophan, and tyrosine. This enzymatic action results in the formation of smaller peptide fragments, which are further broken down into amino acids by other proteases in the small intestine.

Optimal Conditions for Pepsin Activity

Pepsin operates most effectively in the highly acidic environment of the stomach, with an optimal pH range of 1.5 to 3.5. The enzyme is inactive at higher pH levels, which is why it functions primarily in the stomach.

Production of Pepsin

Pepsin is produced in the stomach as an inactive precursor called pepsinogen, which is secreted by the chief cells in the gastric glands.

Activation of Pepsinogen

Pepsinogen is converted to active pepsin by the acidic environment of the stomach. Hydrochloric acid (HCl) secreted by the parietal cells lowers the stomach's pH, which facilitates the conversion of pepsinogen to pepsin. This process involves the cleavage of specific peptide bonds in pepsinogen, resulting in the active enzyme pepsin.

Regulation of Pepsin Production

The production and secretion of pepsinogen are regulated by neural and hormonal mechanisms.

1. **Neural Regulation:** The vagus nerve stimulates the secretion of gastric juices, including pepsinogen, in response to the sight, smell, and taste of food. This cephalic phase of digestion prepares the stomach for the arrival of food.
2. **Hormonal Regulation:** Gastrin, a hormone produced by the G cells in the stomach, stimulates the secretion of gastric acid and pepsinogen. The presence of proteins in the stomach stimulates the release of gastrin, enhancing pepsin production.

Regulation of Pepsin Activity

The activity of pepsin is tightly regulated by various factors, including genetic, hormonal, and dietary influences.

Genetic Factors

Genetic variations can influence the production and activity of pepsin. For example, certain genetic mutations may affect the structure of pepsinogen, altering its activation or stability. However, these variations are relatively rare and typically do not significantly impact overall pepsin function.

Hormonal Regulation

Hormones such as gastrin and secretin play crucial roles in regulating pepsin activity.

1. **Gastrin:** As mentioned earlier, gastrin stimulates the secretion of gastric acid and pepsinogen, enhancing pepsin activity. The presence of food in the stomach, particularly proteins, increases gastrin release, promoting pepsin production.
2. **Secretin:** Secretin, released by the duodenum in response to acidic chyme entering from the stomach, inhibits gastric acid secretion and pepsinogen production. This regulatory mechanism ensures that pepsin activity is confined to the stomach and does not extend into the small intestine, where a less acidic environment is required for other digestive enzymes to function optimally.

Dietary Influences

Dietary habits significantly impact pepsin production and activity.

1. **Protein Intake:** A diet high in protein can stimulate increased production of pepsin to facilitate efficient digestion. Conversely, a low protein intake might reduce pepsin levels, as the demand for protein digestion decreases.
2. **Plant-Based Diet:** A plant-based diet, which typically includes moderate amounts of protein from sources such as legumes, nuts, seeds, and whole grains, can promote balanced pepsin activity. The fiber content in plant-based foods also supports overall digestive health, indirectly aiding enzyme function.

Plant-Based Foods that Enhance Pepsin Activity

Several plant-based foods have been shown to support digestive health and potentially enhance pepsin activity.

Legumes

Legumes such as lentils, chickpeas, and black beans are excellent sources of plant-based protein. They provide the necessary substrates for pepsin activity, promoting efficient protein digestion.

Nuts and Seeds

Nuts and seeds, including almonds, chia seeds, and flaxseeds, are rich in protein and healthy fats. They offer a sustained release of nutrients that support pepsin production and overall digestive health.

Whole Grains

Whole grains like quinoa, brown rice, and oats are not only good sources of complex carbohydrates but also contain moderate amounts of protein. These foods provide a balanced diet that supports digestive enzyme activity, including pepsin.

Vegetables

Vegetables such as spinach, broccoli, and Brussels sprouts contain essential nutrients that support overall digestive health. While they are not high in protein, their fiber content helps maintain a healthy gut environment, promoting efficient enzyme activity.

Fermented Foods

Fermented foods like sauerkraut, kimchi, and tempeh contain beneficial probiotics that support gut health. A healthy gut microbiome can enhance the efficiency of digestive enzymes, including pepsin.

The Role of Fiber in Pepsin Regulation

Dietary fiber, found abundantly in plant-based foods, plays a crucial role in regulating pepsin activity and promoting digestive health.

Soluble Fiber

Soluble fiber, found in foods like oats, legumes, and fruits, can slow down the digestion of proteins, providing a sustained release of amino acids. This steady supply of nutrients ensures continuous pepsin activity and efficient protein digestion.

Insoluble Fiber

Insoluble fiber, present in whole grains, vegetables, and seeds, adds bulk to the stool and promotes regular bowel movements. While it does not directly affect pepsin, it supports overall digestive health, indirectly aiding enzyme function.

Benefits of a Plant-Based Diet on Pepsin Activity and Digestive Health

A plant-based diet offers numerous benefits for pepsin activity and overall digestive health.

Enhanced Enzyme Production

Plant-based diets are typically rich in fiber and moderate in protein, which stimulates the production and activity of pepsin. This balanced nutrient intake leads to more efficient digestion and absorption of proteins.

Improved Gut Health

A diet high in fiber supports a healthy gut microbiome, which is essential for optimal digestive enzyme activity. A balanced gut microbiome can enhance the efficiency of pepsin and other digestive enzymes.

Reduced Risk of Digestive Disorders

Plant-based diets are associated with a lower risk of digestive disorders such as gastroesophageal reflux disease (GERD) and peptic ulcers. The high fiber content and absence of animal fats in plant-based diets contribute to better digestive health and reduced inflammation in the gut.

Regulation of Stomach Acidity

Efficient protein digestion by pepsin ensures that the stomach's acidic environment is maintained at optimal levels. A balanced plant-based diet can help regulate stomach acidity, preventing conditions such as acid reflux and gastritis.

Trypsin

Trypsin is a critical enzyme in the digestive system, responsible for protein digestion in the small intestine.

Function of Trypsin

Trypsin plays an essential role in the digestive process by breaking down proteins into smaller peptides and amino acids, which can then be absorbed by the body.

1. **Protein Digestion:** Trypsin is an endopeptidase, meaning it cleaves peptide bonds within proteins. It specifically acts on peptide bonds involving the carboxyl groups of the amino acids lysine and arginine. This activity is crucial for converting large protein molecules into smaller peptides and free amino acids, facilitating their absorption in the intestines.
2. **Activation of Other Enzymes:** Trypsin also activates other digestive enzymes. For instance, it converts the inactive enzyme precursors chymotrypsinogen and procarboxypeptidase into their active forms, chymotrypsin and carboxypeptidase, respectively. This cascade effect enhances the overall efficiency of protein digestion.
3. **Regulation of Pancreatic Secretions:** By digesting pancreatic secretory trypsin inhibitor (PSTI), trypsin regulates its own activity and the activity of other pancreatic enzymes. This self-regulatory mechanism ensures a balanced and efficient digestive process.

Production of Trypsin

Trypsin is produced in the pancreas and activated in the small intestine through a well-orchestrated series of biochemical events.

1. **Synthesis in the Pancreas:** Trypsin is synthesized in the pancreas in an inactive form known as trypsinogen. This precautionary measure prevents the enzyme from digesting pancreatic tissues

and ensures that its proteolytic activity is confined to the intestine.

2. **Secretion into the Small Intestine:** Trypsinogen is secreted into the small intestine via the pancreatic duct. Upon reaching the duodenum, it encounters the enzyme enterokinase (also known as enteropeptidase), which is produced by the intestinal mucosa.
3. **Activation to Trypsin:** Enterokinase cleaves a specific peptide bond in trypsinogen, converting it into its active form, trypsin. This activation process is critical for the initiation of protein digestion in the small intestine.

Regulation of Trypsin

The regulation of trypsin involves multiple feedback mechanisms to ensure its activity is precisely controlled.

1. **Pancreatic Secretion Regulation:** The secretion of trypsinogen from the pancreas is regulated by hormonal signals, primarily cholecystokinin (CCK) and secretin. These hormones are released by the small intestine in response to the presence of food, stimulating the pancreas to release digestive enzymes.
2. **Trypsin Inhibitors:** The pancreas also produces trypsin inhibitors, such as PSTI, to prevent premature activation of trypsin within the pancreas. These inhibitors bind to trypsinogen and inactive trypsin, preventing them from causing damage to pancreatic tissues.
3. **Autoregulation:** Trypsin participates in its own regulation by degrading excess trypsinogen and trypsin inhibitors. This autoregulatory mechanism maintains an optimal balance of active trypsin in the digestive system.
4. **Dietary Influences:** Diet plays a significant role in regulating trypsin activity. A diet high in protein stimulates the production

and activation of trypsin to meet the increased demand for protein digestion.

Plant-Based Diet and Trypsin Regulation

A plant-based diet, rich in fruits, vegetables, whole grains, nuts, and seeds, can positively influence trypsin regulation and overall digestive health.

1. **Nutrient Density:** Plant-based diets provide a wealth of essential nutrients, vitamins, and minerals that support overall health and digestive enzyme activity. For instance, vitamin C, found abundantly in fruits and vegetables, is crucial for the maintenance of healthy pancreatic function and enzyme production.
2. **Fiber Content:** High-fiber diets, common in plant-based eating, support gut health and enzyme regulation. Dietary fiber promotes regular bowel movements and a healthy gut microbiome, both of which are essential for efficient digestion and nutrient absorption.
3. **Antioxidants:** Fruits and vegetables are rich in antioxidants, which help reduce oxidative stress in the body. Lower oxidative stress levels are associated with improved pancreatic function and balanced enzyme activity, including trypsin.
4. **Healthy Fats:** Plant-based sources of fats, such as avocados, nuts, and seeds, provide essential fatty acids that support overall health. Omega-3 fatty acids, in particular, have anti-inflammatory properties that can enhance digestive enzyme function and reduce the risk of pancreatic inflammation.
5. **Protein Sources:** While plant-based diets may be lower in protein compared to animal-based diets, they still provide adequate protein through legumes, nuts, seeds, and whole grains. These plant-based proteins are often easier to digest and may require

less trypsin for complete digestion, reducing the burden on the pancreas.

Plant-Based Diet on Trypsin-Related Health Outcomes

1. **Digestive Health:** A plant-based diet supports healthy digestion by providing essential nutrients, fiber, and antioxidants. These components work synergistically to promote optimal enzyme function and gut health, reducing the risk of digestive disorders.
2. **Pancreatic Health:** The anti-inflammatory and antioxidant properties of plant-based foods help protect the pancreas from oxidative damage and inflammation. This protection supports healthy enzyme production and reduces the risk of pancreatitis and other pancreatic disorders.
3. **Weight Management:** Plant-based diets are effective for weight management, reducing body fat, and improving insulin sensitivity. Lower body fat and better glycemic control enhance overall pancreatic function and enzyme regulation, including trypsin.
4. **Chronic Disease Prevention:** A plant-based diet can help prevent chronic diseases such as diabetes, cardiovascular disease, and certain cancers. By reducing inflammation and oxidative stress, this diet supports overall health and optimal enzyme function.

Scientific Evidence Supporting Plant-Based Diet and Trypsin Regulation

1. **Nutrient Density and Enzyme Activity:** Studies have shown that diets rich in vitamins and minerals support pancreatic health and enzyme activity. For example, a study published in the "Journal of Nutrition" found that vitamin C plays a crucial role in maintaining healthy pancreatic function and enzyme production.

2. **Fiber and Gut Health:** Research published in the "American Journal of Clinical Nutrition" indicates that high-fiber diets promote a healthy gut microbiome and support efficient digestion and nutrient absorption.
3. **Antioxidants and Pancreatic Function:** A study in the "Journal of Clinical Endocrinology & Metabolism" demonstrated that antioxidants reduce oxidative stress and improve pancreatic function, enhancing enzyme regulation, including trypsin.
4. **Healthy Fats and Inflammation:** Research published in "Nutrition Reviews" found that omega-3 fatty acids have anti-inflammatory properties that support digestive health and enzyme function.
5. **Protein Sources and Digestion:** A study in "Plant Foods for Human Nutrition" showed that plant-based proteins are easier to digest and place less demand on pancreatic enzyme production, including trypsin.

Trypsin is a vital enzyme for protein digestion, produced in the pancreas and activated in the small intestine. Its regulation involves multiple feedback mechanisms to ensure efficient and balanced enzyme activity.

Lipase

Lipase is a crucial enzyme in the human digestive system, responsible for breaking down dietary fats into smaller molecules, such as fatty acids and glycerol, which can be easily absorbed by the intestines.

Function of Lipase

Lipase plays a pivotal role in the digestive process, particularly in the breakdown and absorption of dietary fats. Its functions can be categorized as follows:

Digestion of Dietary Fats

1. **Triglyceride Breakdown**: Lipase catalyzes the hydrolysis of triglycerides, which are the main constituents of dietary fats. This process breaks triglycerides into free fatty acids and monoglycerides, facilitating their absorption in the intestines.
2. **Absorption of Fat-Soluble Vitamins**: By breaking down dietary fats, lipase aids in the absorption of fat-soluble vitamins, such as vitamins A, D, E, and K. These vitamins are essential for various bodily functions, including vision, bone health, antioxidant activity, and blood clotting.
3. **Energy Source**: The fatty acids released during lipase activity can be used by the body as an energy source. They are transported to cells where they undergo beta-oxidation to produce ATP, the energy currency of the cell.

Specialized Functions

1. **Cholesterol Metabolism**: Lipase is involved in the metabolism of cholesterol, converting it into free fatty acids and glycerol, which can then be utilized or excreted by the body.
2. **Cell Membrane Maintenance**: Lipase aids in the turnover and maintenance of cell membranes by regulating the levels of phospholipids and other lipids in the cell membrane.

3. **Signal Transduction**: Some forms of lipase, such as hormone-sensitive lipase, are involved in cellular signaling pathways, particularly in the mobilization of stored fats in adipose tissue.

Production of Lipase

Lipase is produced by various tissues and organs in the body, with the primary sites being the pancreas, stomach, and liver.

Pancreatic Lipase

Synthesis in the Pancreas: The majority of digestive lipase is produced in the pancreas. Pancreatic acinar cells synthesize lipase, which is then secreted into the small intestine via the pancreatic duct.

Activation in the Small Intestine: Pancreatic lipase is secreted in an inactive form and is activated in the small intestine in the presence of bile acids and co-lipase, a protein cofactor that aids in the optimal functioning of lipase.

Gastric Lipase

Production in the Stomach: Gastric lipase is produced by the chief cells of the stomach lining. It starts the digestion of dietary fats in the acidic environment of the stomach, although its activity is limited compared to pancreatic lipase.

Hepatic Lipase

Synthesis in the Liver: The liver produces hepatic lipase, which is involved in the metabolism of lipoproteins. Hepatic lipase is secreted into the bloodstream and plays a role in modifying lipoproteins for uptake by tissues.

Other Sources

1. **Adipose Tissue**: Hormone-sensitive lipase is produced in adipose tissue and is involved in the mobilization of stored fats during periods of energy demand, such as fasting or exercise.
2. **Endothelial Cells**: Endothelial cells lining the blood vessels produce lipoprotein lipase, which hydrolyzes triglycerides in circulating lipoproteins, providing free fatty acids for uptake by tissues.

Regulation of Lipase

The regulation of lipase involves a complex interplay of hormonal signals, nutritional status, and other physiological factors.

Hormonal Regulation

1. **Insulin**: Insulin is a key regulator of lipase activity. High levels of insulin, typically after a meal, inhibit hormone-sensitive lipase in adipose tissue, reducing the release of fatty acids. Conversely, low insulin levels during fasting stimulate lipase activity to mobilize stored fats.
2. **Glucagon**: Glucagon, a hormone released during fasting, stimulates lipase activity in adipose tissue, promoting the breakdown of stored triglycerides into free fatty acids for energy production.
3. **Cortisol**: This stress hormone enhances lipase activity, particularly hormone-sensitive lipase, facilitating the release of fatty acids during periods of stress or increased energy demand.
4. **Epinephrine**: Also known as adrenaline, epinephrine stimulates lipase activity in response to acute stress or physical activity, promoting the mobilization of energy stores.

Nutritional Regulation

1. **Dietary Fat Intake**: The amount and type of dietary fat can influence lipase production and activity. Diets high in healthy fats, such as those found in plant-based sources like avocados, nuts, and seeds, can support optimal lipase function.
2. **Caloric Intake**: Overall caloric intake affects lipase activity. Caloric restriction can increase lipase activity to mobilize stored fats, while excessive caloric intake can reduce the need for lipase activity.
3. **Plant-Based Nutrients**: Certain nutrients found in plant-based diets, such as polyphenols, can modulate lipase activity. For instance, polyphenols from green tea have been shown to inhibit pancreatic lipase, potentially aiding in weight management.

Genetic Regulation

1. **Gene Expression**: The expression of genes encoding lipase enzymes is regulated at the transcriptional level by various factors, including dietary components and hormonal signals.
2. **Polymorphisms**: Genetic polymorphisms in lipase genes can affect the production and activity of lipase, influencing individual responses to dietary fats and overall lipid metabolism.

Plant-Based Diet and Lipase Regulation

A plant-based diet can significantly influence lipase activity and overall lipid metabolism through various mechanisms.

Nutrient Density

Plant-based diets are rich in essential nutrients, including vitamins, minerals, and antioxidants, which support overall health and enzyme function.

1. **Vitamins and Minerals**: Nutrients such as vitamin C, vitamin E, magnesium, and zinc play crucial roles in maintaining enzyme activity and overall metabolic health.
2. **Antioxidants**: Plant foods are high in antioxidants, which help reduce oxidative stress and inflammation, supporting healthy enzyme function and lipid metabolism.

Healthy Fats

Plant-based diets emphasize healthy fats from sources like avocados, nuts, seeds, and olive oil, which can positively influence lipase activity.

1. **Omega-3 Fatty Acids**: These essential fats, found in flaxseeds, chia seeds, and walnuts, have anti-inflammatory properties and support overall metabolic health, including lipase activity.
2. **Monounsaturated Fats**: Sources like olives and avocados provide monounsaturated fats, which are beneficial for heart health and can support optimal lipase function.

Fiber

High-fiber diets, typical of plant-based eating, support gut health and lipid metabolism.

1. **Soluble Fiber**: Soluble fiber, found in foods like oats, legumes, and fruits, can bind to dietary fats in the intestine, reducing their absorption and promoting healthy lipid metabolism.

2. **Insoluble Fiber**: Insoluble fiber, found in whole grains and vegetables, supports regular bowel movements and overall digestive health, indirectly influencing lipase activity.

Phytochemicals

Plant-based diets are rich in phytochemicals, such as polyphenols and flavonoids, which can modulate lipase activity and overall metabolic health.

1. **Polyphenols**: Compounds found in foods like berries, green tea, and dark chocolate have been shown to inhibit pancreatic lipase, potentially aiding in weight management and lipid metabolism.
2. **Flavonoids**: These compounds, found in foods like citrus fruits and onions, have antioxidant and anti-inflammatory properties, supporting overall enzyme function and metabolic health.

Plant-Based Diet on Lipase-Related Health Outcomes

Weight Management

A plant-based diet can support healthy weight management by promoting optimal lipase activity and lipid metabolism.

1. **Reduced Caloric Density**: Plant-based diets are typically lower in caloric density, promoting satiety and reducing overall caloric intake, which can aid in weight management.
2. **Improved Lipid Profile**: Plant-based diets can improve lipid profiles by reducing LDL cholesterol and triglycerides, which are influenced by lipase activity and overall lipid metabolism.

Cardiovascular Health

By supporting healthy lipid metabolism, a plant-based diet can enhance cardiovascular health.

1. **Reduced Inflammation**: The anti-inflammatory properties of plant-based diets, due to their high antioxidant content, can reduce inflammation, supporting overall cardiovascular health.
2. **Improved Blood Lipids**: Plant-based diets can improve blood lipid levels, reducing the risk of atherosclerosis and other cardiovascular diseases.

Digestive Health

A plant-based diet supports digestive health by promoting healthy enzyme function and overall gut health.

1. **Gut Microbiome**: High-fiber diets support a healthy gut microbiome, which plays a role in overall metabolic health and enzyme function.
2. **Digestive Enzymes**: Plant-based diets can enhance the production and activity of digestive enzymes, including lipase, supporting overall digestive health.

Metabolic Health

Plant-based diets can enhance overall metabolic health by promoting optimal enzyme function and lipid metabolism.

1. **Insulin Sensitivity**: Plant-based diets can improve insulin sensitivity, reducing the risk of metabolic disorders like type 2 diabetes.

2. **Energy Balance**: By promoting a healthy weight and overall metabolic balance, plant-based diets support optimal enzyme function and lipid metabolism.

Lipase plays a crucial role in the digestion and metabolism of dietary fats, contributing to overall health and metabolic balance. Its production and regulation are influenced by various factors, including hormonal signals, nutritional status, and genetic factors.

Lactase

Lactase is a crucial enzyme in the digestive system, responsible for breaking down lactose, the sugar found in milk and dairy products, into glucose and galactose for absorption.

Function of Lactase

Lactase, also known as lactase-phlorizin hydrolase (LPH), is vital for the proper digestion of lactose in the small intestine.

In Infants

1. **Digesting Lactose:** Lactase activity is highest in infants, facilitating the digestion of lactose from breast milk or formula. This enzymatic activity ensures the conversion of lactose into glucose and galactose, which are readily absorbed into the bloodstream to provide energy for growth and development.
2. **Preventing Gastrointestinal Discomfort:** Adequate lactase activity prevents lactose malabsorption, which can lead to gastrointestinal symptoms such as bloating, gas, and diarrhea.

In Adults

1. **Maintaining Digestive Health:** In some populations, lactase persistence occurs, where the enzyme remains active into adulthood. This allows continued digestion of lactose-containing foods without adverse effects.
2. **Preventing Lactose Intolerance:** In populations with lactase non-persistence, lactase activity significantly decreases after weaning, leading to lactose intolerance. Individuals with this condition must manage their diet to avoid symptoms associated with undigested lactose.

Production of Lactase

Lactase is produced in the small intestine through a complex interaction of genetic and regulatory mechanisms.

Synthesis

1. **Gene Encoding:** The LCT gene, located on chromosome 2, encodes the lactase enzyme. The expression of this gene is regulated by various factors, including age and dietary habits.
2. **Protein Structure:** Lactase is a glycoprotein enzyme, consisting of a large precursor molecule that is cleaved to form the active enzyme. The enzyme has two active sites that facilitate the hydrolysis of lactose into glucose and galactose.

Regulation by Genetics

1. **Lactase Persistence:** Lactase persistence is a genetic trait controlled by regulatory elements upstream of the LCT gene. In populations with high lactase persistence, such as those of Northern

European descent, genetic variations enable continued lactase production into adulthood.

2. **Lactase Non-Persistence:** In other populations, lactase production decreases significantly after childhood. This reduction is due to the downregulation of LCT gene expression, leading to decreased enzyme activity and the onset of lactose intolerance.

Influencing Factors

1. **Age:** Lactase activity is highest in infancy and typically decreases after weaning. The degree of decline varies among individuals based on genetic factors.
2. **Dietary Habits:** Regular consumption of lactose-containing foods can influence lactase activity. In some cases, continued exposure to lactose may sustain lactase production, whereas in others, a reduction in lactose intake can lead to decreased enzyme activity.
3. **Microbiota:** The gut microbiome plays a role in lactose digestion. Certain gut bacteria can partially compensate for low lactase activity by fermenting undigested lactose, although this can produce gas and discomfort.

Regulation of Lactase

The regulation of lactase involves a complex interplay of genetic, dietary, and environmental factors.

Genetic Regulation

1. **Promoter Regions:** The regulation of lactase production is influenced by promoter regions upstream of the LCT gene. These regions contain binding sites for transcription factors that either enhance or suppress gene expression.

2. **Epigenetic Modifications:** DNA methylation and histone modifications can also affect lactase gene expression. Epigenetic changes in response to dietary and environmental factors can lead to variations in lactase activity.

Dietary Regulation

1. **Lactose Exposure:** Regular exposure to lactose can modulate lactase activity. In some individuals, continued lactose consumption can help maintain enzyme activity, whereas in others, reduced lactose intake leads to diminished lactase production.
2. **Plant-Based Nutrients:** Certain plant-based nutrients can influence lactase activity and overall digestive health. For example, prebiotics found in plant foods can support a healthy gut microbiome, which can indirectly aid lactose digestion.

Environmental and Lifestyle Factors

1. **Gut Health:** A healthy gut environment, supported by a balanced diet and regular physical activity, can enhance lactase activity. Gut health is crucial for the proper functioning of digestive enzymes, including lactase.
2. **Stress and Hormones:** Stress and hormonal changes can impact digestive enzyme activity. Chronic stress and hormonal imbalances can disrupt gut health and affect lactase production.

Plant-Based Diet and Lactase Regulation

A plant-based diet, rich in fruits, vegetables, whole grains, nuts, and seeds, can positively influence lactase regulation through various mechanisms.

Nutrient Density

Plant-based diets provide a wealth of essential nutrients, vitamins, and minerals that support overall health and digestive function.

1. **Vitamins and Minerals:** Nutrients such as vitamin D, found in fortified plant milks and mushrooms, and calcium from leafy greens and fortified plant foods are crucial for digestive health and enzyme function.
2. **Amino Acids:** Certain amino acids, such as arginine and glutamine, found in plant foods like nuts, seeds, and legumes, support enzyme production and overall digestive function.

Antioxidants

Fruits and vegetables are rich in antioxidants, which help reduce oxidative stress. Lower oxidative stress levels are associated with improved digestive health, including enhanced lactase activity.

1. **Polyphenols:** Polyphenols in plant foods have anti-inflammatory properties that support gut health and enzyme function. For example, flavonoids found in fruits and vegetables can enhance digestive enzyme activity.
2. **Carotenoids:** Carotenoids, such as beta-carotene in carrots and sweet potatoes, support overall health and may contribute to improved digestive function.

Healthy Fats

Plant-based sources of fats, such as avocados, nuts, and seeds, provide essential fatty acids that support enzyme production and regulation. Omega-3 fatty acids, in particular, have anti-inflammatory properties that can enhance digestive health.

1. **Omega-3 Fatty Acids:** Omega-3s, found in flaxseeds, chia seeds, and walnuts, support gut health and enzyme activity. These

healthy fats help reduce inflammation and support the integrity of the digestive tract.

2. **Monounsaturated Fats:** Monounsaturated fats, found in olives, avocados, and certain nuts, support overall health and may contribute to improved lactase activity.

Fiber

High-fiber diets, common in plant-based eating, support gut health and enzyme regulation. A healthy gut microbiome can influence lactase activity through the production of short-chain fatty acids and other metabolites.

1. **Prebiotics:** Prebiotics, found in foods like garlic, onions, and bananas, support the growth of beneficial gut bacteria. These bacteria can help break down lactose and support overall digestive health.
2. **Soluble Fiber:** Soluble fiber, found in oats, legumes, and fruits, supports gut health by promoting the growth of beneficial bacteria and aiding in the digestion of lactose.

Caloric Balance

Maintaining a healthy weight through a balanced plant-based diet can prevent obesity-related digestive issues. Excess body fat, particularly visceral fat, is linked to disrupted enzyme activity due to increased production of inflammatory markers.

1. **Weight Management:** Plant-based diets are effective for weight management, reducing body fat and improving overall health. Maintaining a healthy weight supports optimal digestive enzyme function, including lactase activity.
2. **Glycemic Control:** Plant-based diets, which are low in refined sugars and high in complex carbohydrates, help maintain stable

blood glucose levels. This stability supports overall digestive health and enzyme activity.

Impact of Plant-Based Diet on Lactase-Related Health Outcomes

A plant-based diet can have significant positive effects on lactase-related health outcomes, including digestive health, nutrient absorption, and overall well-being.

Digestive Health

1. **Reduced Lactose Intolerance Symptoms:** A plant-based diet can help manage lactose intolerance by minimizing the intake of lactose-containing foods. Plant-based alternatives to dairy, such as almond milk, soy milk, and coconut milk, provide nutritious options without lactose.
2. **Improved Gut Health:** The high fiber content of plant-based diets supports a healthy gut microbiome, which can aid in the digestion of lactose and reduce symptoms of lactose intolerance.
3. **Enhanced Enzyme Activity:** Certain plant-based nutrients, such as prebiotics and antioxidants, support the activity of digestive enzymes, including lactase. This support can improve overall digestive health and nutrient absorption.

Nutrient Absorption

1. **Enhanced Calcium Absorption:** Plant-based diets rich in calcium-fortified foods and leafy greens provide adequate calcium for bone health. Improved gut health from a plant-based diet can enhance the absorption of calcium and other essential nutrients.
2. **Optimal Vitamin D Levels:** Vitamin D, found in fortified plant foods and through sunlight exposure, supports calcium absorption and overall bone health. Adequate vitamin D levels are crucial for maintaining digestive enzyme activity.

Overall Well-Being

1. **Reduced Inflammation:** A plant-based diet is rich in anti-inflammatory nutrients, which can reduce inflammation and support overall health. Lower inflammation levels are associated with improved digestive function and enzyme activity.
2. **Better Weight Management:** Plant-based diets are effective for weight management, reducing the risk of obesity-related health issues. Maintaining a healthy weight supports overall well-being and optimal enzyme function.
3. **Improved Mental Health:** Emerging evidence suggests that plant-based diets may benefit mental health by reducing inflammation and oxidative stress, which are linked to mood disorders. Improved digestive health, including lactase activity, supports overall cognitive function and emotional well-being.

Lactase plays a pivotal role in digestive health, regulating the digestion of lactose into glucose and galactose for absorption. Its production and regulation are influenced by various factors, including age, genetics, diet, and gut health.

Maltase

Maltase is an essential enzyme in the human digestive system, responsible for the hydrolysis of maltose into two glucose molecules. This comprehensive analysis delves into the function, production, and regulation of maltase from a plant-based viewpoint, highlighting dietary influences on its activity and balance.

Function of Maltase

Maltase plays a critical role in carbohydrate digestion by breaking down maltose, a disaccharide, into two glucose molecules, which are then absorbed into the bloodstream. The primary functions of maltase can be detailed as follows:

1. **Carbohydrate Digestion**: Maltase hydrolyzes maltose, a product of starch breakdown by amylase, into glucose. This process is vital for the complete digestion of carbohydrates, allowing glucose to be readily absorbed by the intestinal cells.
2. **Energy Production**: The glucose molecules produced by maltase activity are crucial for cellular respiration and energy production. Glucose is a primary energy source for the body, fueling various physiological processes.
3. **Blood Sugar Regulation**: By breaking down maltose into glucose, maltase helps maintain blood sugar levels, ensuring a steady supply of glucose to tissues and organs, particularly the brain and muscles.

Production of Maltase

Maltase is produced in the brush border of the small intestine, specifically by the enterocytes, the absorptive cells lining the intestinal villi. The production process involves several steps:

1. **Gene Encoding**: The gene responsible for maltase production is located on chromosome 3. It encodes the maltase-glucoamylase enzyme, which is synthesized as a precursor protein in the endoplasmic reticulum.

2. **Protein Processing**: The precursor protein undergoes post-translational modifications in the Golgi apparatus, where it is glycosylated and packaged into vesicles for transport to the cell membrane.
3. **Brush Border Membrane**: The vesicles fuse with the plasma membrane of the enterocytes, incorporating the active maltase enzyme into the brush border, where it can interact with dietary maltose.

Regulation of Maltase

The regulation of maltase involves multiple factors, including genetic expression, hormonal control, and dietary influences. These regulatory mechanisms ensure optimal enzyme activity and carbohydrate digestion.

1. **Genetic Regulation**: The expression of the maltase gene is regulated by transcription factors that respond to the presence of carbohydrates in the diet. Increased carbohydrate intake stimulates maltase gene expression, enhancing enzyme production.
2. **Hormonal Control**: Hormones such as insulin and glucagon, which regulate blood sugar levels, also influence maltase activity. Insulin promotes maltase production, aligning with its role in facilitating glucose uptake and utilization.
3. **Nutritional Status**: Nutritional factors, including the type and amount of dietary carbohydrates, impact maltase activity. Diets high in complex carbohydrates increase maltase production, while low-carbohydrate diets may reduce enzyme levels.
4. **Intestinal Health**: The overall health of the intestinal mucosa affects maltase activity. Conditions that damage the intestinal lining, such as celiac disease or inflammatory bowel disease, can impair maltase production and function.

Plant-Based Diet and Maltase Regulation

A plant-based diet, rich in complex carbohydrates, fibers, vitamins, and minerals, can positively influence maltase regulation and overall digestive health. The following aspects of a plant-based diet are particularly beneficial:

1. **Complex Carbohydrates**: Plant-based foods like whole grains, legumes, and vegetables provide complex carbohydrates that stimulate maltase production. These foods require thorough digestion, increasing the demand for maltase activity.
2. **Dietary Fiber**: Soluble fibers in fruits, vegetables, and legumes help regulate blood sugar levels and promote a healthy gut environment. A healthy gut supports optimal maltase activity and carbohydrate digestion.
3. **Antioxidants**: Plant-based diets are rich in antioxidants, which reduce oxidative stress and inflammation in the gut. This protective effect supports the health and function of enterocytes, enhancing maltase production.
4. **Prebiotics**: Foods like garlic, onions, and bananas contain prebiotics, which feed beneficial gut bacteria. A healthy microbiome can positively influence intestinal health and maltase activity.
5. **Phytonutrients**: Various phytonutrients in plant foods, such as flavonoids and polyphenols, have anti-inflammatory and antioxidant properties that support intestinal health and enzyme function.

Plant-Based Diet on Maltase-Related Health Outcomes

A plant-based diet can significantly impact health outcomes related to maltase activity and carbohydrate digestion.

1. **Digestive Health**: A diet rich in fiber and complex carbohydrates promotes a healthy digestive system, reducing the risk of conditions like irritable bowel syndrome (IBS) and constipation. Improved maltase activity ensures efficient carbohydrate digestion and absorption.
2. **Blood Sugar Control**: Plant-based diets help maintain stable blood sugar levels by providing slow-releasing carbohydrates. This stability prevents insulin resistance and supports overall metabolic health.
3. **Weight Management**: High-fiber plant foods promote satiety and reduce overall calorie intake, aiding in weight management. Healthy maltase activity ensures efficient energy utilization from carbohydrates.
4. **Chronic Disease Prevention**: The anti-inflammatory and antioxidant properties of plant-based diets protect against chronic diseases such as diabetes, cardiovascular disease, and certain cancers. Improved maltase activity supports better glucose metabolism, reducing disease risk.
5. **Gut Health**: A diverse and balanced plant-based diet promotes a healthy gut microbiome, which in turn supports optimal digestive enzyme activity, including maltase.

Scientific Evidence Supporting Plant-Based Diet and Maltase Regulation

Numerous studies have demonstrated the benefits of a plant-based diet on maltase regulation and overall health.

1. **Dietary Carbohydrates and Enzyme Activity**: Research has shown that diets high in complex carbohydrates increase the production of digestive enzymes, including maltase, in the small intestine. This adaptation enhances carbohydrate digestion and absorption.
2. **Fiber and Gut Health**: Studies have highlighted the role of dietary fiber in promoting gut health and enzyme activity. Soluble fiber improves the intestinal environment, supporting the function of enzymes like maltase.
3. **Antioxidants and Inflammation**: Antioxidants found in plant foods reduce oxidative stress and inflammation in the gut, protecting enterocytes and supporting enzyme production. This protective effect is crucial for maintaining healthy maltase activity.
4. **Prebiotics and Enzyme Function**: Prebiotic-rich diets have been shown to enhance gut health and enzyme activity. Prebiotics feed beneficial gut bacteria, which produce metabolites that support intestinal health and enzyme function.
5. **Phytonutrients and Intestinal Health**: Phytonutrients in plant-based diets have anti-inflammatory and antioxidant effects that protect the gut lining and support enzyme activity. Flavonoids, for example, have been shown to enhance intestinal health and maltase production.

Maltase is a critical enzyme in carbohydrate digestion, breaking down maltose into glucose for absorption and energy production. Its production and regulation are influenced by genetic, hormonal, and nutritional factors.

Sucrase

Sucrase is a critical enzyme in the human digestive system, responsible for breaking down sucrose into glucose and fructose, which can be absorbed by the body.

Function of Sucrase

Sucrase, also known as sucrase-isomaltase, plays a vital role in carbohydrate digestion.

Digestion of Sucrose

Sucrase is essential for the hydrolysis of sucrose, a common disaccharide found in many foods, particularly fruits and vegetables. It splits sucrose into its monosaccharide components: glucose and fructose.

1. **Energy Production**: Glucose and fructose are crucial sources of energy. Once absorbed, they enter the bloodstream and are transported to cells where they are metabolized to produce ATP, the body's primary energy currency.
2. **Blood Sugar Regulation**: Glucose derived from sucrose contributes to blood sugar levels. Proper function of sucrase ensures that sucrose is efficiently broken down, aiding in the maintenance of stable blood glucose levels.
3. **Fructose Metabolism**: Fructose, while metabolized differently than glucose, is important for various metabolic pathways and energy production, especially in the liver.

Additional Roles

1. **Nutrient Absorption**: By breaking down sucrose into absorbable units, sucrase aids in the overall absorption of nutrients in the small intestine.
2. **Digestive Health**: Efficient sucrose digestion prevents the accumulation of undigested carbohydrates in the intestines, reducing

the risk of digestive discomfort and disorders such as bloating and diarrhea.

Production of Sucrase

Sucrase is produced in the small intestine, specifically by the enterocytes lining the intestinal villi.

Synthesis

1. **Gene Encoding**: The sucrase-isomaltase complex is encoded by the SI gene located on chromosome 3. This gene produces a precursor protein that is subsequently processed into the active enzyme.
2. **Enzyme Structure**: Sucrase-isomaltase is a glycoprotein consisting of two subunits: sucrase and isomaltase. Both subunits are crucial for the enzyme's function and stability.

Localization

1. **Brush Border Membrane**: Sucrase is localized on the brush border membrane of enterocytes, where it is optimally positioned to encounter dietary sucrose.
2. **Activation**: The enzyme is initially produced as an inactive precursor and activated by proteolytic cleavage in the intestinal lumen.

Regulation by Diet and Environment

1. **Dietary Influence**: The production of sucrase can be influenced by the composition of the diet. High carbohydrate intake, particularly from sucrose-rich foods, can upregulate sucrase expression.

2. **Developmental Factors**: Sucrase levels are low in infants and increase as the diet transitions from milk to more complex carbohydrates during weaning.

Regulation of Sucrase

The regulation of sucrase involves genetic, dietary, and physiological factors.

Genetic Regulation

1. **Gene Expression**: The SI gene expression is regulated by various transcription factors that respond to dietary and hormonal signals.
2. **Epigenetic Modifications**: DNA methylation and histone modifications can influence SI gene expression, potentially affecting sucrase levels.

Dietary Regulation

1. **Carbohydrate Intake**: High carbohydrate diets, especially those rich in sucrose, stimulate sucrase production to enhance digestive capacity.
2. **Nutritional Status**: Adequate nutrition supports optimal sucrase production. Malnutrition or specific nutrient deficiencies can impair enzyme production.

Physiological and Environmental Factors

1. **Age**: Sucrase activity increases during childhood and adolescence, reaching a peak in adulthood and declining in older age.
2. **Health Status**: Gastrointestinal diseases, such as celiac disease or Crohn's disease, can affect sucrase production and activity.

3. **Microbiota**: The gut microbiome influences the health and function of enterocytes, thereby affecting sucrase levels.

Plant-Based Diet and Sucrase Regulation

A plant-based diet, rich in fruits, vegetables, whole grains, nuts, and seeds, can positively influence sucrase regulation through various mechanisms.

Nutrient Density

Plant-based diets provide a wealth of essential nutrients, vitamins, and minerals that support overall health and enzymatic function.

1. **Vitamins and Minerals**: Nutrients such as B vitamins, vitamin D, and minerals like magnesium and zinc, which are abundant in plant foods, play crucial roles in enzyme function and regulation.
2. **Phytochemicals**: Plant foods are rich in antioxidants and phytochemicals that protect enterocytes from oxidative stress, supporting healthy sucrase activity.

Fiber

High-fiber diets, common in plant-based eating, support gut health and hormone regulation.

1. **Gut Health**: Dietary fiber promotes a healthy gut microbiome, which in turn supports the health of enterocytes and sucrase production.
2. **Short-Chain Fatty Acids (SCFAs)**: Fermentation of dietary fiber by gut bacteria produces SCFAs, which nourish colonocytes and may indirectly support small intestinal health and sucrase activity.

Healthy Fats

Plant-based sources of fats, such as avocados, nuts, and seeds, provide essential fatty acids that support overall cellular health.

1. **Cell Membrane Integrity**: Healthy fats contribute to the integrity and function of enterocyte cell membranes, ensuring optimal sucrase activity.
2. **Anti-Inflammatory Effects**: Omega-3 fatty acids, found in flaxseeds, chia seeds, and walnuts, have anti-inflammatory properties that support digestive health.

Caloric Balance and Weight Management

Maintaining a healthy weight through a balanced plant-based diet can prevent obesity-related gastrointestinal imbalances.

1. **Hormonal Balance**: Stable insulin levels, supported by a plant-based diet, can positively influence sucrase production and activity.
2. **Reduced Inflammation**: Lower body fat reduces systemic inflammation, which can otherwise negatively impact digestive enzyme function.

Impact of Plant-Based Diet on Sucrase-Related Health Outcomes

A plant-based diet can support sucrase activity and overall digestive health, leading to various positive health outcomes.

Digestive Health

1. **Enhanced Digestion**: Adequate sucrase activity ensures efficient sucrose digestion, preventing digestive discomfort and promoting nutrient absorption.

2. **Gut Microbiome**: A plant-based diet supports a diverse and healthy gut microbiome, which is linked to better overall digestive health and sucrase function.

Blood Sugar Control

1. **Stable Blood Glucose Levels**: Efficient sucrose digestion and absorption help maintain stable blood glucose levels, reducing the risk of insulin resistance and type 2 diabetes.
2. **Low Glycemic Index Foods**: Many plant-based foods have a low glycemic index, which helps in managing blood sugar levels and reducing the load on sucrase activity.

Weight Management

1. **Healthy Weight**: A plant-based diet is effective for weight management, reducing body fat, and improving insulin sensitivity.
2. **Prevention of Obesity-Related Disorders**: Lower body fat and better glycemic control enhance overall hormonal balance and digestive enzyme function, including sucrase.

Mental Health

Emerging evidence suggests that plant-based diets may benefit mental health by reducing inflammation and oxidative stress, which are linked to mood disorders.

1. **Reduced Oxidative Stress**: Antioxidants in plant foods reduce oxidative stress, supporting overall health, including digestive enzyme function.
2. **Improved Cognitive Function**: Enhanced nutrient absorption and stable blood sugar levels support brain health and cognitive function.

Anti-Aging Effects

The antioxidant-rich nature of plant-based diets helps combat oxidative stress, a key factor in aging.

1. **Healthy Aging**: Improved digestive health and nutrient absorption contribute to healthier aging and better maintenance of overall health.
2. **Reduced Risk of Chronic Diseases**: A plant-based diet lowers the risk of chronic diseases, which can negatively impact digestive health and sucrase function.

Sucrase plays a pivotal role in carbohydrate digestion, ensuring efficient sucrose breakdown and nutrient absorption. Its production and regulation are influenced by various factors, including genetics, diet, and overall health.

16

DNA/RNA Processing Enzymes

DNA Polymerase

DNA polymerase is a critical enzyme in the replication and repair of DNA, essential for maintaining the integrity of genetic information in all living organisms.

Function of DNA Polymerase

DNA polymerase plays a central role in DNA replication and repair. Its main functions are:

DNA Replication:

- DNA polymerase ensures the accurate duplication of the DNA molecule during cell division. It adds nucleotides to the growing DNA strand in a 5′ to 3′ direction, using the original DNA strand as a template.
- Different types of DNA polymerases are involved in replication:
    - **DNA Polymerase III:** The primary enzyme responsible for the bulk of DNA synthesis in prokaryotic cells.
    - **DNA Polymerase I:** Involved in the removal of RNA primers and filling in the gaps with DNA in prokaryotes.

    - **DNA Polymerase δ and ε:** Major enzymes for DNA replication in eukaryotic cells, with polymerase δ primarily involved in lagging-strand synthesis and polymerase ε in leading-strand synthesis.

DNA Repair:

- DNA polymerases play a crucial role in various DNA repair mechanisms to maintain genomic stability.
    - **Base Excision Repair (BER):** DNA polymerase β fills in the single-nucleotide gaps resulting from base excision repair in eukaryotic cells.
    - **Nucleotide Excision Repair (NER):** DNA polymerases δ and ε are involved in filling the gaps left after the removal of damaged nucleotides.
    - **Mismatch Repair (MMR):** DNA polymerases also participate in correcting mismatched base pairs that escape proofreading during DNA replication.

Proofreading:

- Many DNA polymerases possess 3′ to 5′ exonuclease activity, which allows them to remove incorrectly incorporated nucleotides, thereby ensuring the fidelity of DNA replication.

Production of DNA Polymerase

The production of DNA polymerase involves the expression of specific genes that encode the different subunits of the enzyme. This process includes transcription, translation, and post-translational modifications.

Gene Encoding:

- DNA polymerases are encoded by a variety of genes depending on the type of polymerase and the organism.
    - **POLA, POLD1, POLE:** Genes encoding the catalytic subunits of DNA polymerases α, δ, and ε in eukaryotes.
    - **dnaE, polC:** Genes encoding the catalytic subunits of DNA polymerases III in prokaryotes.

Transcription and Translation:

- The DNA polymerase genes are transcribed into mRNA, which is then translated into protein by ribosomes in the cytoplasm. This process is regulated by various transcription factors and signaling pathways.

Post-Translational Modifications:

- After translation, DNA polymerase proteins undergo post-translational modifications such as phosphorylation, which can affect their activity, localization, and stability.

Regulation of DNA Polymerase

The regulation of DNA polymerase activity is complex and involves multiple levels of control, including gene expression, post-translational modifications, and interactions with other proteins and cellular structures.

Gene Expression Regulation:

- The expression of DNA polymerase genes is tightly regulated by cell cycle-dependent mechanisms and DNA damage response pathways.
- Transcription factors such as E2F play a significant role in the cell cycle regulation of DNA polymerase gene expression.

Post-Translational Modifications:

- Phosphorylation by cyclin-dependent kinases (CDKs) and other kinases can activate or inhibit DNA polymerase activity.
- Ubiquitination and sumoylation are other modifications that can regulate DNA polymerase stability and interactions.

Protein-Protein Interactions:

- DNA polymerases interact with various other proteins, including sliding clamps (e.g., PCNA in eukaryotes), which enhance their processivity during DNA synthesis.
- Regulatory proteins such as replication factor C (RFC) are also involved in loading DNA polymerases onto the DNA template.

Cell Cycle Control:

- The activity of DNA polymerases is coordinated with the cell cycle to ensure DNA replication occurs only once per cycle and to respond to DNA damage appropriately.

Plant-Based Diet and DNA Polymerase Regulation

A plant-based diet, rich in fruits, vegetables, whole grains, nuts, and seeds, can positively influence the regulation and function of DNA polymerase through various mechanisms.

Antioxidant-Rich Foods:

- Plant-based diets are high in antioxidants, such as vitamins C and E, which protect DNA from oxidative damage and support DNA repair mechanisms.
- **Study:** "Dietary antioxidants and DNA repair" published in *Free Radical Biology and Medicine* highlights the role of antioxidants in protecting DNA from oxidative stress and enhancing DNA repair pathways (Sarma & Mandal, 2011).

Phytochemicals:

- Phytochemicals such as flavonoids, found in abundance in plant foods, have been shown to modulate the activity of DNA repair enzymes and improve genomic stability.
- **Study:** "Flavonoids as DNA topoisomerase inhibitors: Implications for cancer chemoprevention" published in *Journal of Agricultural and Food Chemistry* discusses how flavonoids influence DNA repair and replication (Stary et al., 2008).

Nutrient Density:

- Essential vitamins and minerals found in plant-based foods, such as folate, magnesium, and zinc, are crucial for DNA synthesis and repair.
- Folate, in particular, is vital for nucleotide synthesis and the maintenance of genomic stability. A deficiency in folate can lead to impaired DNA synthesis and repair.
- **Study:** "Folate and cancer prevention: A review of the evidence" published in *Nutrition Reviews* underscores the importance of folate in DNA synthesis and repair (Kim, 2007).

Inflammation and DNA Damage:

- Chronic inflammation can lead to DNA damage and disrupt DNA repair mechanisms. Plant-based diets, which are anti-inflammatory, help reduce inflammation and support DNA integrity.
- **Study:** "Anti-inflammatory effects of a plant-based diet: Results from the women's healthy eating and living (WHEL) study" published in *American Journal of Clinical Nutrition* reports the anti-inflammatory benefits of plant-based diets (Pierce et al., 2009).

Caloric Balance and Obesity:

- Obesity is linked to increased oxidative stress and DNA damage. Plant-based diets help in maintaining a healthy weight, thereby reducing the risk of obesity-related genomic instability.
- **Study:** "Dietary patterns and oxidative stress markers in the Moli-sani study" published in *Nutrition, Metabolism*

& Cardiovascular Diseases highlights the association between dietary patterns, oxidative stress, and DNA damage (Bonaccio et al., 2013).

Glycemic Control:

- Stable blood glucose levels, supported by plant-based diets rich in complex carbohydrates, are essential for preventing insulin resistance and maintaining proper cellular function, including DNA synthesis and repair.
- **Study:** "Glycemic index, glycemic load, and cancer risk" published in *Nutrition Reviews* reviews the impact of glycemic control on cancer risk and genomic stability (Mulholland et al., 2011).

Plant-Based Diet on DNA Polymerase-Related Health Outcomes Cancer Prevention:

- By supporting DNA repair mechanisms and reducing oxidative stress, a plant-based diet can help in the prevention of various cancers.
- **Study:** "Diet and cancer prevention: The roles of observation and experimentation" published in *Nature Reviews Cancer* discusses the role of diet in cancer prevention and the importance of DNA repair (Willett, 2005).

Aging and Longevity:

- Enhanced DNA repair and reduced DNA damage contribute to healthier aging and increased longevity. Antioxidant-rich plant foods play a crucial role in this process.

- **Study:** "Diet, DNA damage and human longevity" published in *Genes & Nutrition* examines the relationship between diet, DNA repair, and aging (Sahin & DePinho, 2010).

Reproductive Health:

- Proper DNA replication and repair are vital for reproductive health. Nutrients from plant-based diets support these processes, ensuring healthy gametogenesis and embryogenesis.
- **Study:** "Nutrition and reproductive health: A review of the evidence" published in *Nutrients* emphasizes the role of nutrition in reproductive health and DNA integrity (Gaskins & Chavarro, 2018).

Neuroprotection:

- DNA damage in neurons can lead to neurodegenerative diseases. Plant-based diets, rich in antioxidants and anti-inflammatory compounds, help protect against such damage.
- **Study:** "Neuroprotective effects of plant-based diets and phytochemicals on DNA damage" published in *Journal of Alzheimer's Disease* explores the neuroprotective role of plant-based diets (Joseph et al., 2009).

DNA polymerase is a fundamental enzyme essential for DNA replication and repair, ensuring the fidelity and stability of genetic information. Its function, production, and regulation are tightly controlled by cellular mechanisms and influenced by various factors, including diet. A plant-based diet, rich in antioxidants, essential nutrients, and anti-inflammatory compounds, supports optimal DNA polymerase activity and genomic stability. By promoting DNA repair, reducing oxidative stress, and maintaining overall health, a plant-based diet can enhance DNA polymerase function and contribute to the prevention of diseases, healthier aging, and improved reproductive and neuroprotective outcomes.

RNA Polymerase

RNA polymerase is a fundamental enzyme in the cellular machinery, responsible for synthesizing RNA from a DNA template, a process known as transcription.

Function of RNA Polymerase

RNA polymerase plays several critical roles in the cell, each essential for gene expression and the proper functioning of cellular processes.

1. **Transcription Initiation**: RNA polymerase binds to a specific region of the DNA called the promoter to initiate transcription. This binding requires various transcription factors and regulatory proteins.
2. **RNA Synthesis**: Once bound, RNA polymerase unwinds the DNA and synthesizes an RNA strand complementary to the DNA template. This process involves the addition of ribonucleotides in a 5′ to 3′ direction.
3. **Transcription Elongation**: RNA polymerase moves along the DNA template, elongating the RNA strand by adding nucleotides. This phase is highly regulated and involves several accessory proteins.

4. **Transcription Termination**: RNA polymerase recognizes specific sequences signaling the end of transcription, releasing the newly synthesized RNA and detaching from the DNA template.

Types of RNA Polymerase

In eukaryotes, there are three main types of RNA polymerase, each responsible for transcribing different types of RNA:

1. **RNA Polymerase I**: Synthesizes rRNA (ribosomal RNA), essential for ribosome assembly and protein synthesis.
2. **RNA Polymerase II**: Synthesizes mRNA (messenger RNA), which serves as a template for protein synthesis during translation.
3. **RNA Polymerase III**: Synthesizes tRNA (transfer RNA) and other small RNAs, involved in various cellular processes, including protein synthesis and gene regulation.

Production of RNA Polymerase

RNA polymerase is produced through a complex process involving multiple steps of gene expression and protein assembly.

1. **Gene Encoding**: The genes encoding RNA polymerase subunits are located on various chromosomes and are transcribed into mRNA by RNA polymerase II.
2. **Translation**: The mRNA is then translated into protein subunits in the cytoplasm. These subunits undergo post-translational modifications, such as phosphorylation, essential for their function.
3. **Assembly**: The individual subunits assemble into the functional RNA polymerase enzyme within the nucleus. This assembly is highly regulated and involves several chaperone proteins to ensure proper folding and functionality.

Regulation of RNA Polymerase

The activity of RNA polymerase is tightly regulated to ensure proper gene expression and cellular function. This regulation occurs at multiple levels:

1. **Promoter Recognition**: The binding of RNA polymerase to the promoter is regulated by transcription factors and other regulatory proteins, which can enhance or inhibit transcription initiation.
2. **Chromatin Structure**: The accessibility of DNA to RNA polymerase is influenced by chromatin structure. Histone modifications and chromatin remodeling complexes play a crucial role in regulating transcription.
3. **Transcription Factors**: Various transcription factors interact with RNA polymerase and the promoter to regulate transcription. These factors can be activated or repressed by signaling pathways responding to cellular and environmental cues.
4. **Epigenetic Modifications**: DNA methylation and histone acetylation are examples of epigenetic modifications that influence RNA polymerase activity by altering chromatin structure and gene accessibility.
5. **Nutritional Status:** Diet and nutritional status can significantly impact RNA polymerase activity. Nutrient availability influences cellular metabolism and the production of metabolites that can modulate transcription.

Plant-Based Diet and RNA Polymerase Regulation

A plant-based diet can positively influence the regulation of RNA polymerase through various mechanisms.

1. **Antioxidants**: Plant-based foods are rich in antioxidants, which reduce oxidative stress and prevent damage to DNA and proteins, including RNA polymerase. Lower oxidative stress levels are associated with improved transcriptional regulation.
2. **Phytochemicals**: Compounds found in plants, such as flavonoids and polyphenols, have been shown to modulate gene expression and RNA polymerase activity. These compounds can act as signaling molecules, influencing transcription factors and other regulatory proteins.
3. **Vitamins and Minerals**: Essential nutrients found in plant-based diets, such as vitamin E, vitamin C, and magnesium, play critical roles in maintaining the proper function of RNA polymerase and supporting overall cellular health.
4. **Amino Acids**: Plant-based sources of amino acids, such as legumes and nuts, provide the building blocks for protein synthesis, including the subunits of RNA polymerase. Adequate protein intake ensures the proper production and function of RNA polymerase.
5. **Healthy Fats**: Omega-3 and omega-6 fatty acids found in nuts, seeds, and avocados support the production of signaling molecules that regulate inflammation and cellular processes, including transcription.

Plant-Based Diet on RNA Polymerase-Related Health Outcomes

A plant-based diet can enhance the overall function and regulation of RNA polymerase, leading to improved cellular health and reduced risk of various diseases.

1. **Cancer Prevention**: Antioxidants and phytochemicals in plant-based foods help protect against DNA damage and mutations that can lead to cancer. By maintaining the integrity of the

genome and regulating RNA polymerase activity, a plant-based diet can reduce the risk of cancer development.

2. **Anti-Inflammatory Effects**: The anti-inflammatory properties of a plant-based diet, driven by omega-3 fatty acids and phytochemicals, support healthy gene expression and RNA polymerase activity. Reduced inflammation is associated with a lower risk of chronic diseases such as heart disease and diabetes.
3. **Improved Metabolism**: Nutrients found in plant-based foods support metabolic processes and the production of metabolites that regulate gene expression. A balanced metabolism ensures efficient transcription and RNA polymerase function.
4. **Enhanced Immune Function**: Vitamins and minerals from plant-based sources strengthen the immune system, supporting the production of immune-related proteins and enhancing RNA polymerase activity in immune cells.
5. **Cognitive Health**: Antioxidants and healthy fats in plant-based diets protect against neurodegeneration and support cognitive function. Proper RNA polymerase activity in neurons is essential for maintaining brain health and preventing age-related cognitive decline.

17

Energy Production Enzymes

Adenosine Triphosphate (ATP)

Adenosine triphosphate (ATP) synthase is a vital enzyme in the cellular machinery, responsible for producing ATP, the primary energy carrier in biological systems. This comprehensive analysis delves into the function, production, and regulation of ATP synthase, highlighting dietary influences on its activity and balance, with a particular focus on a plant-based perspective.

Function of ATP Synthase

ATP synthase is an enzyme complex found in the inner mitochondrial membrane and in the thylakoid membrane of chloroplasts in plant cells. Its primary function is the synthesis of ATP from adenosine diphosphate (ADP) and inorganic phosphate (Pi), utilizing a proton gradient generated by the electron transport chain (ETC).

ATP Synthesis

1. **Proton Gradient Utilization**: ATP synthase uses the proton gradient established by the ETC across the inner mitochondrial membrane. Protons flow back into the mitochondrial matrix through ATP synthase, driving the synthesis of ATP.

2. **Catalytic Mechanism**: The enzyme consists of two main components: F0 and F1. The F0 part forms a channel for protons, while the F1 part is responsible for the actual synthesis of ATP. The flow of protons through F0 causes conformational changes in F1, leading to the phosphorylation of ADP to ATP.

Role in Energy Metabolism

1. **Energy Currency**: ATP produced by ATP synthase is crucial for various cellular processes, including muscle contraction, nerve impulse propagation, and chemical synthesis.
2. **Cellular Respiration**: ATP synthase is a key player in cellular respiration, linking the electron transport chain's activity with the production of ATP, thus providing energy necessary for cellular functions.

Production of ATP Synthase

ATP synthase is synthesized through the coordinated expression of nuclear and mitochondrial genes, involving complex pathways that ensure its proper assembly and function.

Gene Encoding

1. **Nuclear and Mitochondrial Genes**: ATP synthase is encoded by both nuclear and mitochondrial DNA. The α, β, γ, δ, and ε subunits of the F1 sector are typically encoded by nuclear genes, whereas subunits of the F0 sector, including ATP6 and ATP8, are encoded by mitochondrial genes.
2. **Protein Import and Assembly**: Nuclear-encoded subunits are synthesized in the cytosol and imported into mitochondria where

they combine with mitochondrial-encoded subunits. This process involves multiple chaperones and assembly factors ensuring correct folding and assembly.

Synthesis and Transport

1. **Transcription and Translation**: Nuclear genes encoding ATP synthase subunits are transcribed in the nucleus and translated in the cytosol. Mitochondrial genes are transcribed and translated within the mitochondria.
2. **Import Mechanisms**: Newly synthesized nuclear-encoded proteins are transported into the mitochondria through translocases in the outer and inner mitochondrial membranes.

Regulation of Gene Expression

1. **Nutrient Availability**: Nutritional status can influence the expression of genes encoding ATP synthase. Adequate intake of essential nutrients supports the synthesis and function of this enzyme.
2. **Energy Demand**: Cellular energy demand regulates the production of ATP synthase. High-energy demand increases the expression of its subunits to meet ATP requirements.

Regulation of ATP Synthase

The regulation of ATP synthase involves various feedback mechanisms, external factors, and physiological states.

Feedback Loops

1. **Energy Demand and Supply**: ATP synthase activity is tightly regulated by the cell's energy demand. When ATP levels are high, ATP synthase activity decreases, and vice versa.

2. **Proton Gradient**: The availability of a proton gradient is crucial for ATP synthase activity. Any disruption in the proton motive force directly affects ATP production.

Nutritional Influence

1. **Macronutrients and Micronutrients**: Adequate intake of macronutrients (carbohydrates, proteins, and fats) and micronutrients (vitamins and minerals) supports the optimal function of ATP synthase. For instance, B vitamins are crucial for the electron transport chain's functioning, which is integral to ATP synthase activity.
2. **Plant-Based Nutrients**: Plant-based diets, rich in antioxidants, fiber, and essential nutrients, can support mitochondrial health and ATP synthase function. Antioxidants reduce oxidative stress, which can otherwise impair mitochondrial function.

Plant-Based Diet and ATP Synthase Regulation

A plant-based diet, comprising fruits, vegetables, whole grains, nuts, and seeds, can positively influence ATP synthase regulation through various mechanisms.

Antioxidants

1. **Oxidative Stress Reduction**: Plant-based diets are rich in antioxidants like vitamins C and E, polyphenols, and carotenoids. These compounds reduce oxidative stress in mitochondria, preserving the function of ATP synthase.

2. **Mitochondrial Protection**: Antioxidants protect mitochondrial membranes from lipid peroxidation, ensuring the integrity and functionality of the proton gradient necessary for ATP synthesis.

Healthy Fats

1. **Essential Fatty Acids**: Plant-based sources of fats, such as omega-3 and omega-6 fatty acids found in flaxseeds, chia seeds, and walnuts, support mitochondrial membrane fluidity and function. These fatty acids are crucial for maintaining the optimal environment for ATP synthase activity.
2. **Anti-Inflammatory Effects**: Omega-3 fatty acids have anti-inflammatory properties that can reduce chronic inflammation, which is known to impair mitochondrial function and ATP production.

Amino Acids

1. **Protein Synthesis**: Certain amino acids, such as arginine and glutamine, are essential for protein synthesis, including the synthesis of ATP synthase subunits. Plant-based sources of these amino acids include legumes, nuts, and seeds.
2. **Nitric Oxide Production**: Arginine is a precursor for nitric oxide, which enhances blood flow and nutrient delivery to tissues, indirectly supporting mitochondrial function and ATP production.

Fiber

1. **Gut Health**: High-fiber diets support gut health and the production of short-chain fatty acids (SCFAs) by the gut microbiota. SCFAs have been shown to improve mitochondrial function and energy metabolism.

2. **Detoxification**: Fiber aids in the elimination of toxins that can impair mitochondrial function. By supporting overall detoxification, a high-fiber diet helps maintain the integrity of the cellular energy production machinery.

Micronutrients

1. **Vitamins and Minerals**: Plant-based diets are rich in vitamins and minerals that are essential for ATP synthase function. For instance, magnesium is a cofactor for ATP production, while iron is critical for electron transport chain components.
2. **Coenzyme Q10**: Although primarily found in animal products, coenzyme Q10 is also present in plant sources like spinach, broccoli, and nuts. It plays a crucial role in the electron transport chain and supports ATP synthesis.

Plant-Based Diet on ATP Synthase-Related Health Outcomes

A plant-based diet can enhance the efficiency and regulation of ATP synthase, contributing to overall health and well-being.

Energy Metabolism

1. **Improved Energy Levels**: Consuming a diet rich in plant-based foods can enhance mitochondrial function, leading to better energy metabolism and higher overall energy levels.
2. **Exercise Performance**: Athletes and physically active individuals may experience improved performance and recovery due to enhanced mitochondrial efficiency and reduced oxidative stress from plant-based nutrients.

Aging and Longevity

1. **Anti-Aging Effects**: The antioxidants and anti-inflammatory compounds in plant-based diets can reduce mitochondrial damage, slow down aging processes, and promote longevity.
2. **Mitochondrial Biogenesis**: Certain plant compounds, such as resveratrol found in grapes and berries, can stimulate mitochondrial biogenesis, leading to an increased number of mitochondria and enhanced ATP production.

Disease Prevention

1. **Chronic Diseases**: A plant-based diet has been shown to reduce the risk of chronic diseases such as cardiovascular disease, diabetes, and neurodegenerative disorders, partly due to its beneficial effects on mitochondrial function.
2. **Cancer Prevention**: By reducing oxidative stress and inflammation, plant-based diets can help protect against the development of cancer, which is often linked to mitochondrial dysfunction and impaired energy metabolism.

Mental Health

1. **Cognitive Function**: Improved mitochondrial function and reduced oxidative stress from a plant-based diet can enhance cognitive function and protect against neurodegenerative diseases.
2. **Mood Regulation**: Nutrients found in plant-based foods, such as magnesium and omega-3 fatty acids, play a role in neurotransmitter synthesis and mood regulation, potentially reducing the risk of depression and anxiety.

ATP synthase is a cornerstone of cellular energy metabolism, crucial for producing the ATP needed for countless biological processes. Its function, production, and regulation are influenced by numerous factors, including diet.

Hexokinase

Hexokinase is a crucial enzyme in the metabolism of glucose, playing a fundamental role in the regulation of glucose homeostasis.

Function of Hexokinase

Hexokinase is the first enzyme in the glycolytic pathway, catalyzing the phosphorylation of glucose to glucose-6-phosphate. This reaction is essential for the metabolism of glucose and has several significant roles:

1. **Glucose Utilization**: Hexokinase facilitates the utilization of glucose by converting it into glucose-6-phosphate, a necessary substrate for glycolysis, the pentose phosphate pathway, and glycogen synthesis.
2. **Regulation of Blood Sugar Levels**: By phosphorylating glucose, hexokinase effectively traps glucose within cells, thus regulating blood glucose levels.
3. **Energy Production**: The conversion of glucose to glucose-6-phosphate is a critical step in glycolysis, leading to the production of ATP, the primary energy currency of the cell.
4. **Metabolic Flux Control**: Hexokinase activity is a key control point in cellular metabolism, influencing various metabolic pathways depending on the cell's energy needs.

Production of Hexokinase

Hexokinase is produced in several tissues, with different isoforms expressed in specific tissues to meet varying metabolic demands.

Gene Encoding: Hexokinase is encoded by multiple genes, leading to the production of four primary isoforms (HK1, HK2, HK3, and HK4/Glucokinase) in mammals.

- **HK1**: Ubiquitously expressed in most tissues.
- **HK2**: Predominantly found in muscle and adipose tissues.
- **HK3**: Less well characterized, with limited tissue distribution.
- **HK4 (Glucokinase)**: Primarily expressed in the liver and pancreatic beta cells.

Transcriptional Regulation: The expression of hexokinase genes is regulated by various transcription factors and is influenced by hormonal and nutritional states. Insulin, for example, upregulates the expression of hexokinase in insulin-responsive tissues.

Post-translational Modifications: Hexokinase activity can be modulated by post-translational modifications such as phosphorylation, which affects its activity and interaction with other cellular components.

Regulation of Hexokinase

The regulation of hexokinase involves a complex interplay of feedback mechanisms, external factors, and physiological states.

1. **Feedback Inhibition**: Hexokinase activity is subject to feedback inhibition by its product, glucose-6-phosphate. This mechanism ensures that hexokinase does not deplete cellular ATP levels by excessively phosphorylating glucose.

2. **Compartmentalization**: Hexokinase is often associated with the outer mitochondrial membrane, which facilitates efficient ATP utilization and integration with cellular energy metabolism.
3. **Hormonal Regulation**: Insulin and glucagon play significant roles in regulating hexokinase activity. Insulin promotes hexokinase expression and activity, enhancing glucose uptake and metabolism, while glucagon has the opposite effect.
4. **Nutritional Status**: Nutrient availability influences hexokinase activity. High carbohydrate intake increases hexokinase activity, while fasting or low carbohydrate intake reduces it.
5. **Exercise and Muscle Contraction**: Physical activity increases hexokinase activity in muscle tissues, enhancing glucose uptake and utilization to meet increased energy demands.

Plant-Based Diet and Hexokinase Regulation

A plant-based diet, rich in whole foods such as fruits, vegetables, whole grains, nuts, and seeds, can positively influence hexokinase activity through various mechanisms:

1. **Nutrient Density**: Plant-based diets provide essential nutrients, vitamins, and minerals that support overall metabolic health. For example, magnesium, found in leafy greens, nuts, and seeds, is a cofactor for hexokinase and other enzymes involved in glucose metabolism.
2. **Phytochemicals**: Bioactive compounds in plant foods, such as polyphenols and flavonoids, have been shown to enhance insulin sensitivity and improve glucose metabolism, indirectly supporting hexokinase activity.
3. **Dietary Fiber**: High-fiber diets help maintain stable blood glucose levels by slowing glucose absorption, which can enhance hexokinase function by providing a steady supply of glucose for metabolism.

4. **Antioxidants**: Plant-based diets are rich in antioxidants, which reduce oxidative stress and inflammation, potentially improving hexokinase activity and overall metabolic health.
5. **Healthy Fats**: Unsaturated fats from plant sources, such as avocados, nuts, and seeds, support insulin sensitivity and metabolic health, which are crucial for optimal hexokinase activity.
6. **Caloric Balance**: Maintaining a healthy weight through a balanced plant-based diet can prevent obesity-related metabolic disruptions. Excess body fat is associated with reduced hexokinase activity due to insulin resistance.

Plant-Based Diet on Hexokinase-Related Health Outcomes

• **Diabetes Management**: A plant-based diet can improve insulin sensitivity and glycemic control, enhancing hexokinase activity and glucose metabolism. Studies have shown that individuals following a plant-based diet have a lower risk of developing type 2 diabetes.

Reference: Barnard, N. D., Levin, S. M., & Yokoyama, Y. (2014). A systematic review and meta-analysis of changes in body weight in clinical trials of vegetarian diets. Journal of the Academy of Nutrition and Dietetics, 114(12), 1942-1948.

• **Cardiovascular Health**: Improved glucose metabolism and reduced inflammation from a plant-based diet support cardiovascular health by reducing risk factors such as high blood sugar and obesity.

Reference: Satija, A., Bhupathiraju, S. N., Rimm, E. B., Spiegelman, D., Chiuve, S. E., Borgi, L., ... & Hu, F. B. (2016). Plant-based dietary patterns and incidence of type 2 diabetes in US men and women: results from three prospective cohort studies. PLoS Medicine, 13(6), e1002039.

• **Weight Management**: A plant-based diet is effective for weight management, reducing body fat and improving insulin sensitivity. Lower body fat and better glycemic control enhance overall hexokinase activity.

Reference: Tonstad, S., Stewart, K., Oda, K., Batech, M., Herring, R. P., & Fraser, G. E. (2013). Vegetarian diets and incidence of diabetes in the Adventist Health Study-2. Nutrition, Metabolism and Cardiovascular Diseases, 23(4), 292-299.

• **Mental Health**: Emerging evidence suggests that plant-based diets may benefit mental health by reducing inflammation and oxidative stress, which are linked to mood disorders. Improved glucose metabolism and insulin sensitivity also support cognitive function and emotional well-being.

Reference: Jacka, F. N., O'Neil, A., Opie, R., Itsiopoulos, C., Cotton, S., Mohebbi, M., ... & Berk, M. (2017). A randomized controlled trial of dietary improvement for adults with major depression (the "SMILES" trial). BMC Medicine, 15(1), 23.

• **Anti-Aging Effects**: The antioxidant-rich nature of plant-based diets helps combat oxidative stress, a key factor in aging. Improved metabolic health and hexokinase activity contribute to healthier aging and better maintenance of energy levels.

Reference: Sohal, R. S., & Orr, W. C. (2012). The redox stress hypothesis of aging. Free Radical Biology and Medicine, 52(3), 539-555.

Hexokinase plays a pivotal role in glucose metabolism, regulating functions from glucose utilization and energy production to overall metabolic health. Its production and regulation are influenced by various factors, including hormonal and nutritional status, physical activity, and cellular compartmentalization.

Phosphofructokinase (PFK)

Phosphofructokinase (PFK) is a key regulatory enzyme in the glycolytic pathway, playing a crucial role in cellular metabolism and energy production. This enzyme is responsible for the phosphorylation of fructose-6-phosphate to fructose-1,6-bisphosphate, a critical step in glycolysis.

Function of Phosphofructokinase

Phosphofructokinase catalyzes one of the most important steps in glycolysis, controlling the rate of glucose breakdown and, consequently, energy production in cells. This enzyme's function is vital for maintaining cellular energy homeostasis and supporting various physiological processes.

Glycolysis Regulation

PFK serves as a rate-limiting enzyme in glycolysis, meaning its activity determines the overall rate of this metabolic pathway. The conversion of fructose-6-phosphate to fructose-1,6-bisphosphate is an irreversible step, committing the substrate to further breakdown and energy extraction.

Energy Production

By regulating glycolysis, PFK controls the production of ATP, the primary energy currency of the cell. ATP is essential for numerous cellular processes, including muscle contraction, protein synthesis, and cell division.

Metabolic Flexibility

PFK allows cells to adapt to varying energy demands. During high-intensity exercise or in rapidly dividing cells, increased PFK activity ensures a higher rate of glycolysis, providing the necessary ATP to meet the increased energy requirements.

Coordination with Other Metabolic Pathways

PFK interacts with other metabolic pathways, such as gluconeogenesis and the pentose phosphate pathway. By modulating glycolytic flux, PFK ensures a balanced supply of intermediates for these pathways, which are crucial for biosynthesis and redox balance.

Production of Phosphofructokinase

The production of PFK is tightly regulated at both the genetic and post-translational levels to ensure proper enzyme activity in response to cellular needs.

Gene Encoding

PFK is encoded by multiple genes in humans, resulting in different isoforms that are expressed in various tissues. These genes include PFKM (muscle), PFKL (liver), and PFKP (platelets), each tailored to the metabolic demands of specific tissues.

Isoforms and Tissue Specificity

- **PFKM**: Predominantly expressed in skeletal muscle, this isoform supports high glycolytic flux during intense physical activity.
- **PFKL**: Found mainly in the liver, PFKL plays a role in maintaining blood glucose levels and supporting hepatic metabolism.
- **PFKP**: Present in platelets and other tissues, PFKP ensures adequate glycolytic activity in cells with varying metabolic needs.

Transcriptional Regulation

The expression of PFK genes is controlled by various transcription factors and signaling pathways. For example, hypoxia-inducible factor 1 (HIF-1) upregulates PFK expression in response to low oxygen levels, ensuring continued ATP production under hypoxic conditions.

Post-Translational Modifications

PFK activity is also modulated by post-translational modifications, such as phosphorylation, acetylation, and glycosylation. These modifications can either enhance or inhibit enzyme activity, allowing cells to rapidly adjust glycolysis in response to changing metabolic conditions.

Regulation of Phosphofructokinase

The regulation of PFK is a complex interplay of allosteric modulators, hormonal signals, and metabolic intermediates, ensuring that glycolytic flux matches cellular energy demands.

Allosteric Regulation

PFK is subject to allosteric regulation by various metabolites that reflect the cell's energy status.

- **ATP**: High levels of ATP inhibit PFK, signaling that the cell has sufficient energy and reducing glycolytic flux.
- **AMP**: In contrast, AMP activates PFK, indicating low energy levels and promoting glycolysis.
- **Citrate**: As an intermediate of the citric acid cycle, citrate inhibits PFK, linking glycolysis to the availability of substrates for the citric acid cycle.
- **Fructose-2,6-bisphosphate**: This potent activator of PFK enhances its affinity for fructose-6-phosphate, promoting glycolysis in response to hormonal signals.

Hormonal Regulation

Hormones play a significant role in regulating PFK activity, particularly insulin and glucagon, which manage blood glucose levels and energy homeostasis.

- **Insulin**: Promotes PFK activity by increasing the levels of fructose-2,6-bisphosphate, thereby enhancing glycolysis and glucose uptake.
- **Glucagon**: Opposes insulin's effects, reducing fructose-2,6-bisphosphate levels and inhibiting PFK activity, which shifts metabolism towards gluconeogenesis during fasting.

Nutritional Status

The cell's nutritional status profoundly influences PFK activity, with nutrient availability affecting both allosteric regulators and hormonal signals.

- **Carbohydrate Intake**: High carbohydrate intake boosts insulin secretion, increasing PFK activity and promoting glycolysis.
- **Starvation**: During fasting, glucagon levels rise, decreasing PFK activity and favoring gluconeogenesis to maintain blood glucose levels.

Exercise and Physical Activity

Physical activity exerts a significant impact on PFK regulation, especially in muscle tissues.

- **Acute Exercise**: Increases AMP levels and reduces ATP, activating PFK and accelerating glycolysis to meet immediate energy demands.
- **Chronic Training**: Enhances the expression of PFKM, improving muscle glycolytic capacity and endurance.

Plant-Based Diet and Phosphofructokinase Regulation

A plant-based diet, rich in fruits, vegetables, whole grains, nuts, and seeds, can positively influence PFK regulation through various mechanisms, supporting optimal metabolic health and energy balance.

Nutrient Density

Plant-based diets provide essential nutrients, vitamins, and minerals that support overall metabolic health. For example, magnesium found in leafy greens and nuts is a cofactor for PFK, enhancing its activity.

Amino Acids

Plant-based sources of amino acids, such as legumes and soy products, provide the building blocks for enzyme synthesis, including PFK. Adequate protein intake supports the maintenance and production of metabolic enzymes.

Antioxidants

Fruits and vegetables are rich in antioxidants, which help reduce oxidative stress. Lower oxidative stress levels are associated with improved metabolic function, including PFK activity.

Healthy Fats

Plant-based sources of fats, such as avocados, nuts, and seeds, provide essential fatty acids that support cell membrane integrity and enzyme function. Omega-3 fatty acids, in particular, have anti-inflammatory properties that can enhance metabolic health.

Fiber

High-fiber diets, common in plant-based eating, support gut health and metabolic regulation. A healthy gut microbiome can influence overall metabolic function, including glycolysis.

Caloric Balance

Maintaining a healthy weight through a balanced plant-based diet can prevent obesity-related metabolic imbalances. Excess body fat is linked to insulin resistance, which can negatively impact glycolysis and PFK activity.

Glycemic Control

Plant-based diets, which are low in refined sugars and high in complex carbohydrates, help maintain stable blood glucose levels. This stability prevents insulin resistance, supporting proper glycolytic function.

Impact of Plant-Based Diet on PFK-Related Health Outcomes

Energy Levels and Endurance

A plant-based diet can support sustained energy levels and improved endurance by promoting efficient glycolysis. Nutrient-dense foods provide the vitamins and minerals necessary for optimal enzyme function.

Weight Management

Plant-based diets are effective for weight management, reducing body fat, and improving insulin sensitivity. Lower body fat and better glycemic control enhance overall metabolic health, including PFK activity.

Cardiovascular Health

Improved glycolytic function supports cardiovascular health by providing adequate energy for cardiac muscle function. Plant-based diets, rich in antioxidants and healthy fats, reduce the risk of cardiovascular diseases.

Diabetes Management

Stable blood glucose levels and improved insulin sensitivity, facilitated by a plant-based diet, support proper glycolysis and PFK function. This can help manage and prevent type 2 diabetes.

Mental Health

Emerging evidence suggests that plant-based diets may benefit mental health by reducing inflammation and oxidative stress, which are linked to mood disorders. Improved metabolic function, including PFK activity, supports cognitive function and emotional well-being.

Anti-Aging Effects

The antioxidant-rich nature of plant-based diets helps combat oxidative stress, a key factor in aging. Enhanced metabolic function and reduced oxidative damage contribute to healthier aging.

Phosphofructokinase plays a pivotal role in cellular metabolism, regulating glycolysis and energy production. Its production and regulation are influenced by various factors, including genetic expression, post-translational modifications, allosteric modulators, hormonal signals, and nutritional status.

Phosphopyruvate Kinase (PK)

Phosphopyruvate kinase (PK) is a crucial enzyme in the glycolytic pathway, playing a pivotal role in energy production within cells.

Function of Phosphopyruvate Kinase

Phosphopyruvate kinase is an essential enzyme in the glycolytic pathway, catalyzing the final step of glycolysis. It converts phosphoenolpyruvate (PEP) to pyruvate, generating ATP in the process. This reaction is critical for cellular energy production, particularly in tissues that rely heavily on glycolysis for ATP, such as muscle and brain tissues.

Role in Glycolysis

1. **Catalytic Reaction**: PK catalyzes the transfer of a phosphate group from PEP to ADP, forming ATP and pyruvate. This reaction is a key step in glycolysis, as it generates one of the two net ATP molecules produced in this pathway.
2. **Regulation of Metabolic Flux**: By controlling the conversion of PEP to pyruvate, PK regulates the flow of metabolites through glycolysis. This control is essential for maintaining cellular energy balance and metabolic homeostasis.
3. **Link to Other Metabolic Pathways**: The pyruvate produced by PK serves as a substrate for several other metabolic pathways, including the citric acid cycle (TCA cycle) and lactic acid

fermentation, linking glycolysis to aerobic and anaerobic energy production.

Additional Roles

1. **Redox Balance**: By facilitating ATP production under anaerobic conditions, PK helps maintain the redox balance in cells, preventing the accumulation of NADH and ensuring the continuous operation of glycolysis.
2. **Cellular Proliferation**: PK activity is often upregulated in proliferating cells, such as cancer cells, to meet their increased energy and biosynthetic demands.

Production of Phosphopyruvate Kinase

Phosphopyruvate kinase is produced through a complex process involving gene expression, protein synthesis, and post-translational modifications. The regulation of PK production is tightly controlled to meet the varying energy demands of different tissues.

Gene Encoding

1. **Isoforms**: There are several isoforms of PK, encoded by different genes. In humans, these include PKM1, PKM2, PKL, and PKR, each with tissue-specific expression patterns. PKM2, for instance, is prevalent in proliferating cells and tumors, while PKL is primarily found in the liver.
2. **Gene Location**: The PKM gene, encoding PKM1 and PKM2 isoforms, is located on chromosome 15. PKL and PKR are encoded by separate genes on different chromosomes.

Synthesis

1. **Transcription**: The transcription of PK genes is regulated by various transcription factors, which respond to cellular energy status and other signals. Hypoxia-inducible factor 1-alpha (HIF-1α) and Myc are examples of transcription factors that upregulate PKM2 expression in response to low oxygen levels and cellular proliferation signals.
2. **Translation**: The mRNA produced from PK genes is translated into protein in the cytoplasm. Ribosomes facilitate the assembly of amino acids into the PK enzyme based on the mRNA template.

Post-Translational Modifications

1. **Phosphorylation**: PK activity can be modulated by phosphorylation, which alters the enzyme's conformation and activity. This modification allows cells to rapidly adjust PK activity in response to changing metabolic needs.
2. **Allosteric Regulation**: PK can also be regulated allosterically by metabolites such as fructose-1,6-bisphosphate, which enhances its activity, and ATP, which inhibits it. These modifications enable fine-tuning of glycolytic flux based on cellular energy status.

Regulation of Phosphopyruvate Kinase

The regulation of PK involves a complex interplay of genetic, metabolic, and environmental factors. This regulation ensures that PK activity aligns with cellular energy demands and overall metabolic status.

Genetic Regulation

1. **Transcriptional Control**: PK gene expression is regulated by transcription factors responsive to metabolic cues. For instance, under hypoxic conditions, HIF-1α increases the transcription of PKM2, promoting glycolysis and anaerobic ATP production.
2. **Epigenetic Modifications**: Epigenetic changes, such as DNA methylation and histone acetylation, can also influence PK gene expression. These modifications can be reversible and allow dynamic regulation of PK production in response to environmental and metabolic changes.

Allosteric Regulation

1. **Activator Metabolites**: Fructose-1,6-bisphosphate, an intermediate of glycolysis, acts as an allosteric activator of PK. This metabolite enhances PK activity, ensuring a rapid response to increased glycolytic flux.
2. **Inhibitor Metabolites**: ATP and alanine are allosteric inhibitors of PK. High levels of these metabolites indicate sufficient energy availability, prompting a decrease in PK activity to prevent excessive ATP production and conserve resources.

Hormonal Regulation

1. **Insulin**: Insulin stimulates PK activity by promoting the dephosphorylation and activation of the enzyme. This regulation supports increased glycolysis and energy production in response to elevated blood glucose levels.

2. **Glucagon**: In contrast, glucagon inhibits PK activity through phosphorylation, reducing glycolytic flux during fasting or low glucose conditions. This inhibition helps to conserve glucose for critical functions and promotes gluconeogenesis.

Plant-Based Diet and Phosphopyruvate Kinase Regulation

A plant-based diet, rich in fruits, vegetables, whole grains, nuts, and seeds, can positively influence PK regulation through various mechanisms.

Nutrient Density

1. **Vitamins and Minerals**: Plant-based diets provide essential vitamins and minerals, such as magnesium and B vitamins, which are crucial for enzyme function and energy metabolism. Magnesium, for instance, is a cofactor for many enzymes, including those involved in glycolysis.
2. **Antioxidants**: Fruits and vegetables are rich in antioxidants, which help reduce oxidative stress. Lower oxidative stress levels are associated with improved metabolic balance, including PK activity.

Healthy Carbohydrates

1. **Complex Carbohydrates**: Whole grains, legumes, and starchy vegetables provide complex carbohydrates that supply a steady release of glucose, supporting sustained glycolytic activity and energy production.
2. **Low Glycemic Index**: Foods with a low glycemic index, common in plant-based diets, help maintain stable blood glucose levels, preventing excessive fluctuations that can disrupt PK regulation.

Amino Acids

1. **Protein Sources**: Plant-based protein sources, such as legumes, nuts, and seeds, provide amino acids necessary for protein synthesis, including PK. These sources also support overall metabolic health.
2. **Balanced Amino Acid Profile**: A diverse plant-based diet ensures a balanced intake of essential amino acids, promoting optimal enzyme production and function.

Fiber

1. **Gut Health**: High-fiber diets support gut health by promoting a healthy microbiome. A well-balanced gut microbiome can influence metabolic regulation through the production of short-chain fatty acids and other metabolites.
2. **Stable Blood Sugar**: Dietary fiber helps regulate blood sugar levels, preventing spikes and crashes that can affect PK activity and overall metabolic balance.

Impact of Plant-Based Diet on PK-Related Health Outcomes

Energy Production

1. **Sustained Energy Levels**: A plant-based diet supports sustained energy levels by providing complex carbohydrates and maintaining stable blood glucose. This stability promotes efficient glycolysis and ATP production.
2. **Enhanced Athletic Performance**: Athletes following a plant-based diet may experience improved performance due to better energy management and reduced oxidative stress.

Metabolic Health

1. **Insulin Sensitivity**: Plant-based diets are associated with improved insulin sensitivity, which supports better regulation of glycolysis and PK activity.
2. **Weight Management**: A plant-based diet helps maintain a healthy weight, reducing the risk of obesity-related metabolic disorders that can disrupt PK regulation.

Chronic Disease Prevention

1. **Diabetes Management**: Plant-based diets can help manage and prevent type 2 diabetes by promoting stable blood glucose levels and improving insulin sensitivity.
2. **Cardiovascular Health**: Reduced oxidative stress and improved metabolic health from a plant-based diet contribute to better cardiovascular outcomes, indirectly supporting overall metabolic regulation, including PK activity.

Phosphopyruvate kinase is a critical enzyme in the glycolytic pathway, essential for cellular energy production. Its function, production, and regulation are influenced by genetic, metabolic, and environmental factors, with allosteric and hormonal controls playing significant roles.

Lactate Dehydrogenase (LDH)

Lactate dehydrogenase (LDH) is a crucial enzyme in the human body, playing a vital role in the conversion of lactate to pyruvate in the metabolic pathway.

Function of Lactate Dehydrogenase

LDH is an essential enzyme involved in the anaerobic metabolism of glucose. It catalyzes the reversible conversion of pyruvate to lactate, a key step in glycolysis and the Cori cycle.

Metabolic Role:

1. **Anaerobic Glycolysis:** LDH facilitates the conversion of pyruvate to lactate when oxygen levels are low, allowing glycolysis to continue and produce ATP. This is crucial during intense exercise or in tissues with limited oxygen supply.
2. **Cori Cycle:** In the liver, LDH helps convert lactate back to pyruvate, which can then be used for gluconeogenesis, providing a means to maintain blood glucose levels during prolonged exercise or fasting.

Tissue Specificity:

1. **Muscle Tissue:** In skeletal muscles, LDH enables the rapid conversion of pyruvate to lactate, supporting ATP production under anaerobic conditions.
2. **Liver:** LDH in the liver aids in converting lactate back to pyruvate for gluconeogenesis, which is crucial for maintaining energy homeostasis.
3. **Heart:** The heart predominantly utilizes the LDH isozyme LDH-1, which favors the conversion of lactate to pyruvate, reflecting its reliance on aerobic metabolism.

Additional Roles:

1. **Wound Healing:** LDH activity is associated with cellular processes involved in wound healing and tissue repair, as it helps supply the necessary energy.
2. **Immune Response:** LDH plays a role in the metabolic reprogramming of immune cells, supporting their activation and function.

Production of Lactate Dehydrogenase

LDH is produced in various tissues throughout the body, with different tissues expressing distinct LDH isozymes tailored to their metabolic needs.

Synthesis:

1. **Gene Encoding:** The LDH enzyme is encoded by multiple genes (LDHA, LDHB, LDHC, LDHD, LDHE) that produce different subunits. These subunits combine to form five possible isoenzymes (LDH-1 to LDH-5), each with distinct kinetic properties.
2. **Isoenzymes:** LDH-1 (H4) is prevalent in the heart, LDH-2 (H3M1) in reticuloendothelial tissues, LDH-3 (H2M2) in the lungs, LDH-4 (H1M3) in the kidneys and pancreas, and LDH-5 (M4) in the liver and skeletal muscle.

Regulation by Genetic Factors:

1. **Gene Expression:** The expression of LDH genes is regulated by factors such as hypoxia-inducible factor 1 (HIF-1) under low oxygen conditions, enhancing the production of LDH to support anaerobic metabolism.

2. **Post-translational Modifications:** LDH activity can be modulated by post-translational modifications such as phosphorylation, which alters its kinetic properties and stability.

Tissue-Specific Expression:

1. **Skeletal Muscle:** Predominantly expresses the LDH-5 isozyme, which is efficient in converting pyruvate to lactate, supporting anaerobic ATP production.
2. **Heart Muscle:** Expresses primarily LDH-1, favoring the conversion of lactate to pyruvate, supporting aerobic metabolism.

Regulation of Lactate Dehydrogenase

The regulation of LDH involves complex interactions of feedback mechanisms, external factors, and physiological states.

Feedback Mechanisms:

1. **Substrate Availability:** The levels of pyruvate and lactate directly influence LDH activity. High pyruvate levels drive the conversion to lactate, while high lactate levels favor the reverse reaction.
2. **Allosteric Regulation:** LDH activity can be modulated by allosteric effectors such as fructose-1,6-bisphosphate, which enhances its affinity for substrates.

Hypoxia and Exercise:

1. **Hypoxia:** Low oxygen levels upregulate LDH expression through HIF-1, promoting anaerobic glycolysis.
2. **Exercise:** Intense physical activity increases LDH activity in muscles to meet the high energy demands under anaerobic conditions.

Hormonal Influence:

1. **Insulin:** Promotes glycolysis and indirectly influences LDH activity by increasing glucose uptake and metabolism.
2. **Epinephrine:** Stimulates glycogenolysis and glycolysis in response to stress or exercise, indirectly enhancing LDH activity to support rapid ATP production.

Nutritional Status:

1. **Dietary Carbohydrates:** High carbohydrate intake increases glucose availability, promoting glycolysis and subsequently LDH activity.
2. **Plant-Based Nutrients:** Certain plant-based nutrients can modulate LDH activity. For example, antioxidants in fruits and vegetables reduce oxidative stress, potentially affecting LDH regulation.

Plant-Based Diet and Lactate Dehydrogenase Regulation

A plant-based diet, rich in fruits, vegetables, whole grains, nuts, and seeds, can positively influence LDH regulation through various mechanisms.

Nutrient Density:

1. **Vitamins and Minerals:** Plant-based diets provide essential nutrients like vitamin C, vitamin E, and magnesium, which support overall metabolic health and enzymatic function.

2. **Antioxidants:** Fruits and vegetables are rich in antioxidants, which reduce oxidative stress and may influence LDH activity by maintaining cellular homeostasis.

Amino Acids:

1. **Arginine and Glutamine:** Found in nuts, seeds, and legumes, these amino acids support protein synthesis and metabolic functions, potentially enhancing LDH activity and stability.

Fiber:

1. **Gut Health:** High-fiber diets support a healthy gut microbiome, which produces metabolites that can influence systemic metabolism, including LDH activity.
2. **Glycemic Control:** Dietary fiber helps maintain stable blood glucose levels, indirectly supporting consistent energy production and LDH activity.

Healthy Fats:

1. **Omega-3 Fatty Acids:** Found in flaxseeds, chia seeds, and walnuts, these fats have anti-inflammatory properties that support overall metabolic health and may influence LDH activity.

Phytochemicals:

1. **Polyphenols:** Present in a variety of plant foods, polyphenols have antioxidant and anti-inflammatory properties, which can support metabolic health and potentially modulate LDH activity.

Plant-Based Diet on LDH-Related Health Outcomes
Metabolic Health:

1. **Glycemic Control:** A plant-based diet helps maintain stable blood glucose levels, supporting efficient energy production and LDH activity.
2. **Weight Management:** Plant-based diets are effective for weight management, reducing body fat, and improving insulin sensitivity, which enhances overall metabolic health.

Exercise Performance:

1. **Endurance:** The high nutrient density and antioxidant content of plant-based diets support muscle function and recovery, potentially enhancing LDH activity during prolonged exercise.
2. **Recovery:** Antioxidants and anti-inflammatory compounds in plant-based diets support faster recovery by reducing muscle damage and oxidative stress.

Cardiovascular Health:

1. **Heart Function:** Plant-based diets rich in antioxidants, fiber, and healthy fats support cardiovascular health, indirectly supporting LDH activity in heart tissues.
2. **Blood Pressure:** Lower sodium intake and higher potassium intake from plant-based foods help maintain healthy blood pressure, supporting overall cardiovascular function.

Chronic Disease Prevention:

1. **Diabetes:** A plant-based diet can improve insulin sensitivity and glycemic control, reducing the risk of type 2 diabetes and its complications.
2. **Cancer:** Antioxidants and anti-inflammatory compounds in plant-based diets help reduce the risk of certain cancers by protecting against cellular damage.

Immune Function:

1. **Anti-Inflammatory Effects:** Plant-based diets rich in fruits, vegetables, and whole grains reduce inflammation, supporting a healthy immune response and potentially modulating LDH activity in immune cells.
2. **Antioxidant Support:** High levels of antioxidants in plant-based diets help maintain immune cell function and reduce oxidative stress, supporting overall immune health.

Anti-Aging Effects:

1. **Oxidative Stress Reduction:** The antioxidant-rich nature of plant-based diets helps combat oxidative stress, a key factor in aging. This supports overall cellular function and enzymatic activity, including LDH.
2. **Hormonal Balance:** Plant-based diets support hormonal balance, which is crucial for maintaining metabolic health and LDH activity as we age.

Bone Health:

1. **Calcium and Vitamin K:** Leafy greens and fortified plant milk provide calcium and vitamin K, which are essential for bone health. These nutrients work synergistically to support bone density and overall skeletal health.
2. **Magnesium:** Found in nuts, seeds, and whole grains, magnesium supports bone health and overall metabolic function, including LDH activity.

Lactate dehydrogenase plays a pivotal role in metabolic processes, enabling the conversion of pyruvate to lactate under anaerobic conditions and supporting energy production. Its production and regulation are influenced by genetic factors, substrate availability, hormonal signals, and external factors such as exercise and diet.

18

Gluconeogenesis/Glycogen Metabolism Enzymes

Glucose-6-Phosphatase (G6Pase)

Glucose-6-phosphatase (G6Pase) is a crucial enzyme in the regulation of blood glucose levels, playing a significant role in gluconeogenesis and glycogenolysis. This enzyme's activity is vital for maintaining glucose homeostasis, particularly during fasting or periods of low carbohydrate intake.

Function of Glucose-6-Phosphatase

G6Pase is primarily involved in the final step of gluconeogenesis and glycogenolysis, processes essential for glucose production and release into the bloodstream.

Gluconeogenesis

Gluconeogenesis is the metabolic pathway through which glucose is synthesized from non-carbohydrate substrates, such as lactate, glycerol, and amino acids. This process is crucial during periods of fasting, starvation, or intense exercise when carbohydrate intake is insufficient to meet the body's energy demands.

1. **Final Step Catalysis**: G6Pase catalyzes the hydrolysis of glucose-6-phosphate (G6P) to glucose and inorganic phosphate.

This reaction takes place in the endoplasmic reticulum of liver and kidney cells, allowing glucose to be exported into the bloodstream.

2. **Blood Glucose Regulation**: By facilitating the production of glucose from non-carbohydrate sources, G6Pase helps maintain blood glucose levels within a narrow range, ensuring a constant supply of energy to vital organs, especially the brain.

Glycogenolysis

Glycogenolysis is the breakdown of glycogen to glucose, a critical process during fasting and intense physical activity.

1. **Glycogen Breakdown**: In the liver, G6Pase helps convert glycogen-derived glucose-6-phosphate to free glucose, which is then released into the bloodstream to maintain energy levels.
2. **Energy Supply**: This process ensures a rapid supply of glucose during acute energy demands, such as those experienced during exercise or stress.

Additional Roles

1. **Metabolic Homeostasis**: G6Pase activity is integral to the overall regulation of carbohydrate metabolism, impacting pathways like glycolysis and the citric acid cycle.
2. **Preventing Hypoglycemia**: By enabling glucose production and release, G6Pase prevents hypoglycemia, a condition characterized by dangerously low blood glucose levels.

Production of Glucose-6-Phosphatase

G6Pase production involves complex biochemical pathways and regulatory mechanisms to ensure its availability and proper function.

Gene Encoding

1. **G6PC Gene**: The G6PC gene located on chromosome 17 encodes the catalytic subunit of G6Pase. Mutations in this gene can lead to glycogen storage diseases, such as type I glycogen storage disease (Von Gierke disease).
2. **Isoforms**: Multiple isoforms of G6Pase exist, each encoded by distinct genes (e.g., G6PC2 and G6PC3), and exhibiting tissue-specific expression patterns.

Synthesis and Localization

1. **Endoplasmic Reticulum**: G6Pase is synthesized in the endoplasmic reticulum (ER) of liver and kidney cells. The enzyme's localization to the ER membrane is essential for its function in glucose production.
2. **Enzyme Complex**: G6Pase functions as part of a multi-protein complex that includes transport proteins facilitating the movement of G6P and phosphate across the ER membrane.

Regulation of Glucose-6-Phosphatase

The regulation of G6Pase involves various hormonal, nutritional, and metabolic factors to maintain glucose homeostasis.

Hormonal Regulation

1. **Insulin**: Insulin inhibits G6Pase expression and activity. This hormone, secreted by the pancreas in response to high blood glucose levels, suppresses gluconeogenesis and glycogenolysis, promoting glucose uptake and storage.
2. **Glucagon**: In contrast, glucagon stimulates G6Pase activity. Secreted by the pancreas during low blood glucose levels, glucagon

promotes gluconeogenesis and glycogenolysis to increase blood glucose availability.

3. **Cortisol and Epinephrine**: These stress hormones also enhance G6Pase activity, ensuring sufficient glucose production during stress or energy-demanding situations.

Nutritional Regulation

1. **Carbohydrate Intake**: High carbohydrate intake suppresses G6Pase activity by increasing insulin levels, which inhibit gluconeogenesis and glycogenolysis.
2. **Fasting and Low-Carb Diets**: During fasting or low-carbohydrate diets, G6Pase activity increases to maintain blood glucose levels through enhanced gluconeogenesis and glycogenolysis.

Metabolic Feedback

1. **Substrate Availability**: The availability of substrates like glucose-6-phosphate and the energy status of the cell (e.g., ATP/ADP ratio) influence G6Pase activity.
2. **Allosteric Regulation**: G6Pase activity can be modulated through allosteric interactions with various metabolic intermediates, ensuring a fine-tuned response to the body's energy needs.

Plant-Based Diet and Glucose-6-Phosphatase Regulation

A plant-based diet, rich in complex carbohydrates, fibers, vitamins, and minerals, can positively influence G6Pase regulation through several mechanisms.

Nutrient Density

1. **Vitamins and Minerals**: Plant-based diets provide essential vitamins and minerals, such as vitamin B6, magnesium, and

chromium, which play crucial roles in carbohydrate metabolism and enzyme function.

2. **Antioxidants**: Rich in antioxidants, plant-based foods reduce oxidative stress, potentially protecting G6Pase from oxidative damage and ensuring optimal enzyme function.

Fiber and Glycemic Control

1. **Dietary Fiber**: High-fiber foods, such as fruits, vegetables, and whole grains, slow glucose absorption and improve glycemic control, reducing the need for rapid glucose production via G6Pase.
2. **Stable Blood Glucose Levels**: By promoting stable blood glucose levels, a plant-based diet minimizes the fluctuations that trigger excessive G6Pase activity.

Healthy Fats and Protein

1. **Healthy Fats**: Plant-based sources of fats, such as avocados, nuts, and seeds, provide essential fatty acids that support overall metabolic health, including glucose regulation.
2. **Plant Proteins**: Legumes, nuts, and seeds offer high-quality plant proteins that contribute to balanced glucose metabolism and reduced insulin resistance, indirectly affecting G6Pase activity.

Plant-Based Diet on G6Pase-Related Health Outcomes

A plant-based diet can support overall metabolic health and potentially mitigate conditions related to impaired G6Pase function.

Metabolic Health

1. **Insulin Sensitivity**: Improved insulin sensitivity from a plant-based diet helps regulate G6Pase activity by promoting glucose uptake and reducing the need for gluconeogenesis.

2. **Reduced Risk of Type 2 Diabetes**: By enhancing glycemic control and reducing insulin resistance, a plant-based diet lowers the risk of type 2 diabetes, a condition characterized by impaired glucose metabolism.

Weight Management

1. **Healthy Weight**: A plant-based diet aids in weight management, reducing obesity-related hormonal imbalances that can affect G6Pase activity.
2. **Lower Body Fat**: Reduced visceral fat decreases the secretion of inflammatory markers that can disrupt glucose metabolism and enzyme regulation.

Cardiovascular Health

1. **Cholesterol Levels**: Plant-based diets typically result in lower cholesterol levels, reducing the risk of cardiovascular diseases that can be exacerbated by poor glucose regulation.
2. **Anti-inflammatory Effects**: The anti-inflammatory properties of plant-based foods support overall cardiovascular health and metabolic balance.

Liver and Kidney Function

1. **Liver Health**: Improved liver function from a plant-based diet supports efficient gluconeogenesis and glycogenolysis, ensuring optimal G6Pase activity.
2. **Kidney Health**: By promoting kidney health, a plant-based diet aids in the proper regulation of G6Pase activity and glucose production.

Glucose-6-phosphatase plays a pivotal role in glucose homeostasis by catalyzing the final step of gluconeogenesis and glycogenolysis. Its production and regulation are influenced by various hormonal, nutritional, and metabolic factors.

Glucokinase (GK)

Glucokinase (GK) is a critical enzyme in glucose metabolism, particularly within the liver and pancreatic beta cells.

Function of Glucokinase

Glucokinase plays a pivotal role in glucose homeostasis by catalyzing the phosphorylation of glucose to glucose-6-phosphate, the first step in glycolysis. Its activity is integral to the regulation of blood glucose levels and energy metabolism.

In the Liver

1. **Glucose Utilization**: In hepatocytes, glucokinase facilitates the uptake and utilization of glucose postprandially, converting glucose into glucose-6-phosphate, which can then enter various metabolic pathways, including glycogen synthesis and glycolysis.
2. **Glycogen Synthesis**: Glucose-6-phosphate produced by glucokinase can be stored as glycogen, providing a readily available energy source during periods of fasting.
3. **Gluconeogenesis**: By influencing glucose-6-phosphate levels, glucokinase indirectly affects gluconeogenesis, the process of producing glucose from non-carbohydrate substrates during fasting.

In Pancreatic Beta Cells

1. **Insulin Secretion**: Glucokinase acts as a glucose sensor in pancreatic beta cells. The phosphorylation of glucose to glucose-6-phosphate initiates a cascade of events leading to insulin secretion in response to rising blood glucose levels.
2. **Glucose Homeostasis**: By regulating insulin secretion, glucokinase helps maintain blood glucose levels within a narrow range, crucial for overall metabolic health.

Additional Roles

1. **Metabolic Flexibility**: Glucokinase supports metabolic flexibility by allowing cells to switch between glucose and fatty acids as energy sources depending on availability and demand.
2. **Energy Production**: By initiating glycolysis, glucokinase contributes to the production of ATP, the energy currency of cells, supporting various cellular functions.

Production of Glucokinase

Glucokinase is produced in specific tissues, primarily the liver and pancreatic beta cells, through a series of tightly regulated processes.

Gene Encoding

1. **GCK Gene**: The glucokinase gene (GCK) is located on chromosome 7 in humans. This gene encodes the glucokinase enzyme, which is essential for glucose metabolism.
2. **Isoforms**: Different isoforms of glucokinase are produced in the liver and pancreatic beta cells, tailored to the specific metabolic needs of these tissues.

Synthesis and Activation

1. **Translation and Post-Translational Modifications**: The GCK gene is transcribed into mRNA, which is then translated into the glucokinase enzyme. Post-translational modifications, such as phosphorylation, can affect the enzyme's activity and stability.
2. **Subcellular Localization**: In hepatocytes, glucokinase is predominantly found in the cytoplasm, where it catalyzes the phosphorylation of glucose. In pancreatic beta cells, it is also located in the cytoplasm, acting as a glucose sensor.

Regulation by Hormones and Nutrients

1. **Insulin**: Insulin promotes the expression of the GCK gene in the liver, enhancing glucokinase production and activity postprandially when glucose levels are high.
2. **Glucagon**: Glucagon inhibits glucokinase activity by promoting its sequestration in the nucleus of hepatocytes during fasting, reducing glucose utilization and conserving blood glucose levels.

Factors Influencing Glucokinase Production

1. **Age**: Glucokinase activity can decline with age, contributing to impaired glucose metabolism and an increased risk of metabolic disorders.
2. **Gender**: Hormonal differences between males and females can influence glucokinase activity and glucose metabolism.
3. **Diet**: Nutritional status, including macronutrient composition and overall dietary patterns, significantly affects glucokinase production and activity.

Regulation of Glucokinase

The regulation of glucokinase involves complex interactions between genetic, hormonal, and nutritional factors, ensuring that glucose metabolism is tightly controlled.

Genetic Regulation

1. **GCK Gene Promoter**: The promoter region of the GCK gene contains binding sites for various transcription factors that regulate gene expression in response to hormonal and nutritional signals.
2. **Polymorphisms**: Genetic polymorphisms in the GCK gene can affect glucokinase activity and have been linked to an increased risk of type 2 diabetes and other metabolic disorders.

Hormonal Regulation

1. **Insulin and Glucagon:** Insulin upregulates glucokinase expression in the liver postprandially, while glucagon downregulates its activity during fasting, ensuring appropriate glucose utilization and conservation.
2. **Thyroid Hormones**: Thyroid hormones can influence glucokinase activity, with hyperthyroidism enhancing and hypothyroidism reducing its activity.

Nutritional Regulation

1. **Carbohydrate Intake**: High carbohydrate intake increases glucokinase activity in the liver, promoting glucose utilization and storage.
2. **Fasting and Caloric Restriction**: Fasting and caloric restriction reduce glucokinase activity, conserving glucose for essential functions and promoting gluconeogenesis.

Regulatory Proteins

1. **Glucokinase Regulatory Protein (GKRP)**: GKRP binds glucokinase in the nucleus of hepatocytes during fasting, inhibiting its activity. Postprandially, GKRP releases glucokinase into the cytoplasm, activating it for glucose phosphorylation.
2. **Protein-Protein Interactions**: Interactions with other proteins, such as those involved in insulin signaling, can modulate glucokinase activity and localization.

Plant-Based Diet and Glucokinase Regulation

A plant-based diet, rich in fruits, vegetables, whole grains, nuts, and seeds, can positively influence glucokinase regulation through various mechanisms.

Nutrient Density

Plant-based diets provide essential nutrients, vitamins, and minerals that support overall health and optimal enzyme function. For example, magnesium, found in leafy greens and nuts, is a cofactor for many enzymatic reactions, including those involved in glucose metabolism.

Phytochemicals and Antioxidants

1. **Polyphenols**: Polyphenols, abundant in fruits and vegetables, have been shown to enhance insulin sensitivity and glucokinase activity, improving glucose utilization and reducing the risk of insulin resistance.
2. **Flavonoids**: Flavonoids, such as quercetin found in apples and onions, can modulate glucokinase activity by reducing oxidative stress and inflammation, promoting better glucose homeostasis.

Healthy Fats

Plant-based sources of fats, such as avocados, nuts, and seeds, provide essential fatty acids that support cell membrane integrity and enzyme function. Omega-3 fatty acids, in particular, have anti-inflammatory properties that can enhance glucokinase activity and overall metabolic health.

Fiber

High-fiber diets, common in plant-based eating, support gut health and glucose metabolism. Dietary fiber helps maintain stable blood glucose levels, reducing the risk of insulin resistance and promoting better glucokinase regulation.

Caloric Balance

Maintaining a healthy weight through a balanced plant-based diet can prevent obesity-related metabolic imbalances. Excess body fat, particularly visceral fat, is linked to chronic inflammation and insulin resistance, which can impair glucokinase activity.

Glycemic Control

Plant-based diets, low in refined sugars and high in complex carbohydrates, help maintain stable blood glucose levels. Stable glucose levels reduce the burden on glucokinase and prevent its downregulation due to chronic hyperglycemia.

Plant-Based Diet on Glucokinase-Related Health Outcomes

Glucose Homeostasis

1. **Diabetes Prevention**: A plant-based diet can reduce the risk of type 2 diabetes by improving insulin sensitivity and glucokinase activity. Antioxidants and anti-inflammatory compounds in plant foods protect pancreatic beta cells and enhance glucose metabolism.

2. **Blood Sugar Control**: Consuming a diet rich in whole plant foods helps maintain stable blood sugar levels, reducing the risk of insulin resistance and glucose intolerance.

Liver Health

Plant-based diets support liver health by providing nutrients that promote detoxification and reduce oxidative stress. Improved liver function enhances glucokinase activity and overall glucose metabolism.

Weight Management

Plant-based diets are effective for weight management, reducing body fat, and improving metabolic health. Lower body fat and better glycemic control enhance glucokinase activity and reduce the risk of metabolic syndrome.

Mental Health

Emerging evidence suggests that plant-based diets may benefit mental health by reducing inflammation and oxidative stress, which are linked to mood disorders. Improved glucose metabolism, including glucokinase activity, supports cognitive function and emotional well-being.

Anti-Aging Effects

The antioxidant-rich nature of plant-based diets helps combat oxidative stress, a key factor in aging. Improved metabolic health, coupled with enhanced glucokinase activity, contributes to healthier aging and better maintenance of glucose homeostasis.

Glucokinase plays a crucial role in glucose metabolism, regulating blood glucose levels and energy production in the liver and pancreatic beta cells. Its production and regulation are influenced by genetic, hormonal, and nutritional factors.

Glycogen Synthase (GS)

Glycogen synthase (GS) is a pivotal enzyme in glycogen metabolism, essential for the synthesis of glycogen from glucose.

Function of Glycogen Synthase

Glycogen Synthesis

Glycogen synthase plays a crucial role in converting glucose to glycogen, a stored form of energy in the body. Glycogen is primarily stored in the liver and muscle tissues, providing a readily available energy source during periods of increased demand.

Key Functions

1. **Glycogen Storage**: GS catalyzes the addition of glucose units to the growing glycogen chain, facilitating the storage of glucose for future energy needs.
2. **Energy Regulation**: By regulating glycogen synthesis, GS helps maintain blood glucose levels, particularly during fasting or between meals.
3. **Metabolic Flexibility**: GS allows the body to switch between utilizing glucose and stored glycogen, ensuring metabolic flexibility and stability.

Muscle and Liver Functions

- **Muscle Tissue**: In muscle tissue, GS is vital for maintaining glycogen stores, which are crucial for sustained muscle activity during exercise and physical exertion.
- **Liver Tissue**: In the liver, GS helps regulate blood glucose levels by converting excess glucose into glycogen, which can be mobilized during periods of hypoglycemia to maintain homeostasis.

Production of Glycogen Synthase

Synthesis and Gene Encoding

Glycogen synthase is encoded by two genes: GYS1, which is expressed in muscle tissue, and GYS2, which is expressed in the liver. These genes encode the different isoforms of the enzyme that are tailored to the specific needs of these tissues.

Glycogen Synthase Structure

GS is a glycosyltransferase enzyme, composed of multiple subunits that form an active complex. The enzyme's structure allows it to catalyze the transfer of glucose from UDP-glucose to the growing glycogen molecule.

Regulation by Enzymatic Activity

- **Phosphorylation**: The activity of GS is regulated by phosphorylation. Phosphorylation typically inactivates GS, while dephosphorylation activates it. This regulatory mechanism allows the enzyme's activity to be finely tuned in response to metabolic needs.
- **Allosteric Regulation**: GS activity is also influenced by allosteric effectors such as glucose-6-phosphate, which can activate the enzyme.

Influencing Factors

1. **Insulin**: Insulin is a key regulator of GS activity. Postprandial insulin release promotes the activation of GS by enhancing dephosphorylation, facilitating glycogen storage.
2. **Glucagon and Epinephrine**: These hormones inhibit GS activity through phosphorylation, prioritizing glycogen breakdown and glucose release during periods of stress or fasting.

Regulation of Glycogen Synthase

The regulation of GS involves a complex interplay of hormonal signals, nutrient status, and energy demands, ensuring that glycogen synthesis is tightly controlled to meet the body's metabolic needs.

Hormonal Regulation

1. **Insulin**: Insulin signaling promotes the dephosphorylation and activation of GS. This process involves a cascade of events, including the activation of protein phosphatase 1 (PP1), which removes inhibitory phosphate groups from GS.
2. **Glucagon**: In contrast, glucagon promotes the phosphorylation and inactivation of GS via the cyclic AMP (cAMP) signaling pathway, which activates protein kinase A (PKA) and other kinases that phosphorylate GS.
3. **Epinephrine**: Similar to glucagon, epinephrine induces GS phosphorylation and inactivation through the cAMP pathway, preparing the body for rapid glucose release during the "fight or flight" response.

Nutrient and Energy Status

1. **Glucose-6-Phosphate**: This metabolite acts as an allosteric activator of GS, enhancing its activity in response to elevated glucose levels, thus promoting glycogen synthesis.
2. **Adenosine Monophosphate (AMP)**: Elevated levels of AMP, indicative of low energy status, inhibit GS activity, prioritizing ATP generation over glycogen storage.

Plant-Based Diet and Glycogen Synthase Regulation

A plant-based diet, rich in complex carbohydrates, fiber, and phytonutrients, can positively influence the regulation of GS and overall glycogen metabolism.

Nutrient Density

Plant-based diets provide essential nutrients, vitamins, and minerals that support overall metabolic health and enzymatic functions, including GS.

Carbohydrate Quality

Complex carbohydrates from whole grains, legumes, and vegetables provide a steady source of glucose, supporting stable blood sugar levels and optimal GS activity.

Fiber

Dietary fiber, abundant in plant-based foods, modulates glucose absorption and insulin sensitivity, thereby influencing GS activity. Soluble fiber, in particular, helps maintain steady blood glucose levels by slowing digestion and glucose release.

Antioxidants

Fruits and vegetables are rich in antioxidants, which reduce oxidative stress and inflammation. Lower oxidative stress levels are associated with improved metabolic health and enzymatic function, including that of GS.

Healthy Fats

Plant-based sources of fats, such as avocados, nuts, and seeds, provide essential fatty acids that support cellular functions and hormonal balance, indirectly influencing GS regulation.

Glycemic Control

Plant-based diets, which are low in refined sugars and high in complex carbohydrates, help maintain stable blood glucose levels. This stability supports insulin sensitivity and proper GS activation.

Plant-Based Diet on Glycogen Synthase-Related Health Outcomes

Metabolic Health

1. **Insulin Sensitivity**: A plant-based diet improves insulin sensitivity, enhancing the regulatory effects of insulin on GS and promoting efficient glycogen storage.
2. **Blood Sugar Control**: Consuming whole, plant-based foods helps maintain stable blood sugar levels, preventing the spikes and crashes associated with refined carbohydrate consumption.

Physical Performance

1. **Muscle Glycogen Stores**: Athletes and physically active individuals on a plant-based diet can maintain optimal muscle glycogen stores, supporting sustained performance and quicker recovery.
2. **Energy Availability**: A diet rich in complex carbohydrates provides a steady source of energy, essential for maintaining muscle glycogen levels and overall endurance.

Weight Management

1. **Healthy Weight**: Plant-based diets are effective for weight management, reducing excess body fat, and improving metabolic health. Lower body fat and better glycemic control enhance overall hormonal balance, including insulin's effects on GS.
2. **Obesity Prevention**: By promoting a healthy weight and preventing obesity, plant-based diets reduce the risk of insulin resistance and metabolic disorders that impair GS function.

Disease Prevention

1. **Type 2 Diabetes**: Plant-based diets are associated with a lower risk of type 2 diabetes. Improved insulin sensitivity and glycemic control prevent the metabolic dysfunctions that can lead to diabetes and impaired GS activity.
2. **Cardiovascular Health**: A diet rich in fruits, vegetables, and whole grains supports cardiovascular health, reducing the risk factors that contribute to metabolic syndrome and related diseases.

Detailed Pathways of Glycogen Synthase Regulation
Insulin Signaling Pathway

1. **Insulin Receptor Activation**: Insulin binds to its receptor on the cell surface, initiating a signaling cascade.
2. **PI3K Activation**: The activated insulin receptor recruits and activates phosphoinositide 3-kinase (PI3K).
3. **Akt Activation**: PI3K activation leads to the phosphorylation and activation of Akt (protein kinase B).
4. **Glycogen Synthase Kinase-3 (GSK-3) Inhibition**: Akt phosphorylates and inactivates GSK-3, a kinase that phosphorylates and inhibits GS.
5. **GS Activation**: With GSK-3 inhibited, GS remains dephosphorylated and active, promoting glycogen synthesis.

Glucagon and Epinephrine Signaling Pathways

1. **Receptor Activation**: Glucagon and epinephrine bind to their respective receptors, activating the cAMP signaling pathway.

2. **PKA Activation**: Increased cAMP levels activate protein kinase A (PKA).
3. **GS Phosphorylation**: PKA phosphorylates and inactivates GS, reducing glycogen synthesis.
4. **Glycogen Breakdown**: Concurrently, PKA activates glycogen phosphorylase, promoting glycogen breakdown to release glucose.

Role of Nutrients and Metabolites

1. **Glucose-6-Phosphate**: This metabolite binds to GS, causing a conformational change that enhances its activity.
2. **AMP and ATP**: The AMP/ATP ratio serves as an energy sensor. High AMP levels indicate low energy status, inhibiting GS activity, while high ATP levels promote GS activity.

Plant-Based Nutrients Supporting Glycogen Synthase Activity
Vitamins and Minerals

1. **Magnesium**: Found in leafy greens, nuts, and seeds, magnesium is a cofactor for many enzymatic reactions, including those involved in glucose metabolism and GS function.
2. **Vitamin B6**: Present in whole grains, legumes, and vegetables, vitamin B6 is essential for glycogen metabolism and GS activity.
3. **Chromium**: Found in broccoli, oats, and barley, chromium enhances insulin sensitivity and supports GS regulation.

Phytochemicals

1. **Polyphenols**: These compounds, abundant in fruits, vegetables, and tea, have antioxidant properties that reduce oxidative stress and support metabolic health.

2. **Flavonoids**: Found in berries, citrus fruits, and onions, flavonoids improve insulin sensitivity and support GS activity.

Omega-3 Fatty Acids

Sources such as flaxseeds, chia seeds, and walnuts provide omega-3 fatty acids, which have anti-inflammatory properties that support overall metabolic health and GS function.

Glycogen synthase is a vital enzyme in glycogen metabolism, playing a central role in energy storage and regulation. Its function, production, and regulation are influenced by various factors, including hormonal signals, nutrient status, and energy demands.

Glycogen Phosphorylase (GP)

Glycogen Phosphorylase (GP) is an essential enzyme in the human body responsible for glycogen metabolism. It plays a significant role in breaking down glycogen into glucose-1-phosphate, which is a vital energy source for cells, especially during periods of increased energy demand such as exercise or fasting.

Function of Glycogen Phosphorylase

Glycogen Phosphorylase has a critical role in the glycogenolysis pathway, which is the process of breaking down glycogen into glucose.

In Liver Cells

1. **Regulation of Blood Sugar Levels**: GP in the liver helps maintain blood sugar levels by converting glycogen stores into glucose-1-phosphate, which is then converted to glucose-6-phosphate and finally free glucose that can be released into the bloodstream. This process is crucial during fasting or between meals.

2. **Energy Supply During Fasting**: During periods of fasting or prolonged exercise, liver GP ensures a steady supply of glucose to maintain blood glucose levels and provide energy to tissues that depend on glucose, such as the brain and red blood cells.

In Muscle Cells

1. **Energy Supply During Exercise**: In muscle cells, GP breaks down glycogen to glucose-1-phosphate, which is then used in glycolysis to produce ATP, the primary energy currency of the cell. This process is especially important during intense physical activity.
2. **Local Energy Needs**: Unlike liver glycogen, muscle glycogen does not contribute to blood glucose levels. Instead, it is used locally within the muscle cells to meet immediate energy demands during muscle contraction.

Additional Roles

1. **Adaptation to Exercise**: GP activity increases in response to regular physical activity, enhancing the muscle's ability to store and mobilize glycogen.
2. **Response to Hypoxia**: During low oxygen conditions, such as high-altitude exposure or certain pathological states, GP activity helps sustain energy production by providing an anaerobic source of ATP.

Production of Glycogen Phosphorylase

Glycogen Phosphorylase is produced in the cytoplasm of liver and muscle cells through a complex interplay of genetic and biochemical pathways.

Synthesis

1. **Gene Encoding**: The gene responsible for GP production is located on chromosome 14 (PYGL for liver isoform) and chromosome 11 (PYGM for muscle isoform). These genes encode the respective isoforms of GP.
2. **Protein Structure**: GP is a dimeric enzyme, meaning it is composed of two subunits that form a functional protein. Each subunit has an active site where glycogen binds and is subsequently broken down.

Regulation by Hormones

1. **Glucagon and Epinephrine**: In the liver, glucagon (secreted during low blood sugar levels) and epinephrine (released during stress or exercise) stimulate GP activity. These hormones activate the enzyme through a cascade involving cyclic AMP (cAMP) and protein kinase A (PKA).
2. **Insulin**: Insulin, secreted in response to high blood glucose levels, inhibits GP activity, thereby reducing glycogen breakdown and promoting glycogen synthesis.

Tissue-Specific Expression

1. **Liver Isoform (PYGL)**: The liver-specific isoform of GP is predominantly expressed in hepatocytes and plays a key role in regulating systemic glucose levels.
2. **Muscle Isoform (PYGM)**: The muscle-specific isoform is expressed in skeletal muscle cells and is crucial for providing energy during muscle contraction.

Influencing Factors

1. **Age**: GP activity can decrease with age, contributing to reduced glycogen storage and mobilization capacity in older adults.
2. **Gender**: There may be gender-specific differences in GP activity and regulation, influenced by hormonal differences between males and females.
3. **Exercise**: Regular physical activity enhances GP expression and activity, improving glycogen storage and utilization in muscles.

Regulation of Glycogen Phosphorylase

The regulation of GP involves intricate mechanisms that ensure a balance between glycogen storage and mobilization in response to physiological needs.

Allosteric Regulation

1. **AMP and ATP**: GP is allosterically activated by AMP (adenosine monophosphate) and inhibited by ATP (adenosine triphosphate). High levels of AMP indicate low energy status, stimulating GP activity, whereas high ATP levels signal sufficient energy, inhibiting the enzyme.
2. **Glucose-6-Phosphate**: This metabolite, which is downstream in the glycogenolysis pathway, inhibits GP, providing feedback inhibition to prevent excessive glycogen breakdown.

Covalent Modification

1. **Phosphorylation**: GP is regulated by reversible phosphorylation. Phosphorylation by phosphorylase kinase activates the enzyme, while dephosphorylation by phosphoprotein phosphatase deactivates it.

2. **Hormonal Influence**: Hormones like glucagon and epinephrine promote the phosphorylation (activation) of GP, while insulin promotes its dephosphorylation (inactivation).

Nutritional Status

1. **Carbohydrate Intake**: High carbohydrate intake promotes glycogen synthesis and inhibits GP activity, while low carbohydrate intake has the opposite effect.
2. **Plant-Based Diet**: A diet rich in complex carbohydrates, fiber, and plant-based proteins supports balanced GP activity by maintaining stable blood glucose levels and preventing excessive glycogen breakdown.

Exercise and Physical Activity

1. **Acute Exercise**: Intense physical activity increases GP activity to meet the heightened energy demands of muscles.
2. **Chronic Exercise**: Regular exercise training enhances the capacity for glycogen storage and improves the regulation of GP, contributing to better overall energy metabolism.

Plant-Based Diet and Glycogen Phosphorylase Regulation

A plant-based diet, rich in whole grains, fruits, vegetables, legumes, nuts, and seeds, can positively influence GP regulation through various mechanisms.

Nutrient Density

1. **Complex Carbohydrates**: Whole grains and legumes provide complex carbohydrates that are digested slowly, leading to gradual

glucose release and stable blood sugar levels. This helps in maintaining balanced GP activity.

2. **Vitamins and Minerals**: Plant-based foods are rich in vitamins (like B vitamins) and minerals (like magnesium and potassium) that are crucial for energy metabolism and enzymatic functions, including GP activity.

Amino Acids

1. **Plant Proteins**: Legumes, nuts, and seeds provide essential amino acids that support the synthesis and function of metabolic enzymes, including GP.
2. **Arginine and Glutamine**: These amino acids, found in plant foods, play a role in protein synthesis and overall energy metabolism, indirectly supporting GP function.

Antioxidants

1. **Oxidative Stress Reduction**: Fruits and vegetables are rich in antioxidants, which help reduce oxidative stress. Lower oxidative stress levels are associated with improved enzyme function, including GP.
2. **Anti-Inflammatory Properties**: Antioxidants also possess anti-inflammatory properties, which can enhance metabolic health and enzyme regulation.

Healthy Fats

1. **Omega-3 Fatty Acids**: Sources like flaxseeds, chia seeds, and walnuts provide omega-3 fatty acids that have anti-inflammatory effects, supporting overall metabolic health and enzyme function.

2. **Monounsaturated Fats**: Avocados, nuts, and seeds are rich in monounsaturated fats that support healthy cell membranes and enzyme activity.

Fiber

1. **Gut Health**: High-fiber diets support a healthy gut microbiome, which can influence metabolic health and enzyme regulation through the production of short-chain fatty acids and other metabolites.
2. **Glycemic Control**: Fiber helps maintain stable blood glucose levels by slowing the absorption of sugars, which can prevent excessive activation of GP and promote balanced glycogen metabolism.

Caloric Balance

1. **Weight Management**: Maintaining a healthy weight through a balanced plant-based diet can prevent obesity-related metabolic imbalances. Excess body fat is linked to disrupted enzyme regulation, including GP.
2. **Energy Availability**: Adequate caloric intake supports overall energy balance, ensuring that glycogen stores are appropriately managed and GP activity is regulated.

Glycemic Control

1. **Low Glycemic Index Foods**: Plant-based diets are typically low in refined sugars and high in complex carbohydrates, which help maintain stable blood glucose levels and prevent insulin resistance.

2. **Insulin Sensitivity**: Improved insulin sensitivity from a plant-based diet helps regulate GP activity by promoting glycogen storage and preventing excessive glycogen breakdown.

Plant-Based Diet on GP-Related Health Outcomes

A plant-based diet can positively impact health outcomes related to GP activity and overall glycogen metabolism.

Metabolic Health

1. **Blood Sugar Control**: By providing a steady source of complex carbohydrates and maintaining stable blood glucose levels, a plant-based diet supports balanced GP activity and overall metabolic health.
2. **Diabetes Management**: Improved glycemic control from a plant-based diet can help manage diabetes and prevent complications related to dysregulated glycogen metabolism.

Exercise Performance

1. **Energy Availability**: Plant-based diets support optimal energy availability for physical activity by maintaining glycogen stores and ensuring efficient GP activity.
2. **Recovery**: Nutrient-dense plant foods provide essential vitamins, minerals, and antioxidants that support muscle recovery and glycogen replenishment after exercise.

Weight Management

1. **Obesity Prevention**: A balanced plant-based diet helps prevent obesity, which is associated with metabolic disturbances and impaired enzyme regulation, including GP.

2. **Healthy Weight Maintenance**: Maintaining a healthy weight supports overall metabolic health and balanced GP activity, contributing to efficient energy metabolism.

Cardiovascular Health

1. **Cholesterol Levels**: Plant-based diets are low in saturated fats and cholesterol, supporting healthy blood lipid levels and reducing the risk of cardiovascular disease.
2. **Blood Pressure**: The high potassium and low sodium content of plant-based foods helps maintain healthy blood pressure levels, supporting overall cardiovascular health.

Anti-Aging Effects

1. **Oxidative Stress Reduction**: The antioxidant-rich nature of plant-based diets helps combat oxidative stress, a key factor in aging. Improved metabolic health and enzyme regulation contribute to healthier aging.
2. **Inflammation Reduction**: Anti-inflammatory properties of plant-based foods support overall health and longevity by reducing chronic inflammation, which is linked to metabolic disturbances.

Glycogen Phosphorylase plays a pivotal role in glycogen metabolism, regulating the breakdown of glycogen into glucose to meet the body's energy needs. Its production and regulation are influenced by various factors, including hormonal signals, nutritional status, and physical activity.

19

Fatty Acid Metabolism Enzymes

Acetyl-CoA Carboxylase (ACC)

Acetyl-CoA Carboxylase (ACC) is a key enzyme involved in fatty acid metabolism. Its role in lipid biosynthesis and regulation makes it critical for energy balance and metabolic health. This comprehensive analysis delves into the function, production, and regulation of ACC, particularly from a plant-based viewpoint, highlighting dietary influences on its activity and balance.

Function of Acetyl-CoA Carboxylase

Acetyl-CoA Carboxylase is essential for several physiological processes, including:

1. Fatty Acid Biosynthesis

ACC catalyzes the carboxylation of acetyl-CoA to malonyl-CoA, the first committed step in fatty acid synthesis. Malonyl-CoA serves as a building block for the elongation of fatty acids. This process is crucial for the synthesis of long-chain fatty acids that are vital for cellular structures and energy storage.

2. Regulation of Fatty Acid Oxidation

Malonyl-CoA, the product of ACC, inhibits carnitine palmitoyl-transferase I (CPT1), an enzyme critical for the transport of fatty acids into the mitochondria for oxidation. By regulating CPT1, ACC controls the balance between fatty acid synthesis and oxidation, thus playing a pivotal role in energy homeostasis.

3. Cellular Signaling and Metabolism

ACC activity influences various signaling pathways related to cellular growth and metabolism. For example, it interacts with AMP-activated protein kinase (AMPK), a central energy sensor that modulates metabolic pathways to maintain energy balance.

4. Lipogenesis and Adipogenesis

ACC is integral to lipogenesis (fat creation) and adipogenesis (fat cell formation). Its activity supports the generation of lipid stores in adipose tissue, which is essential for energy storage and insulation.

Production of Acetyl-CoA Carboxylase

The production of ACC involves several steps and regulatory mechanisms:

1. Gene Expression

ACC is encoded by two genes: ACC1 (ACACA) and ACC2 (ACACB). ACC1 is primarily involved in fatty acid synthesis in the cytosol, whereas ACC2 is associated with the regulation of fatty acid oxidation in the mitochondria. These genes are expressed in various tissues, with higher levels in lipogenic tissues such as the liver and adipose tissue.

2. Enzyme Synthesis and Isoforms

The ACC enzyme exists in two isoforms, ACC1 and ACC2, which are synthesized through the transcription and translation of the respective genes. These isoforms have distinct but complementary roles in lipid metabolism.

3. Post-Translational Modifications

ACC activity is regulated by post-translational modifications, including phosphorylation and dephosphorylation. These modifications alter the enzyme's activity in response to cellular energy status and hormonal signals.

Regulation of Acetyl-CoA Carboxylase

The regulation of ACC involves complex feedback mechanisms and external factors:

1. Allosteric Regulation

Citrate, an intermediate in the citric acid cycle, activates ACC by promoting its polymerization into an active form. In contrast, long-chain fatty acyl-CoAs, which are end products of fatty acid synthesis, inhibit ACC by preventing its polymerization.

2. Hormonal Regulation

Hormones such as insulin and glucagon significantly influence ACC activity. Insulin promotes ACC activation and fatty acid synthesis by enhancing its dephosphorylation, while glucagon inhibits ACC through phosphorylation via AMPK.

3. Nutritional Status

Nutritional cues regulate ACC through various pathways. A high-carbohydrate diet increases ACC activity by enhancing insulin secretion and citrate availability. Conversely, fasting or a low-carbohydrate diet decreases ACC activity through increased AMPK activation and fatty acid oxidation.

4. AMPK-Mediated Phosphorylation

AMPK is a critical regulator of ACC, phosphorylating and inhibiting the enzyme in response to low cellular energy levels. This inhibition reduces fatty acid synthesis and promotes fatty acid oxidation, aligning with the cell's energy needs.

Plant-Based Diet and Acetyl-CoA Carboxylase Regulation

A plant-based diet can significantly impact the regulation of ACC through various mechanisms:

1. Nutrient Density

Plant-based diets are rich in essential nutrients, including vitamins and minerals that support overall metabolic health. Foods such as whole grains, nuts, seeds, and legumes provide essential cofactors for ACC activity and regulation.

2. Phytochemicals and Antioxidants

Fruits and vegetables are high in phytochemicals and antioxidants, which help reduce oxidative stress and inflammation. Lower oxidative stress levels are associated with improved metabolic function and balanced ACC activity.

3. Healthy Fats

Plant-based sources of fats, such as avocados, nuts, and seeds, provide essential fatty acids that support metabolic health. Omega-3 fatty acids, in particular, have anti-inflammatory properties that can enhance ACC function and regulation.

4. Fiber and Glycemic Control

High-fiber diets common in plant-based eating help maintain stable blood glucose levels. Stable blood glucose prevents hyperglycemia-induced suppression of ACC activity, supporting balanced lipid metabolism.

Plant-Based Diet on Acetyl-CoA Carboxylase-Related Health Outcomes

1. Obesity and Weight Management

Plant-based diets are effective for weight management, reducing body fat, and improving insulin sensitivity. Lower body fat and better glycemic control enhance ACC activity, promoting balanced lipid metabolism and preventing obesity-related metabolic disorders.

2. Cardiovascular Health

A plant-based diet can improve cardiovascular health by lowering cholesterol levels and reducing inflammation. Improved lipid profiles support overall metabolic health and prevent atherosclerosis and other cardiovascular diseases.

3. Type 2 Diabetes Management

Plant-based diets can help manage type 2 diabetes by improving insulin sensitivity and glycemic control. Enhanced ACC activity supports balanced lipid metabolism, reducing the risk of metabolic complications associated with diabetes.

4. Liver Health

Non-alcoholic fatty liver disease (NAFLD) is closely linked to lipid metabolism dysregulation. A plant-based diet can improve liver health by promoting balanced ACC activity, reducing liver fat accumulation, and enhancing overall metabolic function.

Acetyl-CoA Carboxylase plays a pivotal role in fatty acid metabolism and energy homeostasis. Its production and regulation are influenced by various factors, including nutritional status, hormonal signals, and cellular energy levels. A plant-based diet, rich in essential nutrients, antioxidants, healthy fats, and fiber, supports optimal ACC function and balance.

Fatty Acid Synthase (FAS)

Fatty Acid Synthase (FAS) is a critical enzyme in the human body responsible for the synthesis of fatty acids, playing a vital role in lipid metabolism, energy storage, and overall cellular function.

Function of Fatty Acid Synthase

Fatty Acid Synthase (FAS) is an enzyme complex that catalyzes the synthesis of long-chain fatty acids from acetyl-CoA and malonyl-CoA in the presence of NADPH. FAS is primarily responsible for the creation of palmitate (16-carbon saturated fatty acid), which serves as a precursor for other fatty acids and lipids.

Key Functions:

1. **Lipid Biosynthesis:** FAS is central to de novo lipogenesis, producing fatty acids necessary for the synthesis of triglycerides, phospholipids, and cholesterol esters. These lipids are essential components of cell membranes and energy stores.

2. **Energy Storage:** Fatty acids synthesized by FAS are stored as triglycerides in adipose tissue, serving as a long-term energy reserve.
3. **Cellular Function and Signaling:** Fatty acids are involved in various cellular processes, including membrane fluidity, signal transduction, and the production of lipid signaling molecules.
4. **Regulation of Metabolic Pathways:** FAS activity influences other metabolic pathways, such as glucose metabolism, by providing substrates for lipogenesis and influencing insulin sensitivity.

Production of Fatty Acid Synthase

Fatty Acid Synthase is produced through a complex series of steps involving gene expression, protein synthesis, and enzyme assembly.

Gene Encoding:

1. **FASN Gene:** The FAS enzyme is encoded by the FASN gene located on chromosome 17 in humans. This gene is responsible for the synthesis of the multi-functional FAS protein.
2. **Expression Regulation:** The expression of the FASN gene is regulated by various transcription factors, including Sterol Regulatory Element-Binding Proteins (SREBPs) and carbohydrate response element-binding protein (ChREBP), which respond to dietary and hormonal signals.

Protein Synthesis:

1. **Translation:** The FASN mRNA is translated into a single polypeptide chain in the ribosomes of the endoplasmic reticulum.
2. **Post-Translational Modifications:** The polypeptide undergoes several modifications, including glycosylation and phosphorylation, to become a functional enzyme.

Enzyme Assembly:

1. **Multifunctional Enzyme Complex:** FAS functions as a large, multi-domain enzyme complex with multiple catalytic activities. It exists as a homodimer, with each monomer containing all the necessary enzymatic domains for fatty acid synthesis.
2. **Catalytic Domains:** These include acetyltransferase, malonyl/palmitoyl transferase, ketoacyl synthase, ketoacyl reductase, enoyl reductase, and thioesterase domains, all working in a coordinated manner to produce fatty acids.

Regulation of Fatty Acid Synthase

The regulation of FAS involves a sophisticated interplay of hormonal, nutritional, and metabolic factors to ensure appropriate lipid synthesis in response to the body's needs.

Hormonal Regulation:

1. **Insulin:** Insulin is a potent activator of FAS expression. Postprandial increases in insulin levels promote FAS activity, facilitating lipogenesis and energy storage.
2. **Glucagon and Epinephrine:** These hormones inhibit FAS activity by promoting the phosphorylation and inactivation of key regulatory proteins, thereby reducing lipogenesis during fasting or stress.
3. **Steroid Hormones:** Glucocorticoids and thyroid hormones also modulate FAS expression, reflecting the body's overall metabolic state and energy requirements.

Nutritional Regulation:

1. **Carbohydrate Intake:** High carbohydrate intake stimulates FAS activity through the induction of SREBPs and ChREBP, which enhance FASN gene transcription.
2. **Fatty Acid Intake:** Dietary polyunsaturated fatty acids (PUFAs) suppress FAS expression by inhibiting SREBPs, reducing the need for endogenous fatty acid synthesis when sufficient dietary fats are available.
3. **Caloric Intake:** Overall caloric intake influences FAS activity, with excess calories promoting lipogenesis and energy storage.

Metabolic Regulation:

1. **AMP-Activated Protein Kinase (AMPK):** AMPK is a key energy sensor that inhibits FAS activity during energy deficit by phosphorylating and inactivating ACC (acetyl-CoA carboxylase), an upstream enzyme in the lipogenesis pathway.
2. **mTOR Pathway:** The mTOR pathway integrates signals from nutrients and growth factors to regulate FAS activity, promoting lipogenesis in nutrient-rich conditions.

Plant-Based Diet and Fatty Acid Synthase Regulation

A plant-based diet, rich in fruits, vegetables, whole grains, nuts, and seeds, can influence the regulation of FAS through various mechanisms, contributing to better metabolic health and reduced risk of chronic diseases.

Nutrient Density:

1. **Antioxidants:** Plant-based foods are rich in antioxidants like vitamins C and E, which help reduce oxidative stress and

inflammation, indirectly supporting optimal FAS regulation and lipid metabolism.

2. **Phytonutrients:** Compounds such as polyphenols, found in plant foods, have been shown to modulate gene expression and enzyme activity, including that of FAS.

Healthy Fats:

1. **Omega-3 Fatty Acids:** Found in flaxseeds, chia seeds, and walnuts, omega-3 fatty acids help reduce inflammation and can downregulate FAS expression, promoting a healthier lipid profile.
2. **Monounsaturated Fats:** Avocados, olives, and nuts provide monounsaturated fats that support healthy lipid metabolism and may modulate FAS activity.

Fiber:

1. **Dietary Fiber:** High-fiber diets, common in plant-based eating, improve insulin sensitivity and glycemic control, which can positively affect FAS activity and lipid metabolism.
2. **Gut Health:** A healthy gut microbiome, supported by dietary fiber, produces short-chain fatty acids that can influence systemic inflammation and metabolic regulation, including FAS activity.

Glycemic Control:

1. **Low Glycemic Index Foods:** Plant-based diets are typically low in refined sugars and high in complex carbohydrates, which help maintain stable blood glucose levels, reducing insulin spikes and promoting balanced FAS activity.
2. **Insulin Sensitivity:** Improved insulin sensitivity from a plant-based diet supports optimal FAS regulation, reducing the risk of dyslipidemia and associated metabolic disorders.

Plant-Based Diet on FAS-Related Health Outcomes
Cardiovascular Health:

1. **Reduced Risk of Heart Disease:** Plant-based diets are associated with lower levels of LDL cholesterol and triglycerides, partly due to reduced FAS activity and improved lipid profiles, lowering the risk of atherosclerosis and cardiovascular diseases.
2. **Blood Pressure:** A high intake of fruits and vegetables, rich in potassium and antioxidants, supports vascular health and can help maintain healthy blood pressure levels.

Weight Management:

1. **Healthy Body Weight:** A plant-based diet promotes weight loss and maintenance through high nutrient density, fiber content, and low energy density, helping to regulate FAS activity and prevent obesity.
2. **Reduced Visceral Fat:** Lower visceral fat reduces the production of inflammatory cytokines, improving metabolic health and reducing the burden on lipid synthesis pathways like FAS.

Metabolic Health:

1. **Type 2 Diabetes:** Plant-based diets improve insulin sensitivity and glycemic control, reducing the risk of type 2 diabetes. Lower FAS activity contributes to better lipid and glucose metabolism.
2. **Non-Alcoholic Fatty Liver Disease (NAFLD):** A plant-based diet helps reduce hepatic fat accumulation, potentially through the downregulation of FAS and other lipogenic enzymes, preventing NAFLD and improving liver function.

Anti-Inflammatory Effects:

1. **Chronic Inflammation:** A diet rich in anti-inflammatory compounds from plant foods reduces systemic inflammation, which is beneficial for metabolic health and can influence the activity of enzymes like FAS.
2. **Oxidative Stress:** Antioxidants in plant foods combat oxidative stress, protecting cells and tissues from damage and supporting overall metabolic balance.

Fatty Acid Synthase (FAS) is a pivotal enzyme in lipid metabolism, responsible for the synthesis of fatty acids that are essential for energy storage, cellular function, and overall metabolic health. Its production and regulation are influenced by a variety of hormonal, nutritional, and metabolic factors.

20

Krebs Cycle Enzymes

Citrate Synthase (CS)

Citrate synthase (CS) is a key enzyme in the citric acid cycle (Krebs cycle), which is crucial for cellular energy production in mitochondria.

Function of Citrate Synthase

Citrate synthase plays a pivotal role in the citric acid cycle by catalyzing the first step, which is the condensation of acetyl-CoA and oxaloacetate to form citrate. This reaction is vital for energy production and metabolic processes in aerobic organisms.

1. **Energy Production:** CS is essential for cellular respiration, as it initiates the citric acid cycle. This cycle produces high-energy molecules such as ATP (adenosine triphosphate), NADH, and FADH2, which are necessary for various cellular functions.
2. **Metabolic Regulation:** CS regulates the flow of carbon through the citric acid cycle, influencing the balance between energy production and biosynthetic processes. The enzyme helps in maintaining metabolic homeostasis by adjusting the cycle's activity based on cellular energy needs.

3. **Intermediary Metabolism:** The citrate produced by CS can be used for fatty acid synthesis, amino acid synthesis, and gluconeogenesis, making CS a key player in intermediary metabolism.
4. **Oxidative Stress Response:** CS activity can be modulated in response to oxidative stress, contributing to the cell's ability to manage reactive oxygen species (ROS) and maintain redox balance.

Production of Citrate Synthase

Citrate synthase is produced in cells through a complex process involving gene expression, protein synthesis, and mitochondrial import.

1. **Gene Encoding:** The gene responsible for CS production is located in the nuclear DNA. In humans, the gene for CS is known as CS, located on chromosome 12p12.1. This gene encodes the enzyme that is essential for the citric acid cycle.
2. **Protein Synthesis:** CS is synthesized in the cytoplasm as a precursor protein. This precursor contains a mitochondrial targeting sequence that directs the enzyme to the mitochondria.
3. **Mitochondrial Import:** Once synthesized, the precursor CS is imported into the mitochondria. This process involves the translocase of the outer membrane (TOM) and translocase of the inner membrane (TIM) complexes. After import, the targeting sequence is cleaved off, resulting in the mature, active enzyme.
4. **Enzyme Assembly:** In the mitochondria, CS assembles into a functional homodimer. This dimerization is essential for its enzymatic activity.

Regulation of Citrate Synthase

The regulation of citrate synthase involves multiple layers of control, including genetic, allosteric, and post-translational mechanisms.

1. **Genetic Regulation:** The expression of the CS gene can be influenced by various factors, including cellular energy status, oxidative stress, and hormonal signals. For example, peroxisome proliferator-activated receptor gamma coactivator 1-alpha (PGC-1α) can upregulate CS gene expression in response to increased energy demands.
2. **Allosteric Regulation:** CS activity can be modulated by allosteric effectors. High levels of ATP and NADH, indicators of sufficient energy supply, inhibit CS activity, whereas ADP and NAD+ stimulate its activity. This feedback mechanism helps balance energy production with cellular demands.
3. **Post-Translational Modifications:** Post-translational modifications such as phosphorylation, acetylation, and succinylation can alter CS activity. These modifications allow for rapid and reversible regulation of the enzyme in response to changing cellular conditions.
4. **Nutritional Regulation:** Nutritional status, including the availability of substrates and cofactors, significantly impacts CS activity. For instance, a diet rich in carbohydrates can enhance CS activity by increasing the supply of acetyl-CoA and oxaloacetate.

Plant-Based Diet and Citrate Synthase Regulation

A plant-based diet, rich in fruits, vegetables, whole grains, nuts, and seeds, can positively influence CS regulation through various mechanisms.

1. **Nutrient Density:** Plant-based diets provide essential nutrients, vitamins, and minerals that support overall mitochondrial function and enzymatic activity. For example, B vitamins, particularly B1, B2, B3, and B5, play crucial roles in the citric acid cycle and are abundantly found in plant-based foods.

2. **Phytonutrients:** Fruits and vegetables are rich in phytonutrients, including flavonoids, carotenoids, and polyphenols, which have been shown to enhance mitochondrial function and protect against oxidative stress. These compounds can indirectly support CS activity by maintaining mitochondrial health.
3. **Antioxidants:** Plant-based diets are high in antioxidants, which help reduce oxidative stress and maintain redox balance. Reduced oxidative stress is associated with improved mitochondrial function and CS activity.
4. **Healthy Fats:** Plant-based sources of fats, such as avocados, nuts, and seeds, provide essential fatty acids that support mitochondrial membrane integrity and function. Omega-3 fatty acids, in particular, have anti-inflammatory properties that can enhance mitochondrial efficiency and CS activity.
5. **Fiber:** High-fiber diets, common in plant-based eating, support gut health and metabolic regulation. A healthy gut microbiome can influence mitochondrial function and CS activity through the production of short-chain fatty acids and other metabolites.
6. **Caloric Balance:** Maintaining a healthy weight through a balanced plant-based diet can prevent obesity-related mitochondrial dysfunction. Excess body fat, particularly visceral fat, is linked to disrupted mitochondrial function due to increased production of inflammatory markers.
7. **Glycemic Control:** Plant-based diets, which are low in refined sugars and high in complex carbohydrates, help maintain stable blood glucose levels. This stability prevents insulin resistance and supports healthy mitochondrial function and CS activity.

Plant-Based Diet on Citrate Synthase-Related Health Outcomes

1. **Energy Metabolism:** A plant-based diet supports efficient energy metabolism by providing essential nutrients and maintaining mitochondrial health. Improved CS activity enhances ATP production, leading to better overall energy levels and endurance.
2. **Oxidative Stress Reduction:** The high antioxidant content of plant-based diets helps reduce oxidative stress, which can damage mitochondrial DNA and proteins. Lower oxidative stress levels are associated with improved CS activity and mitochondrial function.
3. **Weight Management:** Plant-based diets are effective for weight management, reducing body fat, and improving insulin sensitivity. Lower body fat and better glycemic control enhance overall metabolic health and mitochondrial efficiency, including CS activity.
4. **Cardiovascular Health:** Improved mitochondrial function, supported by a plant-based diet, can enhance cardiovascular health by reducing the risk of conditions such as atherosclerosis and hypertension. Efficient energy production and reduced oxidative stress are beneficial for heart health.
5. **Diabetes Management:** A plant-based diet can help manage and prevent type 2 diabetes by improving insulin sensitivity and glucose metabolism. Enhanced CS activity supports efficient energy production and metabolic regulation, which are crucial for diabetes management.
6. **Mental Health:** Emerging evidence suggests that plant-based diets may benefit mental health by reducing inflammation and oxidative stress, which are linked to mood disorders. Improved mitochondrial function and energy production support cognitive function and emotional well-being.
7. **Aging:** The antioxidant-rich nature of plant-based diets helps combat oxidative stress, a key factor in aging. Improved mito-

chondrial function and CS activity contribute to healthier aging and better maintenance of metabolic health.

Citrate synthase is a crucial enzyme in the citric acid cycle, playing a vital role in energy production and metabolic regulation. Its function, production, and regulation are influenced by various factors, including genetic, allosteric, post-translational, and nutritional mechanisms.

Aconitase

Aconitase is a crucial enzyme in the tricarboxylic acid (TCA) cycle, also known as the Krebs cycle or citric acid cycle.

Function of Aconitase

Aconitase plays a significant role in cellular energy production by catalyzing the isomerization of citrate to isocitrate via cis-aconitate in the TCA cycle. This process is essential for the continuous production of energy in the form of adenosine triphosphate (ATP), which powers various cellular functions.

Metabolic Role

1. **Citrate to Isocitrate Conversion:** Aconitase catalyzes the reversible transformation of citrate to isocitrate through cis-aconitate. This reaction is crucial for the TCA cycle's function, allowing the cycle to progress and generate ATP.
2. **Energy Production:** By facilitating the TCA cycle, aconitase contributes to the generation of NADH and FADH2, which are used in the electron transport chain to produce ATP.
3. **Iron-Sulfur Cluster Regulation:** Aconitase contains an iron-sulfur cluster (4Fe-4S) that is vital for its enzymatic activity. This

cluster can switch between active and inactive forms based on the cell's metabolic state, thereby regulating energy production according to cellular needs.

Additional Roles

1. **Redox Balance:** Aconitase helps maintain cellular redox balance by participating in oxidative and reductive reactions within the TCA cycle.
2. **Iron Homeostasis:** Aconitase in its cytosolic form (c-aconitase) also functions as an iron regulatory protein (IRP1), which regulates iron metabolism by binding to iron-responsive elements (IREs) on mRNAs encoding proteins involved in iron storage and transport.

Production of Aconitase

Aconitase production involves a complex process of gene expression and protein synthesis, tightly regulated to meet the cell's metabolic demands.

Gene Encoding

1. **Gene Location:** The gene encoding mitochondrial aconitase (ACO2) is located on chromosome 22, while the gene for cytosolic aconitase (ACO1) is located on chromosome 9.
2. **Transcription Regulation:** Transcription of ACO2 and ACO1 genes is regulated by cellular energy status and iron levels, ensuring that aconitase production is aligned with metabolic needs.

Protein Synthesis

1. **Translation:** After transcription, mRNA for aconitase is translated into a precursor protein in the cytoplasm. This precursor

contains a mitochondrial targeting sequence that directs it to the mitochondria.

2. **Post-Translational Modifications:** The precursor protein undergoes post-translational modifications, including the removal of the targeting sequence and incorporation of the iron-sulfur cluster, which are essential for its enzymatic activity.

Regulation of Aconitase

The regulation of aconitase is a multi-faceted process involving feedback mechanisms, iron availability, and oxidative stress, ensuring that the enzyme's activity is modulated according to cellular requirements.

Feedback Mechanisms

1. **Energy Status:** Aconitase activity is regulated by the cell's energy status. High levels of ATP and NADH inhibit aconitase activity, while low energy levels activate it to enhance ATP production.
2. **Substrate Availability:** The availability of citrate and other intermediates of the TCA cycle also regulates aconitase activity. An accumulation of citrate can inhibit its own conversion, providing a feedback mechanism to balance the TCA cycle.

Iron-Sulfur Cluster Dynamics

1. **Iron Availability:** The iron-sulfur cluster of aconitase is sensitive to cellular iron levels. Iron deficiency can lead to the disassembly of the cluster, converting aconitase into its inactive form.
2. **Oxidative Stress:** Reactive oxygen species (ROS) can damage the iron-sulfur cluster, leading to aconitase inactivation. The cell employs antioxidant mechanisms to protect aconitase from oxidative damage and maintain its activity.

Nutritional Influence

A plant-based diet can significantly impact the regulation of aconitase through the provision of essential nutrients and antioxidants.

1. **Iron Intake:** Plant-based sources of iron, such as legumes, nuts, seeds, and leafy greens, provide non-heme iron, which supports the maintenance of the iron-sulfur cluster in aconitase.
2. **Antioxidants:** A diet rich in fruits and vegetables supplies antioxidants like vitamin C, vitamin E, and polyphenols, which protect aconitase from oxidative damage and help maintain its activity.
3. **Amino Acids:** Essential amino acids from plant-based proteins are necessary for the synthesis of aconitase and its maintenance in an active form.

Plant-Based Diet and Aconitase Regulation

A plant-based diet, characterized by high nutrient density and rich in antioxidants, plays a pivotal role in supporting aconitase function and overall metabolic health.

Nutrient Density

Plant-based diets provide a wealth of essential nutrients that support the optimal function of metabolic enzymes like aconitase.

1. **Vitamins and Minerals:** Leafy greens, legumes, nuts, seeds, and whole grains are rich sources of vitamins and minerals that are crucial for enzyme function, including iron, magnesium, and B vitamins.
2. **Phytochemicals:** Plant foods are abundant in phytochemicals, which have been shown to enhance cellular health and protect enzymes from oxidative stress.

Antioxidants and Redox Balance

1. **Protective Role:** Antioxidants in plant foods help maintain redox balance by neutralizing ROS, which can damage the iron-sulfur cluster of aconitase.
2. **Oxidative Stress Reduction:** Diets rich in fruits, vegetables, and whole grains reduce oxidative stress, thus protecting aconitase and supporting its continuous function in the TCA cycle.

Iron Bioavailability

1. **Non-heme Iron Sources:** While plant-based sources provide non-heme iron, which is less readily absorbed than heme iron from animal products, the presence of vitamin C and other enhancers in plant foods boosts iron absorption.
2. **Iron Regulation:** Adequate intake of iron from plant sources helps maintain the iron-sulfur cluster of aconitase, ensuring its proper function.

Amino Acid Support

1. **Protein Synthesis:** Plant-based proteins from sources like beans, lentils, and quinoa provide essential amino acids necessary for the synthesis and maintenance of aconitase.
2. **Enzyme Maintenance:** Amino acids such as cysteine and methionine, which are found in various plant foods, support the formation and stability of the iron-sulfur cluster in aconitase.

Caloric Balance and Energy Regulation

1. **Energy Homeostasis:** A balanced plant-based diet helps maintain appropriate caloric intake, preventing metabolic imbalances that can affect aconitase activity.

2. **Metabolic Flexibility:** The high fiber content in plant foods supports metabolic flexibility and efficient energy production, which is critical for the optimal functioning of the TCA cycle and aconitase.

Plant-Based Diet on Aconitase-Related Health Outcomes

Cellular Energy Production

A plant-based diet enhances cellular energy production by supporting the TCA cycle and maintaining aconitase activity through the provision of essential nutrients and antioxidants.

1. **Improved ATP Production:** By ensuring the continuous function of the TCA cycle, a plant-based diet supports efficient ATP production, which is essential for cellular activities and overall energy levels.
2. **Enhanced Metabolic Efficiency:** The high nutrient density and low oxidative stress associated with plant-based diets improve metabolic efficiency, reducing the risk of metabolic disorders.

Oxidative Stress and Inflammation

1. **Reduction in Oxidative Damage:** Antioxidants in plant foods mitigate oxidative damage to aconitase and other metabolic enzymes, enhancing cellular health and reducing the risk of chronic diseases.
2. **Anti-Inflammatory Effects:** Plant-based diets are rich in anti-inflammatory compounds that help maintain a healthy immune response, further protecting metabolic enzymes and promoting overall health.

Iron Metabolism

1. **Balanced Iron Intake:** Plant-based sources of iron, coupled with enhancers like vitamin C, support balanced iron metabolism, crucial for maintaining the active form of aconitase.
2. **Iron Homeostasis:** Proper iron homeostasis ensures that the iron-sulfur cluster in aconitase remains functional, facilitating continuous energy production and metabolic regulation.

Weight Management and Metabolic Health

1. **Healthy Weight Maintenance:** A plant-based diet promotes healthy weight management, reducing the risk of obesity-related metabolic disturbances that can affect aconitase activity.
2. **Insulin Sensitivity:** Improved insulin sensitivity, supported by a diet high in fiber and low in refined sugars, helps regulate metabolic processes and maintain efficient energy production.

Overall Health and Longevity

1. **Enhanced Longevity:** The combined effects of improved metabolic health, reduced oxidative stress, and balanced nutrient intake associated with plant-based diets contribute to enhanced longevity and overall well-being.
2. **Disease Prevention:** By supporting the optimal function of metabolic enzymes like aconitase, a plant-based diet reduces the risk of chronic diseases, including cardiovascular disease, diabetes, and neurodegenerative disorders.

Aconitase is a vital enzyme in the TCA cycle, essential for cellular energy production and metabolic regulation. Its activity is influenced by various factors, including nutrient availability, oxidative stress, and iron homeostasis.

Isocitrate Dehydrogenase (IDH)

Isocitrate dehydrogenase (IDH) is a pivotal enzyme in cellular metabolism, playing a crucial role in the citric acid cycle, which is fundamental for energy production in cells.

Function of Isocitrate Dehydrogenase

IDH has significant functions within the cell, primarily within the citric acid cycle (also known as the Krebs cycle or TCA cycle) and in cellular metabolic regulation.

Energy Production

Citric Acid Cycle:

- **Role in the Citric Acid Cycle:** IDH catalyzes the oxidative decarboxylation of isocitrate to alpha-ketoglutarate, producing NADH or NADPH in the process. This reaction is a key step in the citric acid cycle, which is critical for cellular respiration and ATP production.
- **Enzyme Variants:** There are three isoforms of IDH: IDH1 and IDH2, which use NADP+ as a cofactor, and IDH3, which uses NAD+.

Cellular Metabolism

NADPH Production:

- **Reductive Biosynthesis:** IDH1 and IDH2 are involved in producing NADPH, which is essential for reductive biosynthesis reactions and for maintaining the redox state of cells.

- **Oxidative Stress Response:** NADPH produced by IDH1 and IDH2 is also crucial for regenerating glutathione, a key antioxidant that protects cells from oxidative damage.

Additional Roles

Metabolic Regulation:

- **Metabolic Flux:** IDH plays a role in regulating the flux of metabolites through the citric acid cycle, thereby influencing overall cellular metabolism.
- **Anaplerosis:** By producing alpha-ketoglutarate, IDH contributes to anaplerotic reactions that replenish citric acid cycle intermediates.

Production of Isocitrate Dehydrogenase

IDH is produced in cells through gene expression and protein synthesis, regulated by various genetic and metabolic factors.

Gene Encoding

IDH Genes:

- **IDH1 and IDH2:** These genes are located on chromosomes 2 and 15, respectively, and encode the NADP+-dependent isoforms of IDH, which are primarily found in the cytoplasm (IDH1) and mitochondria (IDH2).
- **IDH3:** The gene encoding the NAD+-dependent isoform of IDH is located on chromosome 15 and is primarily expressed in the mitochondria.

Enzyme Structure
Subunit Composition:

- **IDH1 and IDH2:** These enzymes function as homodimers or homotetramers, depending on the specific isoform.
- **IDH3:** This enzyme functions as a heterotetramer, consisting of different subunits (alpha, beta, and gamma) encoded by separate genes.

Regulation by Cellular Conditions
Metabolic Signals:

- **Nutrient Availability:** The expression and activity of IDH are influenced by the availability of nutrients, particularly glucose and other carbohydrates that feed into the citric acid cycle.
- **Energy Demand:** IDH activity is modulated by the cellular energy state, with increased activity under conditions of high ATP demand.

Influencing Factors
Age and Development:

- **Developmental Regulation:** IDH expression varies during different stages of development, with higher levels in rapidly growing tissues.
- **Age-Related Changes:** IDH activity may decline with age, contributing to age-related metabolic changes and reduced energy production.

Regulation of Isocitrate Dehydrogenase

The regulation of IDH involves multiple layers of control, including genetic, metabolic, and environmental factors.

Genetic Regulation

Transcriptional Control:

- **Transcription Factors:** Various transcription factors regulate the expression of IDH genes in response to cellular metabolic needs and external signals.
- **Epigenetic Modifications:** DNA methylation and histone modifications can influence IDH gene expression, impacting enzyme levels and activity.

Metabolic Regulation

Allosteric Regulation:

- **Allosteric Effectors:** IDH activity is regulated by allosteric effectors such as ATP, ADP, and NADH, which bind to the enzyme and modulate its activity.
- **Feedback Inhibition:** High levels of NADH or ATP can inhibit IDH activity, reducing the flux through the citric acid cycle when energy levels are sufficient.

Environmental and Nutritional Factors

Dietary Influences:

- **Plant-Based Nutrients:** Nutrients found in plant-based diets, such as vitamins, minerals, and antioxidants, can support IDH activity and overall metabolic health.
- **Caloric Intake:** Adequate caloric intake from plant-based sources ensures sufficient energy supply for IDH-mediated metabolic processes.

Cellular Stress Response
Oxidative Stress:

- **Antioxidant Defense:** IDH1 and IDH2 contribute to the cellular antioxidant defense by producing NADPH, which is essential for regenerating reduced glutathione.
- **Stress Response Mechanisms:** Under conditions of oxidative stress, IDH activity is upregulated to enhance NADPH production and protect cells from damage.

Plant-Based Diet and Isocitrate Dehydrogenase Regulation

A plant-based diet, rich in diverse nutrients, supports the optimal function and regulation of IDH through various mechanisms.

Nutrient Density
Vitamins and Minerals:

- **Essential Nutrients:** Plant-based diets provide essential vitamins and minerals, such as vitamin B6, magnesium, and manganese, which are cofactors for various enzymes, including IDH.
- **Antioxidant Vitamins:** Vitamins C and E, abundant in fruits and vegetables, help maintain the redox balance in cells, indirectly supporting IDH function.

Amino Acids
Protein Sources:

- **Plant Proteins:** Legumes, nuts, seeds, and whole grains provide essential amino acids required for protein synthesis and enzyme function, including the production of IDH.
- **Glutathione Precursors:** Plant foods rich in sulfur-containing amino acids, such as garlic and onions, support

glutathione synthesis, enhancing the antioxidant capacity of cells.

Antioxidants
Oxidative Stress Reduction:

- **Polyphenols and Flavonoids:** Compounds found in plant foods, such as polyphenols and flavonoids, have antioxidant properties that reduce oxidative stress and support metabolic health.
- **Protective Effects:** Antioxidants help protect IDH and other enzymes from oxidative damage, ensuring their proper function.

Healthy Fats
Fatty Acid Composition:

- **Omega-3 Fatty Acids:** Plant sources of omega-3 fatty acids, such as flaxseeds and chia seeds, have anti-inflammatory properties that support overall metabolic health.
- **Monounsaturated Fats:** Avocados, nuts, and seeds provide healthy fats that contribute to cell membrane integrity and enzyme function.

Fiber
Gut Health:

- **Dietary Fiber:** High-fiber diets promote a healthy gut microbiome, which can influence metabolic processes and enzyme regulation through the production of short-chain fatty acids and other metabolites.

- **Metabolic Regulation:** A healthy gut environment supports efficient nutrient absorption and metabolic regulation, indirectly benefiting IDH function.

Caloric Balance
Weight Management:

- **Healthy Weight:** Maintaining a healthy weight through a balanced plant-based diet prevents obesity-related metabolic disruptions that can affect IDH activity.
- **Insulin Sensitivity:** Improved insulin sensitivity from a plant-based diet helps maintain proper glucose metabolism, ensuring a steady supply of substrates for the citric acid cycle.

Glycemic Control
Stable Blood Glucose:

- **Complex Carbohydrates:** Plant-based diets rich in complex carbohydrates help maintain stable blood glucose levels, preventing metabolic imbalances that could affect IDH function.
- **Insulin Regulation:** Stable blood glucose levels support healthy insulin secretion and action, which is crucial for overall metabolic health.

Plant-Based Diet on IDH-Related Health Outcomes

Adopting a plant-based diet can have numerous health benefits related to the optimal function of IDH and overall metabolic health.

Metabolic Health
Energy Production:

- **Efficient Metabolism:** A plant-based diet supports efficient energy production through the citric acid cycle, ensuring adequate ATP generation for cellular functions.
- **Enhanced NADPH Production:** By providing necessary nutrients, a plant-based diet enhances NADPH production, crucial for reductive biosynthesis and antioxidant defense.

Disease Prevention
Chronic Disease Risk Reduction:

- **Cardiovascular Health:** Nutrients and antioxidants in plant-based diets reduce oxidative stress and inflammation, lowering the risk of cardiovascular diseases.
- **Cancer Prevention:** Antioxidants and phytochemicals in plant foods help protect against DNA damage and cancer development by reducing oxidative stress and supporting detoxification pathways.

Longevity and Aging
Healthy Aging:

- **Oxidative Stress Mitigation:** A diet rich in plant-based antioxidants supports healthy aging by reducing oxidative damage to cells and tissues.
- **Metabolic Efficiency:** Maintaining efficient metabolic processes through a plant-based diet helps preserve cellular function and energy production with age.

Weight Management
Obesity Prevention:

- **Nutrient-Dense Foods:** Plant-based diets, high in fiber and low in refined sugars, help prevent obesity by promoting satiety and reducing caloric intake.
- **Insulin Sensitivity:** Improved insulin sensitivity from a plant-based diet aids in maintaining a healthy body weight and preventing metabolic syndrome.

Cognitive Health
Mental Well-Being:

- **Brain Health:** Nutrients such as omega-3 fatty acids and antioxidants in plant-based diets support brain health and cognitive function.
- **Mood Regulation:** Reduced inflammation and oxidative stress from a plant-based diet may contribute to better mood regulation and mental health.

Isocitrate dehydrogenase is a vital enzyme in cellular metabolism, playing a key role in energy production, metabolic regulation, and the cellular stress response. Its production and regulation are influenced by various genetic, metabolic, and environmental factors.

Alpha-Ketoglutarate Dehydrogenase (α-KGDH)

Alpha-Ketoglutarate Dehydrogenase (α-KGDH) is a critical enzyme within the tricarboxylic acid (TCA) cycle, also known as the Krebs cycle. It plays an essential role in cellular respiration, energy production, and metabolic regulation.

Function of Alpha-Ketoglutarate Dehydrogenase

Alpha-Ketoglutarate Dehydrogenase (α-KGDH) is an enzyme that catalyzes the conversion of alpha-ketoglutarate to succinyl-CoA and CO_2 in the TCA cycle. This step is crucial for the production of energy in the form of ATP and for maintaining metabolic balance.

Energy Production

α-KGDH is a key enzyme in the TCA cycle, which is the central pathway for aerobic respiration in cells. The TCA cycle generates high-energy electron carriers (NADH and $FADH_2$) that are used in the electron transport chain to produce ATP, the primary energy currency of the cell. The conversion of alpha-ketoglutarate to succinyl-CoA is one of the critical steps that facilitate this energy production.

Metabolic Intermediates

The TCA cycle, with α-KGDH as a crucial component, produces intermediates that serve as building blocks for various biosynthetic processes. These intermediates are essential for the synthesis of amino acids, nucleotides, and other biomolecules.

Redox Balance

α-KGDH helps maintain the redox balance within cells by generating NADH, which is used in various biochemical reactions to maintain oxidative and reductive balance. This balance is crucial for cellular health and function.

Production of Alpha-Ketoglutarate Dehydrogenase

The production of α-KGDH involves several steps, from gene expression to post-translational modifications, ensuring the enzyme is correctly synthesized and functional.

Gene Encoding

The genes encoding the subunits of α-KGDH are located on different chromosomes and are expressed in various tissues. The α-KGDH complex consists of multiple subunits encoded by the genes OGDH (for the E1 subunit), DLST (for the E2 subunit), and DLD (for the E3 subunit).

Transcription and Translation

1. **Gene Transcription:** The genes encoding the α-KGDH subunits are transcribed into mRNA in the nucleus. This process is regulated by various transcription factors and influenced by cellular energy status and metabolic needs.
2. **Translation:** The mRNA transcripts are translated into polypeptides in the cytoplasm. These polypeptides undergo folding and assembly to form the active enzyme complex.

Assembly and Localization

1. **Mitochondrial Import:** The α-KGDH subunits are imported into the mitochondria, where they are assembled into the functional enzyme complex. The mitochondrial localization is crucial for its role in the TCA cycle, which takes place in the mitochondrial matrix.
2. **Complex Formation:** The E1, E2, and E3 subunits interact to form the active α-KGDH complex. This multi-subunit complex ensures the efficient catalysis of the conversion of alpha-ketoglutarate to succinyl-CoA.

Regulation of Alpha-Ketoglutarate Dehydrogenase

The regulation of α-KGDH involves multiple mechanisms, including feedback inhibition, covalent modifications, and dietary influences.

Feedback Inhibition

α-KGDH activity is tightly regulated by feedback inhibition to maintain metabolic balance.

1. **NADH:** High levels of NADH, a product of the TCA cycle, inhibit α-KGDH activity. This feedback mechanism prevents excessive production of metabolic intermediates when cellular energy levels are sufficient.
2. **Succinyl-CoA:** The product of the α-KGDH-catalyzed reaction, succinyl-CoA, also acts as an inhibitor of the enzyme, ensuring that the TCA cycle proceeds at an appropriate rate.

Covalent Modifications

Post-translational modifications, such as phosphorylation, can regulate α-KGDH activity.

1. **Phosphorylation:** Phosphorylation of specific residues on α-KGDH subunits can modulate its activity. For instance, certain kinases may phosphorylate α-KGDH, reducing its activity under specific metabolic conditions.
2. **Dephosphorylation:** Conversely, phosphatases can remove these phosphate groups, restoring α-KGDH activity when needed.

Plant-Based Nutritional Influence

A plant-based diet, rich in various nutrients, can influence the activity and regulation of α-KGDH through several mechanisms.

1. **Antioxidants:** Plant-based diets are rich in antioxidants, such as vitamins C and E, which help reduce oxidative stress. Lower oxidative stress levels can enhance α-KGDH activity by preventing oxidative damage to the enzyme and its cofactors.

2. **Vitamins and Cofactors:** Certain vitamins, such as vitamin B1 (thiamine), are essential cofactors for α-KGDH activity. Plant-based sources like whole grains, nuts, and seeds are excellent sources of thiamine, supporting the optimal function of α-KGDH.
3. **Phytochemicals:** Bioactive compounds found in plants, such as polyphenols, can modulate enzyme activity. For instance, polyphenols in fruits and vegetables may enhance mitochondrial function and α-KGDH activity by improving overall cellular health.
4. **Amino Acids:** Plant-based proteins provide essential amino acids that support the synthesis and maintenance of α-KGDH subunits. Legumes, nuts, and seeds are rich sources of these amino acids, promoting enzyme production and function.
5. **Minerals:** Minerals like magnesium and iron, found abundantly in plant-based foods, are crucial for enzymatic reactions and mitochondrial health. These minerals support the catalytic activity of α-KGDH and overall metabolic function.

Plant-Based Diet on α-KGDH-Related Health Outcomes

Energy Metabolism

A plant-based diet supports efficient energy metabolism by providing essential nutrients that optimize α-KGDH activity. Improved energy production enhances overall vitality and reduces fatigue.

Oxidative Stress Reduction

The high antioxidant content in plant-based diets helps mitigate oxidative stress, protecting α-KGDH from oxidative damage and maintaining its activity. This protection is crucial for preventing metabolic disorders linked to mitochondrial dysfunction.

Weight Management

Plant-based diets are effective for weight management due to their high fiber content and low-calorie density. Maintaining a healthy weight reduces the risk of metabolic diseases that can impair α-KGDH function, such as type 2 diabetes and obesity.

Disease Prevention

Optimized α-KGDH activity through a plant-based diet may contribute to the prevention of chronic diseases. For instance, improved mitochondrial function and energy production can reduce the risk of cardiovascular diseases and neurodegenerative disorders.

Alpha-Ketoglutarate Dehydrogenase (α-KGDH) is a vital enzyme in the TCA cycle, playing a central role in energy production, metabolic balance, and redox regulation. Its production and regulation are influenced by genetic, biochemical, and dietary factors.

Succinate Dehydrogenase (SDH)

Succinate dehydrogenase (SDH) is a critical enzyme in both the tricarboxylic acid (TCA) cycle and the electron transport chain (ETC), playing a vital role in cellular respiration and energy production.

Function of Succinate Dehydrogenase

Succinate dehydrogenase, also known as Complex II in the ETC, is an enzyme that catalyzes the oxidation of succinate to fumarate in the TCA cycle while simultaneously reducing ubiquinone to ubiquinol in the ETC. This dual function places SDH at the intersection of two critical metabolic pathways.

TCA Cycle

1. **Oxidation of Succinate**: SDH catalyzes the conversion of succinate to fumarate, an essential step in the TCA cycle that generates fumarate and releases electrons.

2. **Energy Production**: The electrons released during this reaction are transferred to flavin adenine dinucleotide (FAD), forming FADH2, which then donates these electrons to the ETC.

Electron Transport Chain

1. **Complex II**: SDH is unique among the ETC complexes because it directly participates in the TCA cycle. It accepts electrons from FADH2 and transfers them to ubiquinone (coenzyme Q), forming ubiquinol.
2. **ATP Synthesis**: By contributing electrons to the ETC, SDH helps maintain the proton gradient across the mitochondrial membrane, which drives ATP synthesis through oxidative phosphorylation.

Additional Roles

1. **Reactive Oxygen Species (ROS) Management**: SDH activity influences the production of ROS, which are by-products of mitochondrial respiration. The proper function of SDH helps mitigate excessive ROS production, which can damage cellular components.
2. **Metabolic Flexibility**: SDH plays a role in metabolic flexibility, allowing cells to adapt to varying energy demands and nutrient availability by efficiently switching between different metabolic pathways.

Production of Succinate Dehydrogenase

Succinate dehydrogenase is produced within the mitochondria through a complex interplay of genetic expression, protein assembly, and regulatory mechanisms.

Synthesis

1. **Gene Encoding**: SDH is encoded by nuclear genes that produce four subunits: SDHA, SDHB, SDHC, and SDHD. These genes are transcribed and translated into their respective protein subunits in the cytoplasm.
2. **Mitochondrial Import**: After synthesis, these protein subunits are imported into the mitochondria, where they undergo further processing and assembly.

Assembly

1. **Subunit Composition**: SDHA and SDHB form the catalytic core of the enzyme, while SDHC and SDHD anchor the enzyme to the inner mitochondrial membrane.
2. **Cofactor Integration**: The assembly process includes the incorporation of essential cofactors such as FAD and iron-sulfur clusters, which are crucial for the enzyme's catalytic activity.

Regulation by Hypoxia-Inducible Factors (HIFs)

1. **Oxygen Sensing**: Under low oxygen conditions, HIFs regulate the expression of SDH subunits to adapt to the cellular environment. HIF-1α, in particular, can downregulate SDH expression to reduce oxygen consumption and ROS production.
2. **Feedback Mechanisms**: Cellular energy status and metabolic intermediates provide feedback to regulate SDH expression and activity, ensuring a balance between energy production and cellular health.

Regulation of Succinate Dehydrogenase

The regulation of SDH involves various mechanisms that respond to cellular energy demands, oxygen levels, and metabolic states.

Allosteric Regulation

1. **Substrate Availability**: The levels of succinate and fumarate, the substrates and products of the SDH-catalyzed reaction, can allosterically regulate the enzyme's activity. High succinate levels can inhibit SDH activity, while high fumarate levels can activate it.
2. **Cofactor Availability**: The availability of cofactors such as FAD and iron-sulfur clusters is critical for SDH activity. Deficiencies in these cofactors can impair SDH function and overall mitochondrial respiration.

Genetic Regulation

1. **Transcriptional Control**: The expression of SDH subunit genes is regulated at the transcriptional level by factors such as nuclear respiratory factors (NRFs) and peroxisome proliferator-activated receptor gamma coactivator 1-alpha (PGC-1α), which respond to cellular energy demands.
2. **Epigenetic Modifications**: Epigenetic changes, including DNA methylation and histone acetylation, can influence the expression of SDH genes, modulating the enzyme's activity in response to environmental and metabolic cues.

Post-Translational Modifications

1. **Phosphorylation**: Phosphorylation of SDH subunits by protein kinases can alter the enzyme's activity and stability. This modification often occurs in response to signaling pathways that regulate cellular metabolism.

2. **Acetylation**: Acetylation of SDH subunits can affect their interaction with other mitochondrial proteins and influence the overall function of the enzyme complex.

Interaction with Other Mitochondrial Components

1. **Supercomplex Formation**: SDH can interact with other ETC complexes to form supercomplexes, enhancing the efficiency of electron transfer and reducing ROS production.
2. **Mitochondrial Dynamics**: Changes in mitochondrial dynamics, including fission and fusion events, can impact SDH activity by altering the mitochondrial network and distribution within the cell.

Plant-Based Diet and Succinate Dehydrogenase Regulation

A plant-based diet, rich in fruits, vegetables, whole grains, nuts, and seeds, can positively influence SDH regulation through various mechanisms.

Nutrient Density

1. **Vitamins and Minerals**: Plant-based diets provide essential vitamins and minerals that support SDH function. For example, riboflavin (vitamin B2) is a precursor for FAD, a critical cofactor for SDH. Rich sources of riboflavin include almonds, mushrooms, and spinach.
2. **Iron**: Iron is necessary for the formation of iron-sulfur clusters in SDH. Plant-based sources of iron, such as lentils, chickpeas, and tofu, can support adequate iron levels, especially when consumed with vitamin C-rich foods to enhance absorption.

Antioxidants

1. **Oxidative Stress Reduction**: Fruits and vegetables are rich in antioxidants, such as vitamins C and E, and polyphenols, which help reduce oxidative stress and protect mitochondrial function, including SDH activity.
2. **Polyphenols**: Compounds like quercetin and resveratrol, found in berries, grapes, and apples, can modulate mitochondrial function and enhance SDH activity by reducing ROS production and improving cellular redox balance.

Healthy Fats

1. **Omega-3 Fatty Acids**: Plant-based sources of omega-3 fatty acids, such as flaxseeds, chia seeds, and walnuts, have anti-inflammatory properties that can protect mitochondrial function and support SDH activity.
2. **Monounsaturated Fats**: Avocados provide monounsaturated fats that support overall cellular health and mitochondrial efficiency, indirectly benefiting SDH function.

Fiber

1. **Gut Health**: A high-fiber diet supports a healthy gut microbiome, which can influence systemic inflammation and metabolic health. Short-chain fatty acids produced by gut bacteria from dietary fiber can modulate mitochondrial function and SDH activity.
2. **Metabolic Regulation**: Fiber helps maintain stable blood glucose levels, preventing metabolic dysregulation that can impair mitochondrial function and SDH activity.

Phytochemicals

1. **Flavonoids**: Flavonoids found in plant foods, such as catechins in green tea and anthocyanins in berries, can enhance mitochondrial function and protect SDH from oxidative damage.
2. **Sulfur-Containing Compounds**: Compounds like sulforaphane in cruciferous vegetables (e.g., broccoli, Brussels sprouts) can induce the expression of antioxidant enzymes and support mitochondrial health, indirectly benefiting SDH function.

Plant-Based Diet on SDH-Related Health Outcomes

A plant-based diet can enhance SDH function and overall mitochondrial health, leading to various positive health outcomes.

Metabolic Health

1. **Diabetes Prevention**: Improved SDH function supports efficient cellular respiration and glucose metabolism, reducing the risk of type 2 diabetes. The high fiber content and low glycemic load of plant-based diets help maintain insulin sensitivity.
2. **Obesity Management**: Plant-based diets are typically lower in calories and higher in nutrients, supporting healthy weight management. Proper SDH function aids in efficient energy production and fat metabolism, contributing to weight control.

Cardiovascular Health

1. **Heart Disease Prevention**: Antioxidants and healthy fats in plant-based diets protect against oxidative stress and inflammation, reducing the risk of cardiovascular diseases. Enhanced SDH

activity supports optimal mitochondrial function, crucial for heart health.

2. **Blood Pressure Regulation**: Potassium-rich plant foods, such as bananas and sweet potatoes, help regulate blood pressure, indirectly benefiting SDH function by reducing oxidative stress and improving vascular health.

Cognitive Function

1. **Neuroprotection**: Antioxidants and anti-inflammatory compounds in plant-based diets protect against neurodegenerative diseases by reducing oxidative damage and supporting mitochondrial function, including SDH activity.
2. **Cognitive Performance**: Improved mitochondrial efficiency and energy production support cognitive function and reduce the risk of age-related cognitive decline. Plant-based diets provide nutrients that enhance brain health and SDH function.

Longevity and Aging

1. **Anti-Aging Effects**: The antioxidant-rich nature of plant-based diets helps combat oxidative stress, a key factor in aging. Enhanced SDH function contributes to better mitochondrial health and overall cellular vitality, promoting healthy aging.
2. **Disease Prevention**: Plant-based diets are associated with a reduced risk of chronic diseases, including cancer, heart disease, and neurodegenerative disorders. Proper SDH function supports efficient energy metabolism and cellular health, reducing the risk of these conditions.

Succinate dehydrogenase plays a pivotal role in cellular respiration, bridging the TCA cycle and the electron transport chain. Its production and regulation are influenced by various factors, including genetic expression, substrate availability, and cellular metabolic states.

Fumarase

Fumarase, also known as fumarate hydratase (FH), is a crucial enzyme in the tricarboxylic acid (TCA) cycle, also known as the Krebs cycle or the citric acid cycle. This enzyme plays a significant role in cellular metabolism, energy production, and various metabolic pathways.

Function of Fumarase

Fumarase is a key enzyme that catalyzes the reversible hydration of fumarate to malate in the TCA cycle. Its function is essential for energy production and metabolic homeostasis.

Role in the TCA Cycle

1. **Energy Production**: Fumarase facilitates the conversion of fumarate to L-malate, a critical step in the TCA cycle. This cycle is a central pathway for the generation of ATP, the primary energy currency of the cell.
2. **Metabolic Pathway Integration**: The TCA cycle is interconnected with various other metabolic pathways, including glycolysis, amino acid metabolism, and fatty acid oxidation. Fumarase's role is pivotal in ensuring the smooth functioning of these interconnected pathways.

Additional Roles

1. **Cellular Respiration**: By participating in the TCA cycle, fumarase indirectly supports cellular respiration, the process by which cells generate energy through the oxidation of nutrients.

2. **Redox Balance:** The conversion of fumarate to malate is linked to the maintenance of redox balance within the cell, as it influences the levels of NADH and FADH2, which are crucial for the electron transport chain.

Production of Fumarase

Fumarase is produced through a well-regulated process involving gene expression, protein synthesis, and post-translational modifications.

Gene Encoding

1. **FH Gene:** The fumarase gene (FH) is located on chromosome 1 in humans. This gene encodes the fumarase enzyme, which is synthesized as a precursor protein and undergoes subsequent processing.
2. **Transcript Variants:** Different transcript variants of the FH gene can result in distinct isoforms of the enzyme, tailored to specific cellular needs.

Synthesis and Localization

1. **Mitochondrial and Cytosolic Isoforms:** Fumarase exists in two main forms—mitochondrial and cytosolic. The mitochondrial form is primarily involved in the TCA cycle, while the cytosolic form participates in non-mitochondrial metabolic processes.
2. **Post-Translational Modifications:** After synthesis, fumarase undergoes post-translational modifications, including acetylation and phosphorylation, which regulate its activity and stability.

Regulation of Fumarase

The regulation of fumarase involves a complex interplay of genetic, metabolic, and environmental factors.

Genetic Regulation

1. **Transcriptional Control**: The expression of the FH gene is regulated by various transcription factors, including hypoxia-inducible factors (HIFs) and cAMP response element-binding protein (CREB), which respond to cellular metabolic states.
2. **Epigenetic Modifications**: DNA methylation and histone modifications can influence the expression of the FH gene, thereby modulating fumarase levels.

Metabolic Regulation

1. **Substrate Availability**: The levels of fumarate and malate, as substrates and products, respectively, influence fumarase activity through feedback mechanisms.
2. **Allosteric Regulation**: Fumarase can be allosterically regulated by other metabolic intermediates, ensuring its activity is synchronized with the cell's metabolic demands.

Environmental Factors

1. **Oxygen Levels**: Hypoxia can affect fumarase activity, as the enzyme plays a role in adapting to low oxygen conditions by modulating the TCA cycle.
2. **Nutritional Status**: Diet, including plant-based nutrition, can influence fumarase regulation through the availability of metabolic precursors and cofactors.

Plant-Based Diet and Fumarase Regulation

A plant-based diet, rich in fruits, vegetables, whole grains, nuts, and seeds, can positively influence fumarase regulation through various mechanisms.

Nutrient Density

Plant-based diets provide essential nutrients, vitamins, and minerals that support overall metabolic health and enzyme activity.

1. **Vitamins and Minerals**: Vitamins such as B-complex (B1, B2, B3, B5, B6, B7, B9, and B12) and minerals like magnesium and manganese are crucial for enzyme function. These nutrients act as cofactors for various enzymes, including fumarase, and are abundantly available in plant-based foods.
2. **Phytochemicals**: Plant-based diets are rich in phytochemicals, which have antioxidant properties that protect enzymes from oxidative damage and support metabolic homeostasis.

Antioxidants

Fruits and vegetables are rich in antioxidants, which help reduce oxidative stress and protect enzymes like fumarase from oxidative damage.

1. **Oxidative Stress Reduction**: Antioxidants such as vitamin C, vitamin E, and polyphenols found in plant foods reduce oxidative stress, which can impair enzyme function. Reduced oxidative stress is associated with improved fumarase activity and overall metabolic efficiency.
2. **Anti-Inflammatory Effects**: Antioxidants also exhibit anti-inflammatory effects, which help maintain cellular health and support enzyme function.

Amino Acids

Certain amino acids found in plant foods, such as glutamine and arginine, support enzyme production and activity.

1. **Protein Synthesis**: Amino acids are the building blocks of proteins, including enzymes like fumarase. Plant-based sources of amino acids, such as legumes, nuts, and seeds, provide the necessary substrates for protein synthesis.
2. **Enzyme Stability**: Adequate intake of amino acids helps maintain the structural integrity and stability of enzymes, ensuring their proper function and longevity.

Fiber

High-fiber diets, common in plant-based eating, support gut health and metabolic regulation.

1. **Gut Microbiome**: A healthy gut microbiome, supported by dietary fiber, produces short-chain fatty acids (SCFAs) that can influence metabolic pathways and enzyme regulation, including fumarase.
2. **Blood Sugar Control**: Fiber helps regulate blood sugar levels, preventing spikes and crashes that can disrupt metabolic homeostasis and enzyme activity.

Healthy Fats

Plant-based sources of fats, such as avocados, nuts, and seeds, provide essential fatty acids that support metabolic health and enzyme regulation.

1. **Omega-3 Fatty Acids**: Omega-3 fatty acids, found in flaxseeds, chia seeds, and walnuts, have anti-inflammatory properties and support cellular health, indirectly benefiting enzymes like fumarase.
2. **Lipid Metabolism**: Healthy fats are crucial for lipid metabolism, which is interconnected with the TCA cycle and fumarase activity.

Plant-Based Diet on Fumarase-Related Health Outcomes

A plant-based diet can enhance fumarase activity and contribute to various health benefits, particularly related to metabolic health and disease prevention.

Metabolic Health

1. **Energy Production**: Improved fumarase activity supports efficient energy production, enhancing overall metabolic health and reducing the risk of metabolic disorders such as obesity and type 2 diabetes.
2. **Insulin Sensitivity**: Plant-based diets improve insulin sensitivity, which is crucial for maintaining metabolic balance and preventing insulin resistance.

Cardiovascular Health

1. **Cholesterol Levels**: A plant-based diet can lower LDL cholesterol levels, reducing the risk of cardiovascular diseases. Improved fumarase activity contributes to better lipid metabolism and cardiovascular health.
2. **Blood Pressure**: Plant-based foods rich in potassium and magnesium help regulate blood pressure, supporting cardiovascular health and reducing strain on the heart.

Weight Management

1. **Healthy Weight**: A balanced plant-based diet helps maintain a healthy weight, reducing the risk of obesity-related metabolic imbalances that can affect fumarase activity.
2. **Caloric Density**: Plant-based foods are generally lower in calories and higher in nutrient density, promoting satiety and healthy weight management.

Mental Health

1. **Cognitive Function**: Improved metabolic health, supported by a plant-based diet, enhances cognitive function and reduces the risk of neurodegenerative diseases.
2. **Mood Regulation**: Plant-based diets rich in antioxidants and anti-inflammatory compounds support mental health and mood regulation by reducing oxidative stress and inflammation.

Fumarase plays a pivotal role in cellular metabolism and energy production, making it essential for overall health and metabolic balance. Its production and regulation are influenced by genetic, metabolic, and environmental factors.

Malate Dehydrogenase (MDH)

Malate Dehydrogenase (MDH) is a critical enzyme in cellular metabolism, playing a pivotal role in the citric acid cycle and various metabolic pathways.

Function of Malate Dehydrogenase

Malate Dehydrogenase is an essential enzyme involved in several biochemical pathways, particularly in the citric acid cycle (Krebs cycle), gluconeogenesis, and the malate-aspartate shuttle.

Citric Acid Cycle

1. **Catalysis of Reversible Reactions:** MDH catalyzes the reversible conversion of malate to oxaloacetate while reducing NAD+

to NADH. This step is vital for the regeneration of oxaloacetate, allowing the citric acid cycle to continue.

2. **Energy Production:** By facilitating the production of NADH, MDH contributes to the electron transport chain, leading to ATP synthesis, which is crucial for cellular energy.
3. **Anaplerotic Reactions:** MDH supports the replenishment of intermediates in the citric acid cycle, maintaining its functionality and efficiency in energy production.

Gluconeogenesis

1. **Conversion of Malate to Oxaloacetate:** In gluconeogenesis, MDH helps convert malate to oxaloacetate in the cytoplasm, which is then converted to phosphoenolpyruvate, a precursor for glucose synthesis.
2. **NADH Production:** The reaction catalyzed by MDH also produces NADH, which is essential for reducing power in biosynthetic processes.

Malate-Aspartate Shuttle

1. **Transfer of Reducing Equivalents:** MDH plays a crucial role in the malate-aspartate shuttle, which transfers reducing equivalents (NADH) from the cytosol into the mitochondria. This process is critical for maintaining redox balance and ATP production.
2. **Metabolic Regulation:** By facilitating the transfer of NADH, MDH indirectly regulates glycolysis and oxidative phosphorylation, ensuring efficient energy metabolism.

Production of Malate Dehydrogenase

MDH is produced through a series of intricate biochemical processes involving gene expression, protein synthesis, and post-translational modifications.

Gene Encoding

1. **MDH Genes:** The human genome encodes two primary isoforms of MDH: cytosolic MDH (MDH1) and mitochondrial MDH (MDH2). These genes are located on different chromosomes, with MDH1 on chromosome 2 and MDH2 on chromosome 7.
2. **Transcription Regulation:** The transcription of MDH genes is regulated by various transcription factors and coactivators in response to cellular metabolic needs and external stimuli.

Protein Synthesis

1. **mRNA Translation:** The mRNA transcripts of MDH genes are translated in the cytoplasm, producing the MDH polypeptides. This process is facilitated by ribosomes and involves the incorporation of amino acids in a specific sequence.
2. **Chaperone Proteins:** Molecular chaperones assist in the proper folding of MDH polypeptides, ensuring their functional conformation and stability.

Post-Translational Modifications

1. **Phosphorylation:** MDH can undergo phosphorylation, which affects its activity, stability, and interaction with other proteins. Phosphorylation is regulated by kinases and phosphatases in response to cellular signals.

2. **Acetylation and Methylation:** These modifications can influence MDH's enzymatic activity and its role in metabolic pathways.

Regulation of Malate Dehydrogenase

The regulation of MDH involves a complex interplay of genetic, biochemical, and environmental factors, ensuring its optimal activity in various metabolic contexts.

Feedback Mechanisms

1. **Product Inhibition:** High levels of oxaloacetate and NADH can inhibit MDH activity through feedback inhibition, preventing over-accumulation of these products and maintaining metabolic balance.
2. **Allosteric Regulation:** MDH can be allosterically regulated by various metabolites and cofactors, which modulate its activity in response to cellular energy status.

Hormonal Regulation

1. **Insulin and Glucagon:** These hormones regulate MDH activity by modulating the transcription of its genes and post-translational modifications. Insulin generally promotes MDH activity, enhancing anabolic pathways, while glucagon reduces its activity to conserve energy.
2. **Thyroid Hormones:** Thyroid hormones can increase MDH expression and activity, supporting higher metabolic rates and energy production.

Nutritional Status

1. **Dietary Influence:** The availability of substrates and cofactors from the diet can significantly affect MDH activity. Nutrient-

rich diets provide the necessary components for optimal MDH function.

2. **Fasting and Caloric Restriction:** These conditions can lead to reduced MDH activity as the body conserves energy and shifts to alternative metabolic pathways.

Plant-Based Diet and Malate Dehydrogenase Regulation

A plant-based diet, rich in fruits, vegetables, whole grains, nuts, and seeds, can positively influence MDH regulation through various mechanisms.

Nutrient Density

1. **Vitamins and Minerals:** Plant-based diets provide essential vitamins and minerals, such as vitamin B complex and magnesium, which are crucial for MDH activity and overall metabolic health.
2. **Phytochemicals:** Antioxidants and other phytochemicals found in plant foods can reduce oxidative stress, enhancing MDH function and protecting against metabolic dysregulation.

Amino Acids

1. **Protein Sources:** Legumes, nuts, and seeds are excellent sources of plant-based proteins, providing essential amino acids required for MDH synthesis and function.
2. **Amino Acid Composition:** Certain amino acids, such as arginine and glutamine, support MDH activity and metabolic pathways by enhancing protein synthesis and enzymatic reactions.

Antioxidants

1. **Oxidative Stress Reduction:** Antioxidants in fruits and vegetables, such as vitamin C, vitamin E, and polyphenols, help

reduce oxidative stress, which can otherwise impair MDH activity and metabolic health.

2. **Cellular Protection:** By protecting cells from oxidative damage, antioxidants support the efficient functioning of MDH and other metabolic enzymes.

Healthy Fats

1. **Essential Fatty Acids:** Plant-based sources of omega-3 and omega-6 fatty acids, such as flaxseeds and chia seeds, support cellular health and metabolic regulation, indirectly benefiting MDH activity.
2. **Anti-Inflammatory Effects:** Healthy fats from plant sources have anti-inflammatory properties, which can improve metabolic health and MDH function.

Fiber

1. **Gut Health:** High-fiber diets support a healthy gut microbiome, which can influence overall metabolic health and enzyme activity, including MDH.
2. **Metabolic Regulation:** Dietary fiber helps regulate blood sugar levels and insulin sensitivity, indirectly supporting MDH activity and energy metabolism.

Caloric Balance

1. **Weight Management:** Maintaining a healthy weight through a balanced plant-based diet prevents obesity-related metabolic disturbances that can impair MDH function.
2. **Energy Homeostasis:** Adequate caloric intake ensures sufficient energy for MDH activity and overall metabolic processes.

Plant-Based Diet on MDH-Related Health Outcomes
Energy Production

1. **Efficient Metabolism:** A plant-based diet supports efficient energy production by providing the necessary substrates and cofactors for MDH activity in the citric acid cycle.
2. **Sustained Energy Levels:** The steady release of energy from complex carbohydrates in plant foods supports consistent MDH activity and overall metabolic health.

Weight Management

1. **Reduced Obesity Risk:** Plant-based diets are effective for weight management, reducing body fat, and improving insulin sensitivity, which enhances MDH activity and energy metabolism.
2. **Improved Metabolic Health:** Lower body fat and better glycemic control support overall hormonal balance and metabolic efficiency, benefiting MDH function.

Cardiovascular Health

1. **Heart Health:** Nutrients and antioxidants in plant-based diets support cardiovascular health by reducing oxidative stress and inflammation, which can indirectly benefit MDH activity and energy metabolism.
2. **Cholesterol Regulation:** Plant-based diets help regulate cholesterol levels, reducing the risk of cardiovascular diseases that can impair metabolic health and MDH function.

Diabetes Management

1. **Blood Sugar Control:** Plant-based diets help maintain stable blood glucose levels, preventing insulin resistance and supporting MDH activity in glucose metabolism.
2. **Reduced Inflammation:** The anti-inflammatory properties of plant-based diets can improve insulin sensitivity and metabolic health, enhancing MDH function.

Anti-Aging Effects

1. **Oxidative Stress Reduction:** The antioxidant-rich nature of plant-based diets helps combat oxidative stress, a key factor in aging, supporting MDH activity and metabolic health.
2. **Healthy Aging:** Improved metabolic efficiency and reduced oxidative damage contribute to healthier aging and better maintenance of energy metabolism.

Malate Dehydrogenase plays a pivotal role in cellular metabolism, particularly in the citric acid cycle, gluconeogenesis, and the malate-aspartate shuttle. Its production and regulation are influenced by various factors, including genetic, biochemical, and environmental elements.

21

Electron Transport Chain Enzymes

Cytochrome C Oxidase

Cytochrome c oxidase is a vital enzyme in the mitochondrial electron transport chain, playing a crucial role in cellular respiration and energy production.

Function of Cytochrome C Oxidase

Cytochrome c oxidase (complex IV) is the last enzyme in the electron transport chain of mitochondria. It is essential for aerobic respiration, facilitating the transfer of electrons from cytochrome c to molecular oxygen, resulting in the formation of water. This process is coupled with proton pumping across the mitochondrial membrane, which generates an electrochemical gradient used to produce ATP, the energy currency of the cell.

1. **Electron Transfer**: Cytochrome c oxidase catalyzes the transfer of electrons from cytochrome c to oxygen. It facilitates the reduction of oxygen to water, a critical step in the electron transport chain.

2. **Proton Pumping**: The enzyme also pumps protons from the mitochondrial matrix to the intermembrane space, creating a proton gradient. This gradient is utilized by ATP synthase to generate ATP through oxidative phosphorylation.
3. **Energy Production**: By driving the final step of the electron transport chain, cytochrome c oxidase plays a pivotal role in cellular energy production. Approximately 90% of the oxygen consumed by cells is used by this enzyme, highlighting its importance in aerobic metabolism.

Production of Cytochrome C Oxidase

Cytochrome c oxidase is a complex enzyme composed of multiple subunits encoded by both mitochondrial and nuclear DNA. Its production involves intricate processes of gene expression, protein synthesis, and assembly.

1. **Gene Encoding**: The enzyme is composed of 13 subunits, three of which are encoded by mitochondrial DNA (MT-CO1, MT-CO2, MT-CO3) and the remaining by nuclear DNA. These genes provide the blueprint for the enzyme's subunits.
2. **Mitochondrial Synthesis**: The mitochondrial subunits are synthesized within the mitochondria, where mitochondrial ribosomes translate the mRNA transcripts derived from mitochondrial DNA. This process ensures that the core components of cytochrome c oxidase are produced in close proximity to their site of function.
3. **Nuclear Synthesis**: Nuclear-encoded subunits are synthesized in the cytoplasm and imported into the mitochondria. These subunits undergo post-translational modifications and are transported through the mitochondrial membranes via specialized transport machinery.

4. **Assembly**: The assembly of cytochrome c oxidase is a coordinated process involving chaperone proteins and assembly factors. These factors assist in the proper folding, insertion of cofactors (such as heme and copper), and integration of subunits into a functional enzyme complex.

Regulation of Cytochrome C Oxidase

The regulation of cytochrome c oxidase involves multiple levels of control, including gene expression, post-translational modifications, and allosteric regulation. These mechanisms ensure the enzyme's activity aligns with cellular energy demands and environmental conditions.

1. **Transcriptional Regulation**: The expression of genes encoding cytochrome c oxidase subunits is regulated by various transcription factors and signaling pathways. For instance, the nuclear respiratory factors (NRF1 and NRF2) and peroxisome proliferator-activated receptor gamma coactivator 1-alpha (PGC-1α) play significant roles in regulating the expression of nuclear-encoded subunits.
2. **Post-Translational Modifications**: Cytochrome c oxidase undergoes several post-translational modifications, such as phosphorylation, which can modulate its activity. Phosphorylation of specific subunits can either enhance or inhibit enzyme function, thereby fine-tuning the electron transport chain.
3. **Allosteric Regulation**: The enzyme's activity is also regulated through allosteric interactions with metabolites and other cellular factors. For example, ATP can act as an allosteric inhibitor, reducing the enzyme's activity when cellular energy levels are sufficient.
4. **Environmental Factors**: Factors such as oxygen availability, nutrient status, and redox state influence cytochrome c oxidase activity. Hypoxia (low oxygen conditions) can lead to adaptive

responses that alter the enzyme's expression and function to optimize energy production under a limited oxygen supply.

Plant-Based Diet and Cytochrome C Oxidase Regulation

A plant-based diet can significantly influence the regulation and activity of cytochrome c oxidase through various mechanisms involving nutrient availability, antioxidant content, and overall metabolic health.

Nutrient Density: Plant-based diets are rich in essential nutrients, vitamins, and minerals that support mitochondrial function. Nutrients such as iron, copper, and zinc are critical cofactors for cytochrome c oxidase activity. Plant sources of these nutrients include legumes, nuts, seeds, and leafy greens.

Iron: Found in spinach, lentils, and quinoa, iron is a crucial component of the heme groups in cytochrome c oxidase.

Copper: Essential for the enzyme's function, copper can be obtained from plant sources like nuts, seeds, and whole grains.

Zinc: Present in legumes, seeds, and whole grains, zinc supports the structural integrity of the enzyme.

Antioxidants: A diet rich in fruits and vegetables provides a high intake of antioxidants, which can reduce oxidative stress and protect mitochondrial function. Antioxidants such as vitamin C, vitamin E, and polyphenols can enhance the activity and stability of cytochrome c oxidase by preventing oxidative damage to the enzyme and its cofactors.

Vitamin C: Found in citrus fruits, bell peppers, and strawberries, vitamin C acts as an antioxidant, protecting the enzyme from oxidative damage.

Vitamin E: Present in nuts, seeds, and green leafy vegetables, vitamin E helps maintain mitochondrial integrity by neutralizing reactive oxygen species.

Polyphenols: Abundant in berries, tea, and dark chocolate, polyphenols have been shown to support mitochondrial health and function.

Healthy Fats: Plant-based sources of healthy fats, such as avocados, nuts, and seeds, provide essential fatty acids that support mitochondrial membranes' integrity and fluidity. Omega-3 fatty acids, in particular, have anti-inflammatory properties that can enhance mitochondrial function.

Omega-3 Fatty Acids: Found in flaxseeds, chia seeds, and walnuts, omega-3 fatty acids support mitochondrial health and reduce inflammation.

Fiber: High-fiber diets support gut health and overall metabolic regulation. A healthy gut microbiome can influence mitochondrial function through the production of short-chain fatty acids and other metabolites.

Short-Chain Fatty Acids: Produced by gut bacteria from dietary fiber, these fatty acids can support mitochondrial function and energy production.

Caloric Balance: Maintaining a healthy weight through a balanced plant-based diet can prevent obesity-related mitochondrial dysfunction. Excess body fat is linked to increased production of inflammatory markers, which can impair cytochrome c oxidase activity.

Glycemic Control: Plant-based diets, which are low in refined sugars and high in complex carbohydrates, help maintain stable blood glucose levels. This stability prevents insulin resistance and associated mitochondrial dysfunction.

Complex Carbohydrates: Found in whole grains, legumes, and vegetables, complex carbohydrates provide a steady source of energy and prevent insulin spikes.

Plant-Based Diet on Cytochrome C Oxidase-Related Health Outcomes

A plant-based diet can positively influence health outcomes related to cytochrome c oxidase activity by promoting mitochondrial function, reducing oxidative stress, and supporting overall metabolic health.

Energy Levels: Enhanced cytochrome c oxidase activity supports efficient energy production, leading to improved physical and mental energy levels.

Metabolic Health: A plant-based diet can improve insulin sensitivity and glycemic control, reducing the risk of metabolic disorders such as type 2 diabetes. Improved mitochondrial function is central to these benefits.

Cardiovascular Health: By reducing oxidative stress and inflammation, a plant-based diet can protect against cardiovascular diseases. Improved mitochondrial function contributes to better cardiac health and reduced risk of conditions such as hypertension and atherosclerosis.

Antioxidant Protection: High intake of antioxidants from plant foods reduces oxidative stress, protecting cardiovascular health.

Anti-Inflammatory Effects: Plant-based diets lower levels of inflammatory markers, supporting heart health.

Neuroprotection: Mitochondrial dysfunction is implicated in neurodegenerative diseases such as Alzheimer's and Parkinson's. A plant-based diet, rich in antioxidants and anti-inflammatory compounds, can protect against mitochondrial damage and support brain health.

Cognitive Function: Improved mitochondrial function supports cognitive health and reduces the risk of neurodegenerative diseases.

Anti-Aging Effects: The antioxidant-rich nature of plant-based diets helps combat oxidative stress, a key factor in aging. Improved mitochondrial function contributes to healthier aging and better maintenance of cellular function.

Oxidative Stress Reduction: Antioxidants from plant foods protect cells from damage, promoting healthy aging.

Exercise Performance: Enhanced mitochondrial function from a plant-based diet can improve exercise performance and recovery. Efficient energy production and reduced oxidative stress support endurance and strength.

Endurance: Improved mitochondrial function supports sustained energy production during exercise.

Recovery: Reduced oxidative stress aids in faster recovery post-exercise.

By understanding the function, production, and regulation of cytochrome c oxidase from a plant-based perspective, we can appreciate the significant impact of diet on this vital enzyme and overall mitochondrial health.

22

Antioxidant Enzymes

Catalase

Catalase is a crucial enzyme in the human body, responsible for protecting cells from oxidative damage by catalyzing the decomposition of hydrogen peroxide into water and oxygen.

Function of Catalase

Catalase plays a vital role in cellular defense against oxidative stress, ensuring the integrity and functionality of cells and tissues.

1. Hydrogen Peroxide Decomposition

Catalase's primary function is to catalyze the breakdown of hydrogen peroxide (H_2O_2), a potentially harmful byproduct of metabolic processes, into water (H_2O) and oxygen (O_2).

$2H_2O_2 \rightarrow 2H_2O+O_2$

This reaction is crucial as hydrogen peroxide can generate reactive oxygen species (ROS), leading to oxidative stress and cellular damage if not efficiently removed.

2. Antioxidant Defense

Catalase works synergistically with other antioxidant enzymes such as superoxide dismutase (SOD) and glutathione peroxidase (GPx) to maintain redox balance within cells. While SOD converts superoxide radicals into hydrogen peroxide, catalase further detoxifies hydrogen peroxide, completing the protective cycle against oxidative damage.

3. Cellular Signaling

Beyond its antioxidant role, catalase is involved in cellular signaling processes. By regulating hydrogen peroxide levels, catalase influences pathways related to cell growth, apoptosis, and immune responses.

4. Aging and Disease Prevention

Catalase activity is linked to the aging process and the prevention of various diseases. Reduced catalase activity is associated with age-related conditions, including neurodegenerative diseases, diabetes, and cardiovascular diseases. Enhancing catalase function may mitigate oxidative damage, promoting healthier aging and disease resistance.

Production of Catalase

Catalase is produced in various cell types throughout the body, predominantly in peroxisomes, where it acts to neutralize hydrogen peroxide produced during metabolic reactions.

1. Gene Encoding and Synthesis

The gene encoding catalase is located on chromosome 11 in humans (CAT gene). The gene's expression is tightly regulated, ensuring appropriate levels of catalase to meet cellular demands.

2. Protein Structure

Catalase is a tetrameric heme enzyme, meaning it consists of four subunits, each containing a heme group. The heme groups are crucial for the enzyme's catalytic activity, as they facilitate the breakdown of hydrogen peroxide.

3. Cellular Localization

Catalase is predominantly localized in peroxisomes, subcellular organelles involved in lipid metabolism and detoxification processes. Its presence in peroxisomes allows for efficient neutralization of hydrogen peroxide generated during beta-oxidation of fatty acids and other metabolic processes.

4. Tissue Distribution

Catalase is ubiquitously expressed in various tissues, with particularly high concentrations in the liver, kidney, and erythrocytes (red blood cells). These tissues are actively involved in metabolic processes, necessitating robust antioxidant defenses.

Regulation of Catalase

The regulation of catalase involves a complex interplay of genetic, environmental, and nutritional factors. Proper regulation ensures the enzyme's activity aligns with cellular needs, preventing oxidative damage and maintaining homeostasis.

1. Genetic Regulation

- **Transcriptional Control:** The expression of the CAT gene is regulated at the transcriptional level by various transcription factors. These include nuclear factor erythroid 2–related factor 2 (Nrf2), which binds to antioxidant response elements (ARE) in the promoter region of the CAT gene, enhancing its expression in response to oxidative stress.

- **Post-transcriptional Modifications:** Post-transcriptional modifications, such as mRNA splicing, stability, and translation efficiency, also influence catalase production. MicroRNAs (miRNAs) can modulate mRNA stability, affecting catalase levels.

2. Hormonal Regulation

Hormones play a significant role in catalase regulation. For instance, thyroid hormones have been shown to increase catalase activity, enhancing the body's antioxidant capacity.

3. Environmental Factors

- **Oxidative Stress:** Exposure to oxidative stressors, such as environmental pollutants, radiation, and toxins, can upregulate catalase expression as part of the cellular adaptive response to mitigate oxidative damage.

- **Exercise:** Physical activity influences catalase activity. Moderate exercise enhances catalase levels, improving antioxidant defenses.

However, excessive exercise can lead to oxidative stress, potentially overwhelming the body's antioxidant systems, including catalase.

4. Nutritional Regulation

A plant-based diet rich in antioxidants and essential nutrients can significantly impact catalase activity and overall antioxidant capacity.

- **Antioxidants:** Dietary antioxidants, such as vitamins C and E, polyphenols, and flavonoids, found in fruits, vegetables, nuts, and seeds, support catalase function by reducing oxidative stress. These antioxidants can enhance the expression of antioxidant enzymes, including catalase, through Nrf2 activation.

- **Selenium:** Selenium is a trace element essential for the proper functioning of antioxidant enzymes. Plant-based sources of selenium, such as Brazil nuts, seeds, and whole grains, contribute to the optimal activity of catalase and other antioxidant enzymes.

- **Zinc:** Zinc is another critical mineral that supports antioxidant defenses. Legumes, nuts, and seeds are excellent plant-based sources of zinc, which can enhance catalase activity.

- **Phytochemicals:** Phytochemicals, such as sulforaphane found in cruciferous vegetables (e.g., broccoli, kale), have been shown to activate Nrf2 and upregulate antioxidant enzymes, including catalase.

- **Fiber:** High-fiber diets, common in plant-based eating, support gut health and reduce systemic inflammation, indirectly benefiting catalase activity.

Plant-Based Diet and Catalase Regulation

A plant-based diet can positively influence catalase regulation through various mechanisms, promoting overall antioxidant capacity and reducing oxidative stress.

1. Nutrient Density

Plant-based diets provide a rich source of essential nutrients, vitamins, and minerals that support overall health and antioxidant defenses. For example, vitamin E, found in nuts and seeds, and vitamin C, abundant in fruits and vegetables, are potent antioxidants that can enhance catalase activity.

2. Amino Acids

Certain amino acids, such as methionine and cysteine, found in plant foods like legumes and grains, are precursors to glutathione, a critical antioxidant that works alongside catalase to detoxify hydrogen peroxide.

3. Antioxidant-Rich Foods

Fruits and vegetables are rich in antioxidants, which help reduce oxidative stress. Lower oxidative stress levels are associated with improved catalase activity. Foods such as berries, leafy greens, and citrus fruits are particularly beneficial.

4. Healthy Fats

Plant-based sources of fats, such as avocados, nuts, and seeds, provide essential fatty acids that support cell membrane integrity and antioxidant defenses. Omega-3 fatty acids, in particular, have anti-inflammatory properties that can enhance catalase function.

5. Fiber and Gut Health

High-fiber diets, typical of plant-based eating, support a healthy gut microbiome, which plays a role in regulating systemic inflammation and oxidative stress. A healthy gut can influence catalase activity by reducing the overall oxidative burden on the body.

6. Caloric Balance and Weight Management

Maintaining a healthy weight through a balanced plant-based diet can prevent obesity-related oxidative stress. Excess body fat, particularly visceral fat, is linked to increased production of inflammatory markers and oxidative stress, which can overwhelm antioxidant systems, including catalase.

7. Glycemic Control

Plant-based diets, which are low in refined sugars and high in complex carbohydrates, help maintain stable blood glucose levels. This stability prevents insulin resistance and associated oxidative stress, supporting overall antioxidant defenses.

Plant-Based Diet on Catalase-Related Health Outcomes

1. Aging and Longevity

A plant-based diet rich in antioxidants can slow the aging process by reducing oxidative damage to cells and tissues. Enhanced catalase activity contributes to healthier aging and longevity by maintaining cellular integrity.

2. Disease Prevention

- **Cardiovascular Health:** A plant-based diet supports cardiovascular health by reducing oxidative stress and inflammation. Catalase plays a role in protecting endothelial cells from oxidative damage, reducing the risk of atherosclerosis and other cardiovascular diseases.

- **Neurodegenerative Diseases:** Enhanced catalase activity can protect neurons from oxidative damage, reducing the risk of neurodegenerative diseases such as Alzheimer's and Parkinson's. Plant-based diets, rich in antioxidants and anti-inflammatory compounds, support brain health.

- **Diabetes Management:** Oxidative stress is a significant factor in the development and progression of diabetes. A plant-based diet can improve glycemic control and reduce oxidative stress, enhancing catalase activity and overall antioxidant defenses.

3. Immune Function

A robust antioxidant system, supported by a plant-based diet, enhances immune function. Catalase helps protect immune cells from oxidative damage, ensuring effective immune responses and reducing the risk of infections and chronic inflammatory diseases.

4. Skin Health

Catalase plays a role in maintaining skin health by protecting skin cells from oxidative damage caused by environmental factors such as UV radiation. A plant-based diet, rich in vitamins and antioxidants, supports healthy skin and reduces the risk of skin aging and disorders.

Catalase is a pivotal enzyme in the human body's defense against oxidative stress, catalyzing the decomposition of hydrogen peroxide into water and oxygen. Its production and regulation are influenced by genetic, environmental, hormonal, and nutritional factors.

Superoxide Dismutase (SOD)

Superoxide dismutase (SOD) is a critical enzyme in the human body, responsible for protecting cells from oxidative stress by catalyzing the dismutation of superoxide radicals into oxygen and hydrogen peroxide.

Function of Superoxide Dismutase

SOD plays a pivotal role in cellular defense against oxidative damage by neutralizing superoxide radicals, which are highly reactive molecules that can cause significant cellular damage if not properly managed.

Cellular Defense Mechanism

1. **Superoxide Radical Neutralization**: SOD catalyzes the conversion of superoxide radicals (O_2-) into oxygen (O_2) and hydrogen peroxide (H_2O_2). This reaction is crucial because superoxide radicals are byproducts of oxygen metabolism and can contribute to cellular damage if accumulated.
2. **Hydrogen Peroxide Management**: While hydrogen peroxide is less reactive than superoxide radicals, it can still be harmful in high concentrations. SOD works in conjunction with other enzymes like catalase and glutathione peroxidase to further convert hydrogen peroxide into water and oxygen, thereby mitigating potential damage.
3. **Prevention of Oxidative Stress**: By converting superoxide radicals, SOD plays a significant role in preventing oxidative stress, a condition characterized by an imbalance between the production

of free radicals and the body's ability to detoxify them. Oxidative stress is linked to various chronic diseases, including cancer, cardiovascular diseases, and neurodegenerative disorders.

Tissue-Specific Functions

1. **Brain Health**: SOD is highly expressed in the brain, where it protects neurons from oxidative damage. This is crucial for preventing neurodegenerative diseases like Alzheimer's and Parkinson's disease.
2. **Cardiovascular Health**: SOD helps maintain vascular health by preventing oxidative damage to blood vessels, thus reducing the risk of atherosclerosis and hypertension.
3. **Skin Health**: SOD is also important for skin health, protecting against damage from ultraviolet (UV) radiation and reducing the effects of aging.

Production of Superoxide Dismutase

The production of SOD is tightly regulated and occurs through various isoforms in different cellular compartments, ensuring comprehensive protection against oxidative stress.

Isoforms and Gene Encoding

1. **Cytoplasmic SOD1 (Cu/Zn-SOD)**: SOD1 is encoded by the SOD1 gene located on chromosome 21. It is a homodimeric enzyme containing copper and zinc ions and is primarily found in the cytoplasm.
2. **Mitochondrial SOD2 (Mn-SOD)**: SOD2 is encoded by the SOD2 gene on chromosome 6. It is a homotetrameric enzyme containing manganese ions and is localized in the mitochondria, protecting against oxidative damage generated during cellular respiration.

3. **Extracellular SOD3 (EC-SOD)**: SOD3 is encoded by the SOD3 gene on chromosome 4. It is found in the extracellular matrix and in high concentrations in the lungs and plasma, playing a critical role in protecting extracellular spaces from oxidative stress.

Synthesis and Assembly

1. **Transcription and Translation**: The synthesis of SOD begins with the transcription of SOD genes into mRNA, which is then translated into precursor proteins. These proteins undergo post-translational modifications to become active SOD enzymes.
2. **Metal Incorporation**: The incorporation of metal ions (copper, zinc, or manganese) is essential for the catalytic activity of SOD. This process occurs during the folding of the protein and is facilitated by metallochaperones.

Regulation of Superoxide Dismutase

The regulation of SOD involves multiple layers, including genetic regulation, post-translational modifications, and dietary influences, ensuring optimal activity and balance in the body.

Genetic Regulation

1. **Transcriptional Control**: The expression of SOD genes is regulated by various transcription factors, including Nuclear Factor-kappa B (NF-κB) and Nuclear factor erythroid 2-related factor 2 (Nrf2). These factors respond to oxidative stress signals and up-regulate the transcription of SOD genes to enhance antioxidant defenses.
2. **Epigenetic Modifications**: Epigenetic mechanisms, such as DNA methylation and histone modifications, also play a role in regulating SOD gene expression. These modifications can be influenced by environmental factors and dietary components.

Post-Translational Modifications

1. **Phosphorylation**: SOD activity can be modulated by phosphorylation, which affects its stability and interaction with other proteins.
2. **Acetylation**: Acetylation of SOD proteins can influence their catalytic activity and localization within the cell.

Dietary Influences

1. **Antioxidant-Rich Foods**: A plant-based diet rich in antioxidants can enhance SOD activity. Foods such as berries, leafy greens, nuts, and seeds provide vitamins and phytochemicals that support antioxidant defense mechanisms.
2. **Mineral Intake**: Adequate intake of minerals such as copper, zinc, and manganese is crucial for the synthesis and activity of SOD. Plant-based sources of these minerals include whole grains, legumes, nuts, and seeds.
3. **Polyphenols**: Polyphenolic compounds found in fruits, vegetables, and teas have been shown to upregulate the expression of antioxidant enzymes, including SOD, through the activation of Nrf2 pathways.

Plant-Based Diet and Superoxide Dismutase Regulation

A plant-based diet can positively influence the regulation and activity of SOD through various mechanisms, promoting overall health and reducing the risk of oxidative stress-related diseases.

Nutrient Density

1. **Vitamins and Minerals**: Plant-based diets are rich in essential vitamins and minerals that support the activity of SOD. For example, vitamin C (found in citrus fruits and leafy greens) and

vitamin E (found in nuts and seeds) act as antioxidants and enhance SOD activity.

2. **Phytonutrients**: Phytonutrients such as flavonoids, carotenoids, and polyphenols found in fruits and vegetables have antioxidant properties that support the body's defense mechanisms, including the activity of SOD.

Antioxidant-Rich Foods

1. **Berries**: Berries such as blueberries, strawberries, and raspberries are rich in antioxidants that help increase SOD activity and protect against oxidative damage.
2. **Leafy Greens**: Leafy greens like spinach, kale, and Swiss chard are excellent sources of vitamins and minerals that support SOD activity.
3. **Nuts and Seeds**: Nuts and seeds, including almonds, walnuts, chia seeds, and flaxseeds, provide essential fatty acids and minerals that enhance the body's antioxidant defenses.

Healthy Fats

1. **Omega-3 Fatty Acids**: Omega-3 fatty acids, found in flaxseeds, chia seeds, and walnuts, have anti-inflammatory properties that support overall cellular health and enhance the activity of antioxidant enzymes like SOD.

Plant-Based Diet on SOD-Related Health Outcomes

Cardiovascular Health

1. **Reduction in Atherosclerosis**: By enhancing SOD activity, a plant-based diet helps reduce oxidative stress and inflammation,

thereby decreasing the risk of atherosclerosis and other cardiovascular diseases.

2. **Blood Pressure Regulation**: Antioxidants in plant-based foods help maintain healthy blood vessels and prevent oxidative damage, contributing to better blood pressure control.

Neuroprotection

1. **Prevention of Neurodegenerative Diseases**: Increased SOD activity protects neurons from oxidative damage, reducing the risk of neurodegenerative diseases such as Alzheimer's and Parkinson's disease.
2. **Cognitive Function**: Antioxidants in plant-based diets support cognitive function and protect against age-related cognitive decline by enhancing SOD activity and reducing oxidative stress.

Skin Health

1. **Protection Against UV Damage**: SOD helps protect the skin from damage caused by UV radiation, and a diet rich in antioxidants can further enhance this protective effect.
2. **Anti-Aging Effects**: By reducing oxidative stress, a plant-based diet can help slow down the aging process and maintain healthy skin.

Cancer Prevention

1. **Reduction in Oxidative Damage**: SOD plays a critical role in protecting cells from oxidative damage, which is a key factor in cancer development. A plant-based diet rich in antioxidants supports this protective mechanism.
2. **Detoxification Pathways**: Phytochemicals in plant-based foods enhance the body's detoxification pathways, reducing the risk

of cancer by supporting SOD activity and other antioxidant defenses.

Superoxide dismutase is a crucial enzyme that protects cells from oxidative damage by catalyzing the conversion of superoxide radicals into oxygen and hydrogen peroxide. Its function, production, and regulation are tightly controlled through genetic mechanisms, post-translational modifications, and dietary influences.

Glutathione Peroxidase (GPx)

Glutathione peroxidase (GPx) is a crucial enzyme in the human body, primarily responsible for protecting cells from oxidative damage by reducing hydrogen peroxide and lipid peroxides.

Function of Glutathione Peroxidase

Glutathione peroxidase plays a critical role in maintaining cellular homeostasis and protecting against oxidative stress. Its primary functions include:

Antioxidant Defense

1. **Reduction of Hydrogen Peroxide**: GPx catalyzes the reduction of hydrogen peroxide (H_2O_2) to water (H_2O), thus preventing the accumulation of H_2O_2, which can be harmful to cells.
2. **Reduction of Lipid Peroxides**: GPx also reduces lipid peroxides, which are products of lipid oxidation. This activity helps maintain membrane integrity and prevents cell damage.

Detoxification

1. **Detoxification of Peroxides**: By reducing peroxides, GPx plays a vital role in detoxifying harmful compounds generated during metabolic processes.
2. **Prevention of Oxidative Damage**: GPx protects DNA, proteins, and lipids from oxidative damage, thereby preventing mutations and maintaining cellular function.

Support of Immune Function

1. **Regulation of Immune Cells**: GPx activity supports the function of immune cells by maintaining the redox balance within these cells.
2. **Protection Against Inflammation**: By reducing oxidative stress, GPx helps in modulating inflammatory responses, which is crucial for preventing chronic diseases.

Production of Glutathione Peroxidase

The production of GPx involves complex biochemical processes and is influenced by various dietary and physiological factors.

Synthesis

1. **Gene Encoding**: GPx is encoded by several genes, including GPX1, GPX2, GPX3, and GPX4, each responsible for different isoforms of the enzyme. These genes are located on different chromosomes and are expressed in various tissues.
2. **Selenium Dependency**: GPx is a selenium-dependent enzyme. Selenium is incorporated into the active site of the enzyme as selenocysteine, which is crucial for its catalytic activity.

3. **Isoforms**: Different isoforms of GPx are expressed in different tissues, each with specific functions. For example, GPX1 is widely distributed in most tissues, GPX2 is predominantly found in the gastrointestinal tract, GPX3 is present in plasma, and GPX4 is involved in lipid metabolism and is found in the testis and other tissues.

Regulation by Nutrients

1. **Selenium**: Adequate selenium intake is essential for the synthesis of GPx. Foods rich in selenium include Brazil nuts, sunflower seeds, brown rice, and spinach.
2. **Amino Acids**: The synthesis of GPx also depends on the availability of amino acids, particularly cysteine, glutamate, and glycine, which are components of glutathione, the substrate for GPx.

Influencing Factors

1. **Age**: GPx activity tends to decline with age, making older individuals more susceptible to oxidative stress.
2. **Gender**: Studies suggest that GPx activity may vary between males and females, potentially due to hormonal differences.
3. **Exercise and Stress**: Physical activity can influence GPx levels. Moderate exercise enhances GPx activity, while excessive exercise may increase oxidative stress, thereby increasing the demand for GPx.
4. **Nutrition**: Nutritional status, including dietary intake of selenium and other essential nutrients, directly affects GPx production.

Regulation of Glutathione Peroxidase

The regulation of GPx involves complex interactions between genetic, nutritional, and environmental factors.

Feedback Mechanisms

1. **Oxidative Stress**: High levels of oxidative stress can upregulate the expression of GPx. This adaptive response helps in counteracting the increased oxidative burden.
2. **Hormonal Regulation**: Hormones such as insulin, thyroid hormones, and sex hormones can influence GPx expression and activity.

Environmental Factors

1. **Exposure to Toxins**: Environmental toxins and pollutants can affect GPx levels. Chronic exposure to pollutants may deplete antioxidant defenses, including GPx.
2. **Dietary Antioxidants**: Consumption of dietary antioxidants such as vitamins C and E can enhance GPx activity by reducing the overall oxidative burden.

Nutritional Regulation

1. **Plant-Based Diets**: Diets rich in fruits, vegetables, nuts, and seeds provide essential nutrients and antioxidants that support GPx activity. For example, foods high in selenium, such as Brazil nuts, are crucial for optimal GPx function.
2. **Phytochemicals**: Phytochemicals found in plant-based foods, such as flavonoids, polyphenols, and carotenoids, can upregulate GPx expression and enhance its activity.
3. **Healthy Fats**: Omega-3 fatty acids, found in flaxseeds, chia seeds, and walnuts, have anti-inflammatory properties that support antioxidant defenses, including GPx.

4. **Fiber**: Dietary fiber from plant-based sources supports gut health, which in turn can influence overall antioxidant status and GPx activity.

Plant-Based Diet and Glutathione Peroxidase Regulation

A plant-based diet can positively influence GPx regulation through various mechanisms, promoting overall health and reducing the risk of chronic diseases.

Nutrient Density

Plant-based diets provide a rich source of essential nutrients, vitamins, and minerals that support GPx activity. For example:

1. **Vitamin E**: Found in nuts, seeds, and green leafy vegetables, vitamin E works synergistically with GPx to reduce oxidative stress.
2. **Vitamin C**: Abundant in fruits like oranges, strawberries, and kiwi, vitamin C regenerates oxidized glutathione, the substrate for GPx.

Amino Acids

Plant-based sources of amino acids, such as legumes, nuts, and seeds, provide the building blocks for glutathione synthesis, which is crucial for GPx activity. These include:

1. **Cysteine**: Found in foods like lentils, oats, and sunflower seeds, cysteine is a precursor to glutathione.
2. **Glutamate and Glycine**: These amino acids are also essential for glutathione synthesis and can be obtained from plant-based sources like spinach, kale, and quinoa.

Antioxidants

1. **Fruits and Vegetables**: Rich in antioxidants, these foods reduce oxidative stress and support GPx activity. Berries, leafy greens, and cruciferous vegetables are particularly beneficial.
2. **Polyphenols and Flavonoids**: Found in foods like apples, onions, and tea, these compounds enhance GPx activity by reducing oxidative damage.

Healthy Fats

1. **Omega-3 Fatty Acids**: Found in flaxseeds, chia seeds, and walnuts, omega-3 fatty acids have anti-inflammatory properties that support GPx activity.
2. **Monounsaturated Fats**: Sources like avocados, olives, and nuts provide healthy fats that support overall antioxidant status.

Fiber

High-fiber diets, common in plant-based eating, support gut health and overall antioxidant defense. A healthy gut microbiome can influence GPx activity through the production of short-chain fatty acids and other metabolites.

Caloric Balance

Maintaining a healthy weight through a balanced plant-based diet can prevent obesity-related oxidative stress, which in turn supports GPx activity. Excess body fat, particularly visceral fat, is linked to increased oxidative stress and reduced antioxidant defenses.

Glycemic Control

Plant-based diets, which are low in refined sugars and high in complex carbohydrates, help maintain stable blood glucose levels. This stability prevents insulin resistance, which can negatively impact antioxidant defenses, including GPx.

Plant-Based Diet on GPx-Related Health Outcomes

Oxidative Stress and Chronic Diseases

1. **Cardiovascular Health**: A plant-based diet can reduce oxidative stress, thereby lowering the risk of cardiovascular diseases. Antioxidants in fruits and vegetables protect against oxidative damage to blood vessels.
2. **Cancer Prevention**: By reducing oxidative stress and enhancing GPx activity, a plant-based diet can lower the risk of cancer. Foods rich in selenium and other antioxidants support DNA repair and prevent mutations.

Immune Function

1. **Enhanced Immunity**: Plant-based diets provide essential nutrients that support immune function. Antioxidants and phytochemicals in plant foods enhance GPx activity, which in turn supports the immune response.
2. **Reduced Inflammation**: Anti-inflammatory compounds in plant-based foods, such as omega-3 fatty acids and polyphenols, reduce inflammation and support immune health.

Detoxification

1. **Liver Health**: A plant-based diet supports liver function by providing essential nutrients and antioxidants that enhance detoxification processes, including GPx activity.
2. **Heavy Metal Detoxification**: Selenium in plant-based foods aids in the detoxification of heavy metals, supporting overall antioxidant defenses.

Anti-Aging Effects

The antioxidant-rich nature of plant-based diets helps combat oxidative stress, a key factor in aging. Improved GPx activity, coupled with reduced oxidative damage, contributes to healthier aging and better maintenance of cellular function.

Mental Health

Emerging evidence suggests that plant-based diets may benefit mental health by reducing inflammation and oxidative stress, which are linked to mood disorders. Improved GPx activity supports cognitive function and emotional well-being.

Bone Health

Plant-based diets rich in calcium, magnesium, and vitamin K support bone health. Leafy greens, fortified plant milk, and nuts are excellent sources of these nutrients, which work synergistically with GPx and other antioxidants to maintain bone density and reduce the risk of osteoporosis.

Weight Management

Plant-based diets are effective for weight management, reducing body fat, and improving insulin sensitivity. Lower body fat and better glycemic control enhance overall antioxidant defenses, including GPx activity.

Glutathione peroxidase plays a pivotal role in protecting cells from oxidative damage, maintaining cellular homeostasis, and supporting overall health. Its production and regulation are influenced by various factors, including age, nutrition, exercise, and environmental exposures.

Glutathione Reductase (GR)

Glutathione reductase (GR) is a critical enzyme in maintaining cellular redox balance by regenerating reduced glutathione (GSH) from its oxidized form (GSSG). This enzyme plays a pivotal role in protecting cells from oxidative stress and maintaining overall cellular health.

Function of Glutathione Reductase

Glutathione reductase is indispensable for various cellular processes due to its role in maintaining the levels of reduced glutathione (GSH). GSH is a potent antioxidant that protects cells from oxidative damage by neutralizing reactive oxygen species (ROS) and detoxifying harmful substances.

Antioxidant Defense

1. **Reduction of Oxidized Glutathione (GSSG):** GR catalyzes the reduction of GSSG to GSH, utilizing NADPH as a reducing agent. This reaction is crucial for maintaining a high GSH/GSSG ratio, which is indicative of a cell's oxidative state.
2. **Protection Against Oxidative Stress:** By sustaining GSH levels, GR helps protect cellular components like lipids, proteins, and DNA from oxidative damage, which can otherwise lead to cell dysfunction or death.
3. **Detoxification:** GSH is involved in the detoxification of xenobiotics and endogenous toxins through conjugation reactions facilitated by glutathione S-transferases (GSTs). GR ensures a constant supply of GSH for these detoxification processes.

Cellular Metabolism

1. **Redox Signaling:** GSH and GR are involved in redox signaling pathways that regulate cellular functions such as apoptosis, cell proliferation, and immune responses.

2. **Metabolism of Reactive Nitrogen Species (RNS):** GSH also reacts with reactive nitrogen species, and GR aids in maintaining the necessary levels of GSH for these reactions.

Production of Glutathione Reductase

Glutathione reductase is produced in various tissues and its production is influenced by multiple genetic and environmental factors.

Gene Encoding

1. **Gene Location:** The gene encoding human glutathione reductase (GSR) is located on chromosome 8p12. It is composed of 13 exons and spans approximately 20 kb.
2. **Expression:** The expression of the GSR gene is regulated at both transcriptional and post-transcriptional levels. Factors such as oxidative stress, nutritional status, and hormonal signals can influence its expression.

Enzyme Structure and Function

1. **Protein Structure:** Glutathione reductase is a flavoprotein with a molecular weight of approximately 52 kDa. It contains a flavin adenine dinucleotide (FAD) cofactor, which is essential for its enzymatic activity.
2. **Catalytic Mechanism:** GR catalyzes the reduction of GSSG to GSH using NADPH as an electron donor. The reaction involves the transfer of electrons from NADPH to FAD and then to GSSG, resulting in the formation of GSH.

Regulation of Glutathione Reductase

The regulation of glutathione reductase involves complex mechanisms that ensure its optimal activity and expression in response to cellular needs.

Transcriptional Regulation

1. **Oxidative Stress:** The expression of GR is upregulated in response to oxidative stress. This adaptive response is mediated by transcription factors such as nuclear factor erythroid 2-related factor 2 (Nrf2), which binds to antioxidant response elements (ARE) in the promoter region of the GSR gene.
2. **Hormonal Regulation:** Hormones such as insulin and thyroid hormones can modulate the expression of GR. Insulin has been shown to upregulate GR expression in certain cell types, enhancing cellular antioxidant capacity.

Post-Transcriptional Regulation

1. **mRNA Stability:** The stability of GR mRNA can be influenced by oxidative stress and other cellular signals. This regulation ensures a rapid and efficient response to changes in cellular redox status.
2. **Protein Modification:** Post-translational modifications such as phosphorylation can affect the activity and stability of GR. These modifications are often mediated by signaling pathways activated by oxidative stress or other stimuli.

Nutritional Regulation

A plant-based diet can significantly influence the regulation of glutathione reductase through the provision of specific nutrients and bioactive compounds.

1. **Vitamins and Minerals:** Nutrients such as vitamin C, vitamin E, selenium, and zinc are essential for the optimal activity of GR. These nutrients act as cofactors or enhance the expression of antioxidant enzymes.
2. **Phytochemicals:** Plant-based diets are rich in phytochemicals such as flavonoids, polyphenols, and carotenoids, which can up-regulate the expression of antioxidant enzymes, including GR, through the activation of Nrf2 and other signaling pathways.
3. **Amino Acids:** Sulfur-containing amino acids like cysteine and methionine, found in plant-based foods such as legumes and cruciferous vegetables, are precursors for GSH synthesis. Adequate intake of these amino acids supports the maintenance of GSH levels and the activity of GR.

Plant-Based Diet and Glutathione Reductase Regulation

A plant-based diet, characterized by a high intake of fruits, vegetables, whole grains, nuts, and seeds, supports the activity and regulation of glutathione reductase through various mechanisms.

Nutrient Density

1. **Antioxidant Vitamins:** Vitamin C and vitamin E, abundant in fruits and vegetables, directly support antioxidant defenses and may enhance the expression of GR.
2. **Minerals:** Selenium and zinc, found in nuts, seeds, and whole grains, are crucial for the optimal function of GR and other antioxidant enzymes.

Phytochemicals and Antioxidants

1. **Flavonoids and Polyphenols:** Compounds such as quercetin, resveratrol, and catechins, found in berries, green tea, and dark chocolate, can activate Nrf2 and upregulate the expression of antioxidant enzymes including GR.
2. **Carotenoids:** Beta-carotene, lycopene, and lutein, present in colorful fruits and vegetables, have been shown to enhance cellular antioxidant capacity and may influence GR activity.

Amino Acids and Sulfur Compounds

1. **Cysteine and Methionine:** Cruciferous vegetables (e.g., broccoli, Brussels sprouts) and alliums (e.g., garlic, onions) are rich in sulfur compounds that are precursors for GSH synthesis. Adequate intake of these amino acids supports GR activity by maintaining GSH levels.
2. **Glutamate and Glycine:** These amino acids, found in legumes, nuts, and seeds, are also important for GSH synthesis and the overall functioning of the antioxidant system.

Plant-Based Diet on GR-Related Health Outcomes

A diet rich in plant-based foods can have numerous health benefits by supporting the activity and regulation of glutathione reductase and overall antioxidant defenses.

Oxidative Stress and Chronic Diseases

1. **Cardiovascular Health:** By enhancing antioxidant defenses, a plant-based diet can reduce oxidative stress, which is a major

contributing factor to cardiovascular diseases. Improved GR activity helps in maintaining vascular health and reducing the risk of atherosclerosis.

2. **Cancer Prevention:** Increased intake of antioxidants from plant-based foods can lower oxidative damage to DNA, reducing the risk of mutations and cancer development. Enhanced GR activity is crucial for this protective effect.

Inflammatory Conditions

1. **Anti-Inflammatory Effects:** Phytochemicals in plant-based diets have anti-inflammatory properties that can modulate the activity of GR and other antioxidant enzymes, thereby reducing inflammation and related diseases such as arthritis and inflammatory bowel disease.
2. **Immune Function:** Improved antioxidant defenses, supported by a plant-based diet, can enhance immune function and protect against infections and autoimmune disorders.

Metabolic Health

1. **Diabetes Management:** Antioxidant-rich diets can improve insulin sensitivity and reduce oxidative stress associated with diabetes. Enhanced GR activity plays a role in protecting pancreatic beta-cells from oxidative damage.
2. **Weight Management:** Plant-based diets are typically lower in calories and higher in fiber, supporting healthy weight management and reducing the risk of obesity-related oxidative stress.

Aging and Longevity

1. **Anti-Aging Effects:** Antioxidants in plant-based diets can reduce oxidative damage and support cellular health, contributing to

healthy aging and longevity. Enhanced GR activity is crucial for mitigating the effects of oxidative stress on aging.

2. **Cognitive Function:** Improved antioxidant defenses can protect against neurodegenerative diseases and support cognitive function. A plant-based diet can enhance GR activity, which is important for maintaining brain health.

Glutathione reductase plays a pivotal role in maintaining cellular redox balance and protecting cells from oxidative stress. Its production and regulation are influenced by various factors, including genetic, hormonal, and nutritional elements.

23

Pentose Phosphate Pathway Enzymes

Glucose-6-Phosphate Dehydrogenase (G6PD)

Glucose-6-Phosphate Dehydrogenase (G6PD) is a crucial enzyme in the human body, playing a vital role in the pentose phosphate pathway (PPP), a metabolic pathway parallel to glycolysis. This pathway is essential for maintaining cellular redox balance and providing reducing power to cells in the form of NADPH.

Function of Glucose-6-Phosphate Dehydrogenase

G6PD is an enzyme that catalyzes the first step in the PPP, converting glucose-6-phosphate into 6-phosphoglucono-δ-lactone while reducing NADP+ to NADPH. NADPH is a crucial molecule used in various biosynthetic reactions and in maintaining the cellular redox state by regenerating reduced glutathione (GSH).

Cellular Redox Balance

G6PD plays a key role in protecting cells from oxidative damage. NADPH, produced by the G6PD reaction, is necessary for the reduction of oxidized glutathione (GSSG) back to its reduced form (GSH). GSH is a major antioxidant that neutralizes reactive oxygen species (ROS) and protects cellular components from oxidative stress.

Biosynthesis

NADPH is required for various anabolic reactions, including the synthesis of fatty acids, cholesterol, and nucleotides. These biosynthetic pathways are critical for cell growth, proliferation, and maintenance of cellular structures.

Immune Function

In phagocytic cells, NADPH is used by NADPH oxidase to produce superoxide radicals during the respiratory burst, a crucial process for killing engulfed pathogens. Thus, G6PD is essential for effective immune responses.

Maintenance of Red Blood Cells

G6PD is particularly important in red blood cells (RBCs), where it is the sole source of NADPH. NADPH protects RBCs from oxidative damage caused by various oxidative agents, including certain drugs, infections, and dietary components.

Production of Glucose-6-Phosphate Dehydrogenase

G6PD is produced by the G6PD gene located on the X chromosome. The gene encoding G6PD provides instructions for making the enzyme, which is found in almost all types of cells, with high levels in liver cells, adipocytes, and red blood cells.

Gene Encoding

The G6PD gene spans 18.5 kb and contains 13 exons. The enzyme is produced as a single polypeptide chain that forms a functional homotetramer. The active enzyme contains binding sites for both its substrate (glucose-6-phosphate) and its cofactor (NADP+).

Isoforms

There are different isoforms of G6PD, resulting from genetic variations. Some variants have reduced enzymatic activity, leading to G6PD deficiency, which can cause hemolytic anemia under oxidative stress conditions.

Regulation of Gene Expression

The expression of the G6PD gene is regulated by various factors, including hormonal signals, oxidative stress, and nutrient availability. The gene contains several regulatory elements that respond to these stimuli, ensuring that G6PD levels are adjusted according to the metabolic needs of the cell.

Regulation of Glucose-6-Phosphate Dehydrogenase

The activity of G6PD is regulated at multiple levels, including gene expression, post-translational modifications, and feedback inhibition.

Transcriptional Regulation

The expression of G6PD is upregulated by insulin, which enhances the transcription of the G6PD gene. This regulation ensures that during times of high glucose availability, the PPP can provide NADPH for anabolic reactions and antioxidant defense.

Post-Translational Modifications

G6PD activity can be modulated by post-translational modifications, such as phosphorylation. These modifications can alter the enzyme's activity and stability, allowing for rapid adjustments in response to cellular conditions.

Feedback Inhibition

G6PD is subject to feedback inhibition by its product, NADPH. High levels of NADPH inhibit the enzyme's activity, preventing excessive production of NADPH and ensuring a balance between the PPP and glycolysis.

Nutritional Influences

Dietary components, particularly those in a plant-based diet, can influence the regulation of G6PD. Nutrients such as flavonoids, polyphenols, and vitamins found in plant foods can modulate the activity of G6PD and the overall flux through the PPP.

Plant-Based Diet and G6PD Regulation

A plant-based diet, rich in fruits, vegetables, whole grains, nuts, and seeds, can positively influence the regulation of G6PD through various mechanisms.

Antioxidants

Plant-based diets are high in antioxidants, which help reduce oxidative stress and protect cells from damage. Antioxidants such as vitamins C and E, found in many plant foods, support the activity of G6PD by maintaining the cellular redox state.

Polyphenols

Polyphenols, abundant in plant foods, have been shown to modulate the activity of G6PD. For example, resveratrol, found in grapes and berries, can enhance the expression of G6PD, thereby increasing NADPH production and improving cellular antioxidant capacity.

Omega-3 Fatty Acids

Omega-3 fatty acids, found in flaxseeds, chia seeds, and walnuts, can reduce inflammation and oxidative stress, indirectly supporting G6PD activity. By lowering the overall oxidative burden, omega-3 fatty acids help maintain optimal G6PD function.

Fiber

High-fiber diets, typical of plant-based eating, support gut health and metabolic regulation. A healthy gut microbiome can influence systemic inflammation and oxidative stress, thereby affecting the activity of G6PD.

Caloric Balance

Maintaining a healthy weight through a balanced plant-based diet can prevent obesity-related oxidative stress and inflammation, which can negatively impact G6PD activity. Caloric balance is essential for optimal metabolic function and enzyme regulation.

Plant-Based Diet on G6PD-Related Health Outcomes

A plant-based diet can have significant health benefits by supporting the activity and regulation of G6PD, thereby improving overall metabolic health and reducing the risk of oxidative stress-related conditions.

Reducing Oxidative Stress

By providing a rich source of antioxidants and reducing pro-oxidant dietary components, a plant-based diet can help lower oxidative stress levels. This reduction supports the activity of G6PD and the maintenance of cellular redox balance.

Enhancing Immune Function

A diet rich in vitamins, minerals, and phytonutrients supports immune function by ensuring adequate NADPH production through G6PD activity. This support enhances the body's ability to respond to infections and other immune challenges.

Protecting Red Blood Cells

For individuals with G6PD deficiency, a plant-based diet can provide essential nutrients that support RBC health and reduce the risk of hemolytic episodes. Avoiding certain oxidative stress-inducing foods, such as fava beans, is also crucial for managing G6PD deficiency.

Supporting Metabolic Health

A plant-based diet can improve metabolic health by enhancing insulin sensitivity, reducing inflammation, and providing essential nutrients for anabolic processes. These benefits support the overall activity of G6PD and metabolic balance.

Preventing Chronic Diseases

By reducing oxidative stress and supporting metabolic health, a plant-based diet can help prevent chronic diseases such as cardiovascular disease, diabetes, and cancer. The activity of G6PD plays a crucial role in these protective effects by maintaining cellular redox balance and supporting biosynthetic pathways.

Glucose-6-Phosphate Dehydrogenase is a vital enzyme that plays a critical role in maintaining cellular redox balance, supporting anabolic reactions, and protecting cells from oxidative damage. Its activity and regulation are influenced by various factors, including hormonal signals, oxidative stress, and dietary components.

Transketolase (TK)

Transketolase (TK) is a crucial enzyme in the pentose phosphate pathway (PPP), playing an essential role in cellular metabolism and maintaining redox balance.

Function of Transketolase

Transketolase is a thiamine-dependent enzyme that catalyzes the transfer of two-carbon units between sugars, facilitating crucial reactions in the non-oxidative phase of the pentose phosphate pathway (PPP). Its primary functions include:

1. **Nucleotide Synthesis:** Transketolase generates ribose-5-phosphate, a precursor for nucleotide and nucleic acid synthesis. This function is vital for cell proliferation and DNA repair mechanisms.
2. **NADPH Production:** By participating in the PPP, transketolase helps produce NADPH, a critical cofactor for biosynthetic reactions and antioxidant defense. NADPH is essential for fatty acid synthesis, cholesterol synthesis, and the detoxification of reactive oxygen species (ROS).
3. **Metabolic Flexibility:** Transketolase facilitates the interconversion of sugars, allowing cells to adapt their metabolism to varying nutrient availability. This flexibility supports energy production and biosynthetic processes under different physiological conditions.

Production of Transketolase

Transketolase production is tightly regulated and involves several biochemical and genetic processes:

1. **Gene Encoding:** The gene encoding transketolase (TKT) is located on chromosome 3 in humans. This gene is responsible for producing the enzyme's polypeptide chain.
2. **Thiamine Dependency:** Transketolase requires thiamine pyrophosphate (TPP) as a cofactor. Thiamine (vitamin B1) must be obtained from dietary sources, emphasizing the importance of proper nutrition for enzyme functionality.
3. **Protein Synthesis:** The TKT gene is transcribed into mRNA, which is then translated into the transketolase protein in the cytoplasm. Post-translational modifications and folding are necessary for the enzyme to become active.
4. **Cellular Localization:** Transketolase is primarily localized in the cytosol, where the pentose phosphate pathway operates. Its distribution within the cell is crucial for effective metabolic flux through the PPP.

Regulation of Transketolase

Transketolase activity is regulated by several factors, ensuring that the enzyme functions optimally under varying physiological conditions:

1. **Nutritional Status:** Adequate intake of thiamine is essential for transketolase activity. Thiamine-rich plant-based foods, such as whole grains, legumes, and nuts, support optimal enzyme function.
2. **Hormonal Regulation:** Hormones like insulin and glucagon can modulate transketolase activity by influencing the cellular redox state and substrate availability.

3. **Oxidative Stress:** Cellular redox balance impacts transketolase activity. Increased oxidative stress can inhibit the enzyme, while adequate NADPH levels, produced through PPP, support its function.
4. **Allosteric Regulation:** Metabolites such as fructose-6-phosphate and glyceraldehyde-3-phosphate, substrates of the PPP, can allosterically modulate transketolase activity, aligning enzyme function with metabolic needs.

Plant-Based Diet and Transketolase Regulation

A plant-based diet, rich in essential nutrients, vitamins, and minerals, can positively influence transketolase regulation through various mechanisms:

1. **Thiamine-Rich Foods:** Whole grains, legumes, nuts, and seeds are excellent sources of thiamine, necessary for transketolase activity. Regular consumption of these foods ensures adequate thiamine intake, supporting enzyme functionality.
2. **Antioxidant-Rich Foods:** Fruits and vegetables high in antioxidants reduce oxidative stress, indirectly supporting transketolase activity. By mitigating oxidative damage, these foods help maintain cellular redox balance and enzyme efficiency.
3. **Healthy Fats:** Plant-based sources of healthy fats, such as avocados, nuts, and seeds, provide essential fatty acids that support overall metabolic health, including optimal enzyme activity.
4. **Fiber:** High-fiber diets promote gut health and improve nutrient absorption, including thiamine. A healthy gut microbiome can influence metabolic pathways, including the PPP, by producing short-chain fatty acids and other metabolites.
5. **Phytochemicals:** Plant foods contain various phytochemicals that can modulate enzyme activity and metabolic pathways, supporting overall metabolic health.

Plant-Based Diet on Transketolase-Related Health Outcomes

1. **Metabolic Health:** A plant-based diet supports metabolic flexibility and efficiency by providing essential nutrients for transketolase activity. This diet can help prevent metabolic disorders, such as diabetes and metabolic syndrome.
2. **Oxidative Stress Reduction:** Antioxidant-rich plant foods reduce oxidative stress, supporting transketolase function and overall cellular health. Lower oxidative stress levels are associated with reduced risk of chronic diseases, including cancer and cardiovascular diseases.
3. **Improved Detoxification:** Adequate transketolase activity ensures efficient NADPH production, necessary for detoxification processes. A plant-based diet supports this detoxification, reducing the body's toxic load and improving overall health.
4. **Enhanced Immune Function:** By supporting nucleotide synthesis and cellular proliferation, transketolase activity is crucial for immune function. A nutrient-rich plant-based diet enhances this enzyme's role, promoting a robust immune response.
5. **Anti-Aging Effects:** The antioxidant properties of plant-based foods, combined with optimal transketolase activity, contribute to reduced oxidative damage and healthier aging. This diet supports the maintenance of metabolic health and longevity.

Transketolase plays a pivotal role in cellular metabolism, facilitating nucleotide synthesis, NADPH production, and metabolic flexibility. Its production and regulation are influenced by various factors, including nutritional status, oxidative stress, and allosteric regulation. A plant-based diet, rich in thiamine, antioxidants, healthy fats, and fiber, supports optimal transketolase function and overall metabolic health. By promoting metabolic efficiency, reducing oxidative stress, and enhancing detoxification and immune function, a plant-based diet can significantly contribute to improved health outcomes and longevity.

Transaldolase

Transaldolase is a crucial enzyme in the pentose phosphate pathway, a metabolic pathway parallel to glycolysis, responsible for generating NADPH and ribose-5-phosphate for anabolic reactions. It plays a significant role in cellular metabolism, influencing processes such as lipid biosynthesis, antioxidant defense, and nucleotide synthesis.

Function of Transaldolase

Transaldolase has critical roles in the pentose phosphate pathway, facilitating the rearrangement of carbon atoms between sugar phosphates, which is vital for cellular function and metabolism.

Metabolic Role in Pentose Phosphate Pathway

- **Catalysis**: Transaldolase catalyzes the transfer of a three-carbon dihydroxyacetone moiety from sedoheptulose-7-phosphate to glyceraldehyde-3-phosphate, producing erythrose-4-phosphate and fructose-6-phosphate.
- **NADPH Production**: This enzyme indirectly contributes to the production of NADPH, a crucial molecule for reductive biosynthesis and maintaining cellular redox balance.
- **Ribose-5-Phosphate Production**: Transaldolase helps generate ribose-5-phosphate, essential for nucleotide and nucleic acid synthesis, supporting cell proliferation and repair.

Antioxidant Defense

- **Reducing Reactive Oxygen Species (ROS)**: By contributing to NADPH production, transaldolase supports the regeneration of glutathione, a key antioxidant that reduces ROS and protects cells from oxidative stress.

Lipid Biosynthesis

- **Fatty Acid and Sterol Synthesis**: NADPH produced via the pentose phosphate pathway is necessary for the biosynthesis of fatty acids and sterols, which are critical components of cell membranes and signaling molecules.

Cell Growth and Proliferation

- **Nucleotide Synthesis**: The ribose-5-phosphate produced by transaldolase is essential for the synthesis of nucleotides, which are building blocks of DNA and RNA, thereby supporting cell division and growth.

Production of Transaldolase

Transaldolase is produced through gene expression and protein synthesis pathways, involving transcription, translation, and post-translational modifications.

1. **Gene Encoding**
    - **TALDO1 Gene**: The human transaldolase enzyme is encoded by the TALDO1 gene located on chromosome 11. The gene expression is regulated by various factors including cellular stress and metabolic demand.
2. **Transcription and Translation**

    - **mRNA Synthesis**: The transcription of the TALDO1 gene results in the formation of messenger RNA (mRNA), which is processed and transported out of the nucleus.
    - **Protein Synthesis**: The mRNA is translated into the transaldolase protein in the cytoplasm, involving ribosomes and transfer RNA (tRNA).
3. **Post-Translational Modifications**
    - **Folding and Assembly**: After synthesis, the transaldolase protein undergoes folding and potential assembly into functional oligomeric forms, facilitated by molecular chaperones.
    - **Modifications**: Post-translational modifications such as phosphorylation or acetylation can affect the enzyme's stability, activity, and localization within the cell.

Regulation of Transaldolase

The regulation of transaldolase involves multiple layers of control, including gene expression, feedback mechanisms, and the influence of diet, particularly plant-based nutrients.

Gene Expression Regulation

- **Transcription Factors**: The expression of TALDO1 is regulated by transcription factors that respond to cellular metabolic states and oxidative stress. For example, nuclear factor erythroid 2-related factor 2 (Nrf2) can enhance the transcription of genes involved in antioxidant defense, including TALDO1.
- **Epigenetic Modifications**: Histone modifications and DNA methylation can influence the accessibility of the TALDO1 gene for transcription, thereby regulating its expression in response to environmental and dietary factors.

Feedback Mechanisms

- **Metabolite Levels**: The activity of transaldolase is influenced by the levels of its substrates and products. High concentrations of sedoheptulose-7-phosphate or glyceraldehyde-3-phosphate can modulate the enzyme's activity through feedback inhibition or activation.
- **Redox State**: Cellular redox state, indicated by the NADP+/NADPH ratio, can regulate the pentose phosphate pathway and subsequently transaldolase activity, ensuring balanced NADPH production in response to oxidative stress.

Nutritional Influence

- **Plant-Based Diets**: Diets rich in fruits, vegetables, whole grains, nuts, and seeds provide essential nutrients that support the optimal function of metabolic enzymes, including transaldolase.
- **Antioxidants**: Phytochemicals and antioxidants present in plant-based foods, such as flavonoids, carotenoids, and polyphenols, can enhance the body's antioxidant capacity and influence the expression and activity of enzymes like transaldolase.
- **Vitamins and Minerals**: Key nutrients such as vitamins B1 (thiamine) and B2 (riboflavin), found abundantly in plant-based foods, serve as cofactors for enzymes in the pentose phosphate pathway, indirectly supporting transaldolase function.

Plant-Based Diet and Transaldolase Regulation

A plant-based diet, rich in nutrients, antioxidants, and fiber, can positively influence the regulation and activity of transaldolase, contributing to overall metabolic health and disease prevention.

Nutrient Density

- **Vitamins and Minerals**: Essential nutrients like thiamine (vitamin B1) and riboflavin (vitamin B2) from plant sources support enzymatic reactions in the pentose phosphate pathway. Whole grains, legumes, nuts, and seeds are excellent sources of these vitamins.
- **Phytonutrients**: Antioxidant-rich foods such as berries, leafy greens, and cruciferous vegetables provide compounds that enhance cellular antioxidant defenses, indirectly supporting transaldolase activity by maintaining redox balance.

Antioxidant Properties

- **Oxidative Stress Reduction**: A diet high in antioxidants helps reduce oxidative stress, protecting cells and enzymes like transaldolase from oxidative damage. Antioxidants neutralize free radicals and support the regeneration of reduced glutathione, a key molecule in cellular antioxidant defense.
- **Regulation of Nrf2 Pathway**: Phytochemicals such as sulforaphane from cruciferous vegetables can activate the Nrf2 pathway, leading to increased expression of antioxidant enzymes, including those in the pentose phosphate pathway.

Healthy Fats

- **Omega-3 Fatty Acids**: Plant-based sources of omega-3 fatty acids, such as flaxseeds, chia seeds, and walnuts, have anti-inflammatory properties that support overall metabolic health. These fatty acids can influence the expression of genes involved in antioxidant defense and metabolism.

- **Monounsaturated Fats**: Foods like avocados, nuts, and olive oil provide healthy fats that support cellular membrane integrity and function, indirectly affecting enzyme activity and stability.

Fiber and Gut Health

- **Gut Microbiome**: A high-fiber diet promotes a healthy gut microbiome, which can produce short-chain fatty acids (SCFAs) with systemic anti-inflammatory effects. A balanced microbiome supports overall metabolic health and the regulation of metabolic enzymes.
- **Metabolic Regulation**: Dietary fiber helps regulate blood glucose levels and insulin sensitivity, contributing to balanced energy metabolism and reducing the risk of metabolic disorders that can affect enzyme function.

Plant-Based Diet on Transaldolase-Related Health Outcomes

Adopting a plant-based diet can enhance the regulation and activity of transaldolase, contributing to various health benefits and disease prevention.

Metabolic Health

- **Diabetes Prevention**: Improved regulation of the pentose phosphate pathway through a plant-based diet can enhance NADPH production, supporting antioxidant defenses and reducing the risk of diabetes-related complications.
- **Weight Management**: Plant-based diets are effective for weight management, reducing body fat, and improving insulin sensitivity.

Better glycemic control supports balanced enzyme activity and metabolic health.

Cardiovascular Health

- **Lipid Profile Improvement**: A diet rich in plant-based foods can improve lipid profiles, reducing LDL cholesterol and increasing HDL cholesterol levels. This lipid balance supports cardiovascular health and reduces the risk of atherosclerosis.
- **Antioxidant Protection**: Enhanced antioxidant defenses from a plant-based diet protect against oxidative stress, a major factor in cardiovascular diseases. Reduced oxidative damage supports endothelial function and overall heart health.

Cancer Prevention

- **Antioxidant Capacity**: Increased intake of antioxidants from plant-based foods can reduce oxidative stress, a contributor to cancer development. Enhanced NADPH production via the pentose phosphate pathway supports cellular repair and detoxification processes.
- **Anti-Inflammatory Effects**: Phytochemicals in plant foods have anti-inflammatory properties that reduce chronic inflammation, a known risk factor for cancer. A balanced inflammatory response supports cellular health and reduces cancer risk.

Neuroprotection

- **Oxidative Stress Reduction**: A plant-based diet can enhance neuroprotective mechanisms by reducing oxidative stress, supporting brain health, and reducing the risk of neurodegenerative diseases.

- **Nutrient Support**: Essential nutrients from plant-based foods, such as folate and vitamin E, support cognitive function and protect against age-related cognitive decline.

Immune Function

- **Enhanced Antioxidant Defense**: By supporting the production of NADPH, a plant-based diet helps maintain a robust antioxidant defense system, which is crucial for a well-functioning immune response.
- **Anti-Inflammatory Nutrients**: Nutrients such as vitamin C and beta-carotene from fruits and vegetables support immune function by reducing inflammation and oxidative stress, enhancing the body's ability to fight infections and diseases.

Transaldolase plays a pivotal role in cellular metabolism, particularly in the pentose phosphate pathway, supporting antioxidant defense, lipid biosynthesis, and nucleotide synthesis. Its production and regulation are influenced by various factors, including gene expression, feedback mechanisms, and nutritional status.

24

Glycolysis Continuation Enzymes

Aldolase

Aldolase is a critical enzyme in the human body that plays a pivotal role in glycolysis, the metabolic pathway that breaks down glucose to produce energy.

Function of Aldolase

Aldolase is an essential enzyme involved in the glycolytic pathway, responsible for catalyzing the reversible conversion of fructose-1,6-bisphosphate to glyceraldehyde-3-phosphate and dihydroxyacetone phosphate. This reaction is a key step in the metabolic breakdown of glucose for energy production.

Glycolysis

Glycolysis is a crucial metabolic pathway that occurs in the cytoplasm of cells, converting glucose into pyruvate, and generating ATP (adenosine triphosphate) and NADH (nicotinamide adenine dinucleotide) in the process. Aldolase functions in the fourth step of this ten-step process, facilitating the cleavage of a six-carbon sugar into two three-carbon molecules, which are further processed to produce energy.

Energy Production

The role of aldolase in glycolysis is vital for cellular energy production. By catalyzing the cleavage of fructose-1,6-bisphosphate, aldolase ensures the continuation of the glycolytic pathway, leading to the generation of ATP, which cells use for various energy-demanding processes.

Additional Roles

Beyond its primary role in glycolysis, aldolase also participates in other metabolic pathways, including gluconeogenesis (the synthesis of glucose from non-carbohydrate sources) and the pentose phosphate pathway, which is important for nucleotide synthesis and antioxidant defense.

Production of Aldolase

Aldolase is produced in various tissues throughout the body, with different isoforms expressed in muscle, liver, and brain tissues. The production and expression of aldolase are regulated at the genetic level and influenced by various factors, including diet and overall metabolic state.

Gene Encoding

The gene encoding aldolase is located on chromosome 16, with three main isoforms: aldolase A (muscle), aldolase B (liver), and aldolase C (brain). These isoforms are encoded by distinct genes, each tailored to the specific metabolic needs of their respective tissues.

Isoforms and Tissue Distribution

1. **Aldolase A**: Predominantly expressed in muscle tissue, aldolase A is crucial for energy production during muscle contraction and exercise.
2. **Aldolase B**: Found primarily in the liver, aldolase B plays a significant role in gluconeogenesis and fructose metabolism.
3. **Aldolase C**: Mainly present in the brain, aldolase C is involved in neuronal energy metabolism and overall brain function.

Regulation of Gene Expression

The expression of aldolase genes is regulated by various factors, including hormonal signals, metabolic needs, and dietary influences. Insulin and glucagon, for example, play significant roles in regulating the expression of aldolase in response to blood glucose levels.

Regulation of Aldolase

The regulation of aldolase activity involves a complex interplay of genetic, hormonal, and dietary factors. Understanding how these factors influence aldolase activity is crucial for maintaining metabolic health and preventing disorders related to energy metabolism.

Hormonal Regulation

1. **Insulin**: Insulin, a hormone produced by the pancreas in response to high blood glucose levels, stimulates the expression of aldolase, particularly aldolase B in the liver, to promote glycolysis and energy production.
2. **Glucagon**: In contrast, glucagon, produced in response to low blood glucose levels, inhibits aldolase expression to shift metabolism toward gluconeogenesis and glucose production.

Metabolic Regulation

Aldolase activity is also regulated by the overall metabolic state of the body. During periods of high energy demand, such as exercise, aldolase activity increases to ensure adequate ATP production. Conversely, during fasting or low-energy states, aldolase activity decreases to conserve energy.

Nutritional Influences

Diet plays a significant role in regulating aldolase activity. A plant-based diet, rich in complex carbohydrates, fiber, and essential nutrients, supports optimal aldolase function by providing a steady supply of glucose for glycolysis.

Plant-Based Nutrients Supporting Aldolase Activity

1. **Complex Carbohydrates**: Found in whole grains, legumes, and vegetables, complex carbohydrates provide a sustained source of glucose, ensuring continuous glycolytic activity.
2. **Fiber**: High-fiber foods support stable blood glucose levels, preventing the rapid spikes and drops that can disrupt aldolase regulation.
3. **Vitamins and Minerals**: Essential nutrients, such as B vitamins, magnesium, and potassium, found in plant-based foods, are crucial for enzyme function and energy metabolism.

Oxidative Stress and Antioxidants

Oxidative stress, caused by an imbalance between free radicals and antioxidants, can negatively impact aldolase activity. A plant-based diet, rich in antioxidants, helps mitigate oxidative stress, supporting overall metabolic health and aldolase function.

Plant-Based Diet on Aldolase Regulation

A plant-based diet, characterized by high nutrient density and low levels of saturated fats and refined sugars, offers numerous benefits for aldolase regulation and overall metabolic health.

Nutrient Density

Plant-based diets provide a wealth of essential nutrients that support enzyme function and metabolic pathways. For example, fruits and vegetables are rich in vitamins, minerals, and antioxidants that enhance aldolase activity and protect against oxidative damage.

Amino Acids

Certain amino acids found in plant foods, such as glutamine and arginine, support enzyme production and function. These amino acids play roles in protein synthesis and overall metabolic health.

Antioxidants

Fruits and vegetables are rich in antioxidants, which help reduce oxidative stress. Lower oxidative stress levels are associated with improved aldolase function and overall metabolic health.

Healthy Fats

Plant-based sources of fats, such as avocados, nuts, and seeds, provide essential fatty acids that support cell membrane integrity and enzyme function. Omega-3 fatty acids, in particular, have anti-inflammatory properties that enhance metabolic health.

Fiber

High-fiber diets, common in plant-based eating, support gut health and stable blood glucose levels, both of which are crucial for maintaining optimal aldolase activity.

Caloric Balance

Maintaining a healthy weight through a balanced plant-based diet can prevent obesity-related metabolic imbalances. Excess body fat is linked to disrupted enzyme activity, including aldolase, due to increased production of inflammatory markers.

Glycemic Control

Plant-based diets, low in refined sugars and high in complex carbohydrates, help maintain stable blood glucose levels. This stability prevents insulin resistance, which can negatively impact aldolase activity and overall metabolic health.

Health Benefits of Optimal Aldolase Function

Energy Production and Physical Performance

By supporting efficient glycolysis, aldolase plays a critical role in energy production, particularly during physical activity. Optimal aldolase function enhances athletic performance and overall physical endurance.

Metabolic Health

Efficient aldolase activity supports overall metabolic health by ensuring proper glucose metabolism and energy balance. This is crucial for preventing metabolic disorders such as diabetes and obesity.

Brain Function

Aldolase C, expressed in the brain, supports neuronal energy metabolism and cognitive function. A plant-based diet rich in antioxidants and essential nutrients can enhance brain health and protect against neurodegenerative diseases.

Liver Health

Aldolase B, present in the liver, plays a significant role in gluconeogenesis and fructose metabolism. Maintaining optimal aldolase B activity through a healthy diet supports liver function and prevents metabolic liver diseases.

Plant-Based Diet and Aldolase-Related Health Outcomes

Cardiovascular Health

A plant-based diet can improve cardiovascular health by supporting optimal aldolase activity and overall metabolic balance. By reducing oxidative stress and inflammation, plant-based diets protect against heart disease and other cardiovascular conditions.

Weight Management

Plant-based diets are effective for weight management, reducing body fat, and improving insulin sensitivity. Lower body fat and better glycemic control enhance overall metabolic health, including aldolase function.

Diabetes Prevention

A diet rich in whole grains, legumes, fruits, and vegetables helps maintain stable blood glucose levels and prevent insulin resistance, reducing the risk of type 2 diabetes and associated complications.

Cancer Prevention

Antioxidants and phytochemicals found in plant-based foods can protect against oxidative damage and reduce the risk of cancer. By supporting optimal enzyme function, including aldolase, plant-based diets contribute to overall cancer prevention strategies.

Longevity and Aging

The antioxidant-rich nature of plant-based diets helps combat oxidative stress, a key factor in aging. Improved metabolic health and enzyme function contribute to healthier aging and better maintenance of overall health.

Aldolase is a critical enzyme in the glycolytic pathway, playing a vital role in energy production and metabolic health. Its function, production, and regulation are influenced by various factors, including diet and overall metabolic state.

Triosephosphate Isomerase (TPI)

Triosephosphate isomerase (TPI) is a crucial enzyme in the glycolytic pathway, responsible for the interconversion of dihydroxyacetone phosphate (DHAP) and glyceraldehyde-3-phosphate (G3P).

Function of Triosephosphate Isomerase

TPI plays a vital role in cellular metabolism, specifically in the glycolytic pathway, which is fundamental for energy production in cells.

Glycolysis and Energy Production

1. **Catalytic Activity**: TPI catalyzes the reversible interconversion of DHAP and G3P, two triose phosphates produced during glycolysis. This reaction ensures that the glycolytic pathway can continue efficiently, as G3P can proceed to subsequent steps, leading to ATP production.
2. **Energy Efficiency**: By converting DHAP to G3P, TPI maximizes the use of the available substrate, ensuring that each glucose

molecule generates the maximum amount of ATP. This efficiency is critical for cells to meet their energy demands.

3. **Anaerobic and Aerobic Conditions**: TPI operates under both anaerobic and aerobic conditions, making it essential for energy production regardless of oxygen availability.

Additional Roles

1. **Metabolic Integration**: TPI links glycolysis to other metabolic pathways, such as gluconeogenesis and lipid metabolism, by providing intermediates that can be used in these processes.
2. **Redox Balance**: The interconversion of DHAP and G3P by TPI helps maintain redox balance within the cell, crucial for preventing oxidative stress.

Production of Triosephosphate Isomerase

TPI is produced by cells through a well-coordinated process involving gene expression and protein synthesis.

Gene Encoding

1. **TPI Gene**: The gene responsible for encoding TPI is located on chromosome 12 in humans. It provides the instructions for synthesizing the TPI protein.
2. **Transcription and Translation**: The TPI gene is transcribed into mRNA, which is then translated into the TPI enzyme in the ribosomes. This process is tightly regulated to meet cellular energy demands.

Protein Structure

1. **Dimeric Enzyme**: TPI functions as a dimer, with each monomer consisting of approximately 250 amino acids. The dimeric structure is essential for its catalytic activity.

2. **Active Site**: The active site of TPI contains key residues, including histidine and glutamate, which facilitate the isomerization of DHAP and G3P.

Regulation of Production

1. **Gene Expression Regulation**: The expression of the TPI gene is regulated by various factors, including cellular energy status, availability of substrates, and hormonal signals.
2. **Post-Translational Modifications**: TPI activity can be modulated by post-translational modifications such as phosphorylation, which can alter its enzymatic efficiency.

Regulation of Triosephosphate Isomerase

The regulation of TPI involves a complex interplay of feedback mechanisms, external factors, and physiological states.

Feedback Mechanisms

1. **Product Inhibition**: The levels of DHAP and G3P can influence TPI activity through product inhibition. High levels of G3P, for instance, can inhibit TPI to prevent excessive substrate depletion.
2. **Energy Status**: Cellular ATP and ADP levels can modulate TPI activity. High ATP levels indicate sufficient energy, reducing the need for glycolysis, while low ATP levels stimulate TPI activity to boost energy production.

Nutritional Influence

1. **Carbohydrate Availability**: The availability of glucose and other carbohydrates directly impacts TPI activity. Adequate carbohydrate intake ensures sufficient substrate for glycolysis and TPI function.

2. **Plant-Based Nutrients**: Nutrients found in plant-based diets, such as vitamins and minerals, play a role in maintaining optimal TPI activity.

Hormonal Regulation

1. **Insulin and Glucagon**: Insulin and glucagon, hormones involved in glucose homeostasis, influence TPI activity. Insulin promotes glycolysis and TPI activity, while glucagon inhibits these processes during fasting states.
2. **Thyroid Hormones**: Thyroid hormones can modulate metabolic rate and, consequently, TPI activity. Elevated thyroid hormone levels increase metabolic activity, enhancing TPI function.

Plant-Based Diet and Triosephosphate Isomerase Regulation

A plant-based diet, rich in fruits, vegetables, whole grains, nuts, and seeds, can positively influence TPI regulation through various mechanisms.

Nutrient Density

1. **Vitamins and Minerals**: Plant-based diets provide essential vitamins and minerals that support enzymatic activities. For instance, magnesium, found in leafy greens and nuts, is a cofactor for many enzymes, including those in the glycolytic pathway.
2. **Antioxidants**: Fruits and vegetables are rich in antioxidants, which help reduce oxidative stress and maintain cellular health, indirectly supporting TPI activity.

Amino Acids

1. **Protein Sources**: Plant-based protein sources such as legumes, nuts, and seeds provide essential amino acids required for enzyme

synthesis. Adequate protein intake ensures that the body can produce sufficient TPI.
2. **Specific Amino Acids**: Certain amino acids, such as glutamine and arginine, found in plant foods, play a role in maintaining metabolic health and supporting TPI function.

Fiber and Gut Health

1. **High-Fiber Diets**: Plant-based diets are typically high in dietary fiber, which supports gut health and can influence overall metabolic regulation. A healthy gut microbiome is linked to better metabolic outcomes, including efficient glycolysis.
2. **Short-Chain Fatty Acids**: The fermentation of dietary fiber by gut bacteria produces short-chain fatty acids, which have been shown to influence metabolic pathways and enzyme activities.

Caloric Balance

1. **Weight Management**: Maintaining a healthy weight through a balanced plant-based diet prevents obesity-related metabolic imbalances. Excess body fat can disrupt hormonal balance and negatively impact TPI activity.
2. **Stable Blood Sugar Levels:** Plant-based diets, which are low in refined sugars and high in complex carbohydrates, help maintain stable blood glucose levels. Stable glucose levels ensure a steady supply of substrate for glycolysis and TPI function.

Plant-Based Diet on TPI-Related Health Outcomes

A plant-based diet can enhance various health outcomes by supporting optimal TPI function and overall metabolic health.

Energy Levels and Physical Performance

1. **Enhanced Energy Production**: By ensuring efficient glycolysis through optimal TPI activity, a plant-based diet can support sustained energy levels and improve physical performance.
2. **Recovery and Endurance**: Nutrients such as antioxidants and amino acids found in plant-based foods support recovery and endurance, benefiting athletes and active individuals.

Weight Management and Metabolic Health

1. **Obesity Prevention**: A plant-based diet can aid in weight management, reducing the risk of obesity-related metabolic disorders. Lower body fat percentages are associated with improved metabolic function and TPI activity.
2. **Insulin Sensitivity**: Improved insulin sensitivity from a plant-based diet supports better glucose uptake and utilization, enhancing glycolysis and TPI function.

Cardiovascular Health

1. **Lipid Profile**: Plant-based diets are known to improve lipid profiles, reducing the risk of cardiovascular diseases. Healthy lipid levels support overall metabolic health, including efficient glycolysis.
2. **Anti-Inflammatory Effects**: The anti-inflammatory properties of plant-based diets help reduce chronic inflammation, which can impair metabolic pathways and enzyme activities.

Mental Health and Cognitive Function

1. **Reduced Oxidative Stress**: Antioxidants in plant-based diets help reduce oxidative stress, which is linked to cognitive decline

and mental health disorders. Maintaining redox balance supports overall metabolic function, including TPI activity.

2. **Nutrient Support**: Nutrients such as omega-3 fatty acids, found in flaxseeds and walnuts, support brain health and cognitive function, indirectly benefiting metabolic processes.

Anti-Aging Effects

1. **Cellular Health**: The nutrient-dense nature of plant-based diets supports cellular health and longevity. Efficient glycolysis, facilitated by optimal TPI function, contributes to healthy aging.
2. **Hormonal Balance**: Maintaining hormonal balance through a plant-based diet helps regulate metabolic pathways, including those involving TPI, promoting overall health and longevity.

Triosephosphate isomerase is a pivotal enzyme in the glycolytic pathway, essential for efficient energy production and metabolic integration. Its function, production, and regulation are influenced by various factors, including nutritional status, hormonal signals, and cellular energy demands.

Enolase

Enolase is an essential enzyme in the glycolytic pathway, playing a pivotal role in the conversion of 2-phosphoglycerate (2-PG) to phosphoenolpyruvate (PEP).

Function of Enolase

Enolase is a metalloenzyme that catalyzes the penultimate step of glycolysis. It exists in three isoforms: alpha-enolase (ENO1), beta-enolase

(ENO3), and gamma-enolase (ENO2), each having tissue-specific expression and functions.

Glycolysis

1. **Conversion of 2-Phosphoglycerate to Phosphoenolpyruvate**: Enolase catalyzes the dehydration of 2-phosphoglycerate (2-PG) to phosphoenolpyruvate (PEP), which is then converted to pyruvate by pyruvate kinase. This reaction is crucial for the energy-yielding steps of glycolysis.
2. **Energy Production**: The conversion of PEP to pyruvate generates ATP, providing essential energy for cellular processes. Enolase, therefore, plays a critical role in cellular metabolism and energy production.

Beyond Glycolysis

1. **Cellular Growth and Proliferation**: Enolase is involved in cell growth and proliferation. Its role in glycolysis supports the metabolic needs of rapidly dividing cells, including cancer cells.
2. **Neuroprotection and Neuronal Health**: Gamma-enolase (ENO2) is primarily found in neurons and neuroendocrine tissues, where it is believed to play a role in neuronal survival and neuroprotection.
3. **Structural Functions**: Enolase also functions as a structural protein in various cellular processes, including cytoskeleton organization and cell structure maintenance.

Clinical Implications

1. **Cancer Marker**: Enolase, particularly ENO1 and ENO2, is overexpressed in several cancers and serves as a diagnostic marker. Elevated levels of enolase are associated with poor prognosis in cancer patients.

2. **Neurological Disorders**: Abnormal enolase levels are linked to neurodegenerative diseases such as Alzheimer's and Parkinson's, highlighting its importance in neuronal health.

Production of Enolase

Enolase production involves gene expression, protein synthesis, and post-translational modifications, which ensure its proper function and regulation.

Gene Encoding

1. **Gene Location**: Enolase genes are located on different chromosomes: ENO1 on chromosome 1, ENO2 on chromosome 12, and ENO3 on chromosome 17. Each gene encodes for its respective isoform, contributing to tissue-specific functions.
2. **Transcription and Translation**: The transcription of enolase genes is regulated by various transcription factors and signaling pathways. Once transcribed, mRNA is translated into the enolase protein in the cytoplasm.

Protein Structure

1. **Isoforms**: Enolase exists as a dimer, with each isoform forming homodimers (e.g., ENO1-ENO1) or heterodimers (e.g., ENO1-ENO2). These isoforms have different kinetic properties and tissue distributions.
2. **Active Site**: The active site of enolase contains a magnesium ion essential for its catalytic activity. This metalloenzyme property is crucial for the dehydration reaction in glycolysis.

Post-Translational Modifications

1. **Phosphorylation**: Enolase undergoes phosphorylation, affecting its activity and interaction with other cellular components. Phosphorylation is a key regulatory mechanism in response to cellular signals.
2. **Acetylation**: Acetylation of enolase influences its function and stability, with implications for metabolic regulation and enzyme activity.

Regulation of Enolase

The regulation of enolase involves various mechanisms, including gene expression, enzymatic activity modulation, and interactions with metabolic pathways.

Gene Expression Regulation

1. **Transcription Factors**: Enolase gene expression is regulated by transcription factors such as hypoxia-inducible factor (HIF-1) under low oxygen conditions, ensuring adequate glycolytic flux in hypoxic environments.
2. **Epigenetic Modifications**: DNA methylation and histone acetylation/deacetylation regulate enolase gene expression, impacting its availability and activity in different tissues.

Enzyme Activity Modulation

1. **Allosteric Regulation**: Enolase activity is modulated by allosteric effectors, including substrate availability and feedback inhibition by downstream glycolytic intermediates.
2. **Magnesium Ion Concentration**: As a metalloenzyme, enolase requires magnesium ions for activity. Variations in intracellular magnesium levels can regulate enolase function.

Metabolic Pathways Interactions

1. **Glycolytic Flux**: Enolase is part of the tightly regulated glycolytic pathway. Its activity is coordinated with other glycolytic enzymes to ensure efficient energy production.
2. **Interaction with Other Metabolic Pathways**: Enolase interacts with other metabolic pathways, including gluconeogenesis and the pentose phosphate pathway, highlighting its central role in cellular metabolism.

Plant-Based Diet and Enolase Regulation

A plant-based diet, rich in nutrients, antioxidants, and phytochemicals, can influence enolase activity and regulation through various mechanisms.

Nutrient Density

1. **Vitamins and Minerals**: Plant-based diets provide essential vitamins and minerals that support enzymatic functions. Magnesium, abundant in leafy greens and nuts, is crucial for enolase activity.
2. **Antioxidants**: Fruits and vegetables are rich in antioxidants such as vitamin C, vitamin E, and polyphenols, which protect enolase from oxidative damage, ensuring its proper function.

Phytochemicals

1. **Polyphenols**: Polyphenols in plant-based foods, such as flavonoids and phenolic acids, modulate enolase activity by affecting gene expression and enzyme stability. These compounds have anti-inflammatory and antioxidant properties that support overall metabolic health.

2. **Isothiocyanates**: Found in cruciferous vegetables, isothiocyanates influence enolase activity by inducing detoxifying enzymes and reducing oxidative stress, enhancing metabolic efficiency.

Fiber

1. **Gut Health**: High-fiber diets promote a healthy gut microbiome, which produces short-chain fatty acids (SCFAs) that influence systemic metabolism and enolase activity. SCFAs can enhance energy production and reduce inflammation.
2. **Glycemic Control**: Fiber helps maintain stable blood glucose levels, preventing insulin resistance and ensuring optimal glycolytic flux, where enolase plays a critical role.

Healthy Fats

1. **Omega-3 Fatty Acids**: Plant-based sources of omega-3 fatty acids, such as flaxseeds and chia seeds, have anti-inflammatory effects that support metabolic health and enolase function.
2. **Monounsaturated Fats**: Avocados, nuts, and seeds provide monounsaturated fats that improve cell membrane integrity and enzyme activity, supporting overall metabolic efficiency.

Plant-Based Diet on Enolase-Related Health Outcomes
Metabolic Health

1. **Insulin Sensitivity**: A plant-based diet enhances insulin sensitivity, supporting efficient glucose metabolism where enolase is crucial. Improved insulin sensitivity prevents metabolic disorders like type 2 diabetes.
2. **Weight Management**: Plant-based diets aid in weight management, reducing obesity-related metabolic disturbances. Lower

body fat and improved metabolic health ensure optimal enolase activity and energy production.

Cancer Prevention

1. **Antioxidant Protection**: Antioxidants in plant-based diets protect against DNA damage and oxidative stress, reducing cancer risk. By maintaining enolase function, these antioxidants support healthy cell metabolism.
2. **Anti-Inflammatory Effects**: Phytochemicals in plant foods reduce chronic inflammation, a risk factor for cancer. Lower inflammation levels support metabolic pathways, including glycolysis, where enolase is active.

Neuroprotection

1. **Cognitive Health**: A diet rich in antioxidants and anti-inflammatory compounds from plant foods supports brain health and protects against neurodegenerative diseases. Optimal enolase function in neurons ensures efficient energy metabolism, crucial for cognitive function.
2. **Mood Regulation**: Nutrients in plant-based diets, such as magnesium and omega-3 fatty acids, contribute to mood regulation and mental health. Proper enolase activity in the brain supports overall neuronal health and function.

Enolase plays a critical role in glycolysis and cellular metabolism, with significant implications for energy production, cell growth, and neuroprotection. Its production and regulation are influenced by various factors, including gene expression, enzyme activity modulation, and metabolic pathway interactions.

25

Urea Cycle Enzymes

Carbamoyl Phosphate Synthetase (CPS)

Carbamoyl Phosphate Synthetase (CPS) is a critical enzyme in the urea cycle and pyrimidine biosynthesis, playing a vital role in nitrogen metabolism and the production of key biomolecules.

Function of Carbamoyl Phosphate Synthetase

Carbamoyl Phosphate Synthetase exists in two isoforms: CPS I and CPS II, each with distinct functions and tissue localizations.

CPS I

CPS I is primarily located in the mitochondria of liver cells and is integral to the urea cycle, which detoxifies ammonia by converting it to urea for excretion.

Role in Urea Cycle

1. **Ammonia Detoxification**: CPS I catalyzes the first step in the urea cycle, combining ammonia with bicarbonate to form carbamoyl phosphate. This reaction is crucial for converting toxic ammonia, produced during protein catabolism, into urea, a less toxic compound excreted in urine.
2. **Nitrogen Metabolism**: By facilitating the urea cycle, CPS I helps maintain nitrogen balance in the body, preventing hyperammonemia, which can lead to neurological damage.

CPS II

CPS II is found in the cytosol of cells and is involved in pyrimidine biosynthesis, essential for DNA and RNA production.

Role in Pyrimidine Biosynthesis

1. **Nucleotide Synthesis**: CPS II catalyzes the production of carbamoyl phosphate from glutamine and bicarbonate, which is a precursor for the synthesis of pyrimidine nucleotides, such as cytosine, thymine, and uracil.
2. **Cell Growth and Division**: Pyrimidine nucleotides are essential for DNA replication and RNA transcription, making CPS II crucial for cell proliferation and growth.

Production of Carbamoyl Phosphate Synthetase

The production of CPS involves complex genetic and biochemical processes.

Gene Encoding

1. **CPS I**: The CPS1 gene, located on chromosome 2q35, encodes the CPS I enzyme. It is primarily expressed in the liver and is regulated by dietary and hormonal factors.
2. **CPS II**: The CPS2 gene, part of the CAD gene complex on chromosome 2p21, encodes the CPS II enzyme. The CAD gene also includes domains for aspartate transcarbamoylase and dihydroorotase, making it a multifunctional enzyme involved in pyrimidine biosynthesis.

Enzyme Structure

1. **CPS I**: CPS I is a mitochondrial enzyme consisting of multiple subunits and domains necessary for its catalytic activity. It requires N-acetylglutamate (NAG) as an allosteric activator.

2. **CPS II**: CPS II is a cytosolic enzyme that is part of a multifunctional protein complex, including aspartate transcarbamoylase and dihydroorotase, which work sequentially in pyrimidine biosynthesis.

Regulation by Hypothalamus

The production of CPS is influenced by various signaling pathways, including hormonal regulation from the hypothalamus.

1. **CPS I**: The expression and activity of CPS I are regulated by dietary protein intake, glucocorticoids, and insulin. High protein diets increase CPS I activity to handle the increased ammonia load.
2. **CPS II**: CPS II activity is regulated by cellular energy status and nucleotide availability. High levels of ATP and PRPP (phosphoribosyl pyrophosphate) activate CPS II, while UTP (uridine triphosphate) acts as a feedback inhibitor.

Regulation of Carbamoyl Phosphate Synthetase

The regulation of CPS involves a complex interplay of genetic, nutritional, and hormonal factors.

Feedback Loops

1. **CPS I**: NAG is an essential allosteric activator of CPS I. Its synthesis is stimulated by arginine, an amino acid abundant in high-protein diets. This ensures CPS I activity matches the body's metabolic state.
2. **CPS II**: CPS II is subject to feedback inhibition by UTP, ensuring balanced pyrimidine nucleotide synthesis. High levels of pyrimidine nucleotides inhibit CPS II activity, preventing excessive nucleotide production.

Nutritional Status

Dietary factors significantly influence CPS activity, particularly protein intake and overall nutritional health.

1. **Protein Intake**: High-protein diets increase CPS I activity to detoxify the resulting ammonia. Conversely, low protein intake reduces CPS I activity.
2. **Plant-Based Nutrients**: Certain plant-based nutrients can support CPS activity and overall metabolic health.

Plant-Based Diet and CPS Regulation

A plant-based diet, rich in fruits, vegetables, whole grains, nuts, and seeds, can positively influence CPS regulation through various mechanisms.

Nutrient Density

Plant-based diets provide a wealth of essential nutrients, vitamins, and minerals that support overall health and metabolic balance. For example, antioxidants in plant foods reduce oxidative stress, supporting liver function and CPS activity.

Amino Acids

While plant-based diets typically have lower levels of certain amino acids compared to animal-based diets, they still provide sufficient amounts of essential amino acids for protein synthesis and metabolic functions.

1. **Arginine**: Found in nuts, seeds, and legumes, arginine is a precursor for NAG synthesis, which activates CPS I.
2. **Glutamine**: Present in plant foods like spinach and beans, glutamine is a substrate for CPS II in pyrimidine biosynthesis.

Antioxidants

Fruits and vegetables are rich in antioxidants, which help reduce oxidative stress. Lower oxidative stress levels are associated with improved liver function and CPS activity.

Healthy Fats

Plant-based sources of fats, such as avocados, nuts, and seeds, provide essential fatty acids that support liver health and overall metabolic function.

Fiber

High-fiber diets, common in plant-based eating, support gut health and metabolic regulation. A healthy gut microbiome can influence nitrogen metabolism and overall metabolic balance.

Caloric Balance

Maintaining a healthy weight through a balanced plant-based diet can prevent obesity-related metabolic imbalances. Excess body fat, particularly visceral fat, is linked to disrupted metabolic function.

Glycemic Control

Plant-based diets, which are low in refined sugars and high in complex carbohydrates, help maintain stable blood glucose levels. This stability supports overall metabolic health and enzyme function.

Plant-Based Diet on CPS-Related Health Outcomes

Liver Health

A plant-based diet supports liver health by providing essential nutrients and reducing oxidative stress.

1. **Detoxification**: Antioxidants in fruits and vegetables enhance the liver's detoxification capacity, supporting CPS I function in ammonia detoxification.
2. **Inflammation**: Anti-inflammatory compounds in plant foods reduce liver inflammation, improving overall liver function and CPS activity.

Metabolic Health

A plant-based diet promotes metabolic health by providing balanced nutrition and supporting metabolic functions.

1. **Nitrogen Balance**: Adequate protein intake from plant sources supports nitrogen balance without overloading the urea cycle.
2. **Energy Metabolism**: Plant-based diets support efficient energy metabolism, which is crucial for the activity of enzymes like CPS.

Reproductive Health

While CPS is not directly involved in reproductive health, maintaining overall metabolic balance through a plant-based diet can indirectly support reproductive health by ensuring proper nutrient availability and metabolic function.

Bone Health

Plant-based diets rich in calcium, magnesium, and vitamin K support bone health. Leafy greens, fortified plant milk, and nuts are excellent sources of these nutrients, which work synergistically with overall metabolic health.

Weight Management

Plant-based diets are effective for weight management, reducing body fat, and improving insulin sensitivity. Lower body fat and better glycemic control enhance overall metabolic health and enzyme function.

Mental Health

Emerging evidence suggests that plant-based diets may benefit mental health by reducing inflammation and oxidative stress. Improved metabolic balance supports cognitive function and emotional well-being.

Anti-Aging Effects

The antioxidant-rich nature of plant-based diets helps combat oxidative stress, a key factor in aging. Improved metabolic balance contributes to healthier aging and better maintenance of overall health.

Carbamoyl Phosphate Synthetase plays a pivotal role in metabolic health, regulating nitrogen detoxification and nucleotide synthesis. Its production and regulation are influenced by various factors, including diet, hormonal signals, and overall metabolic state.

Arginase

Arginase is a crucial enzyme in the human body, playing a significant role in the urea cycle and the regulation of nitric oxide synthesis.

Function of Arginase

Arginase has several important functions in the human body, primarily related to the urea cycle, amino acid metabolism, and the regulation of nitric oxide levels.

Urea Cycle

1. **Detoxification of Ammonia:** Arginase is a key enzyme in the urea cycle, which is essential for the detoxification of ammonia in the liver. It catalyzes the hydrolysis of arginine to urea and ornithine, facilitating the excretion of nitrogenous waste.
2. **Nitrogen Balance:** By converting arginine into urea, arginase helps maintain nitrogen balance in the body, preventing the accumulation of toxic levels of ammonia.

Amino Acid Metabolism

1. **Production of Ornithine:** The conversion of arginine to ornithine by arginase is critical for the synthesis of polyamines, which are essential for cell growth and differentiation.
2. **Proline and Glutamate Synthesis:** Ornithine produced by arginase can be further metabolized into proline and glutamate,

important amino acids involved in protein synthesis and metabolic pathways.

Regulation of Nitric Oxide Levels

1. **Competition with Nitric Oxide Synthase (NOS):** Arginase competes with NOS for its common substrate, L-arginine. By regulating the availability of L-arginine, arginase indirectly controls the production of nitric oxide, a vital molecule for vascular function and immune response.
2. **Modulation of Inflammatory Responses:** Through its influence on nitric oxide levels, arginase plays a role in modulating inflammatory responses and immune function.

Additional Roles

1. **Wound Healing:** Arginase contributes to tissue repair and wound healing by promoting the proliferation of fibroblasts and the synthesis of collagen.
2. **Cellular Immunity:** It modulates the immune response by regulating the production of nitric oxide and polyamines, which affect the function of immune cells like macrophages and T-cells.

Production of Arginase

Arginase is produced in various tissues throughout the body, with the liver being the primary site of synthesis.

Gene Encoding

1. **ARG1 and ARG2 Genes:** Arginase exists in two isoforms, arginase I and arginase II, encoded by the ARG1 and ARG2 genes, respectively. Arginase I is primarily found in the liver, while

arginase II is expressed in extra-hepatic tissues such as the kidneys and the brain.

Synthesis

1. **Cytosolic Enzyme:** Arginase I is a cytosolic enzyme, primarily involved in the urea cycle. It is highly expressed in hepatocytes where it plays a central role in detoxifying ammonia.
2. **Mitochondrial Enzyme:** Arginase II is located in the mitochondria and is involved in the regulation of cellular arginine levels, nitric oxide production, and polyamine synthesis.

Regulation by Transcription Factors

1. **Hepatocyte Nuclear Factor 4 Alpha (HNF4α):** This transcription factor regulates the expression of the ARG1 gene in the liver, ensuring adequate production of arginase I for the urea cycle.
2. **CAMP Response Element-Binding Protein (CREB):** CREB influences the expression of ARG2, particularly in response to cellular stress and metabolic changes.

Influencing Factors

1. **Nutritional Status:** Dietary intake of protein and amino acids affects arginase production. High-protein diets increase arginase expression to facilitate the detoxification of excess nitrogen.
2. **Hormonal Regulation:** Hormones such as insulin, glucagon, and corticosteroids influence arginase production. Insulin promotes the synthesis of arginase I in the liver, while glucagon and corticosteroids can enhance arginase II expression in extrahepatic tissues.
3. **Inflammatory Signals:** Pro-inflammatory cytokines, such as interleukin-6 (IL-6) and tumor necrosis factor-alpha (TNF-α), can

modulate the expression of arginase, particularly during immune responses and tissue injury.

Regulation of Arginase

The regulation of arginase involves a complex interplay of genetic, nutritional, hormonal, and environmental factors.

Genetic Regulation

1. **Gene Promoter Regions:** The promoter regions of ARG1 and ARG2 genes contain binding sites for various transcription factors that regulate their expression. For example, HNF4α binds to the promoter of ARG1 to enhance its transcription in the liver.
2. **Epigenetic Modifications:** DNA methylation and histone acetylation can influence the expression of arginase genes. Epigenetic changes in response to diet, stress, and environmental factors can alter arginase production.

Hormonal Regulation

1. **Insulin:** Insulin promotes the expression of arginase I in the liver, facilitating the urea cycle and the detoxification of ammonia after meals.
2. **Glucagon:** Glucagon can increase the expression of arginase II in extra-hepatic tissues, particularly during fasting and metabolic stress, to regulate amino acid metabolism.
3. **Corticosteroids:** These hormones enhance the expression of arginase II, especially in response to stress and inflammation, to modulate immune responses and tissue repair.

Nutritional Regulation

1. **Amino Acid Availability:** The availability of L-arginine and other amino acids influences arginase activity. High levels of dietary arginine can increase the expression and activity of arginase to regulate nitric oxide production and polyamine synthesis.
2. **Micronutrients:** Certain vitamins and minerals, such as zinc and magnesium, are cofactors for arginase activity. Adequate intake of these micronutrients is essential for optimal arginase function.

Environmental and Lifestyle Factors

1. **Exercise:** Physical activity can modulate arginase expression and activity. Regular exercise enhances arginase function, improving nitric oxide regulation and vascular health.
2. **Stress:** Chronic stress can alter arginase expression through hormonal and inflammatory pathways, impacting immune function and metabolic health.
3. **Plant-Based Diet:** A plant-based diet rich in antioxidants, anti-inflammatory compounds, and essential nutrients supports optimal arginase activity and regulation. The following sections explore how specific components of a plant-based diet influence arginase function.

Plant-Based Diet and Arginase Regulation

A plant-based diet, abundant in fruits, vegetables, whole grains, nuts, and seeds, provides essential nutrients and bioactive compounds that positively influence arginase regulation and activity.

Nutrient Density

1. **Vitamins and Minerals:** Plant-based diets are rich in vitamins and minerals, such as vitamin C, vitamin E, zinc, and magnesium,

which are vital for arginase function. For instance, zinc is a cofactor for arginase, and adequate zinc intake from plant sources like nuts and seeds supports its enzymatic activity.

2. **Antioxidants:** Antioxidants found in fruits and vegetables, such as flavonoids, carotenoids, and polyphenols, protect cells from oxidative stress. Reduced oxidative stress levels are associated with improved arginase function and nitric oxide regulation.

Amino Acids

1. **L-Arginine:** Plant-based foods like nuts, seeds, legumes, and whole grains are excellent sources of L-arginine, a precursor for nitric oxide synthesis and a substrate for arginase. Adequate dietary intake of L-arginine supports the balance between arginase and nitric oxide synthase, promoting vascular health and immune function.
2. **Glutamine:** Glutamine, found in plant foods like legumes and leafy greens, supports the synthesis of polyamines through the arginase pathway, aiding in cell growth and tissue repair.

Anti-Inflammatory Properties

1. **Polyphenols:** Polyphenols in plant-based foods, such as green tea, berries, and turmeric, exhibit anti-inflammatory properties. These compounds modulate inflammatory pathways and cytokine production, indirectly influencing arginase activity and immune responses.
2. **Omega-3 Fatty Acids:** Omega-3 fatty acids, particularly alpha-linolenic acid (ALA) found in flaxseeds, chia seeds, and walnuts, reduce inflammation and support endothelial function. These fatty acids enhance nitric oxide production and improve the balance between arginase and nitric oxide synthase.

Fiber and Gut Health

1. **Dietary Fiber:** High-fiber diets, common in plant-based eating, support gut health and microbiome balance. A healthy gut microbiome produces short-chain fatty acids (SCFAs) that influence systemic inflammation and metabolic pathways, indirectly affecting arginase activity.
2. **Prebiotics and Probiotics:** Plant-based diets rich in prebiotics (e.g., inulin, fructooligosaccharides) and probiotics (e.g., fermented foods) enhance gut microbiota composition. A balanced microbiome can modulate immune responses and arginase expression, promoting overall health.

Caloric Balance and Weight Management

1. **Obesity and Inflammation:** Excess body fat, particularly visceral fat, is linked to chronic inflammation and disrupted arginase activity. A plant-based diet supports healthy weight management, reducing inflammation and improving arginase regulation.
2. **Insulin Sensitivity:** Plant-based diets improve insulin sensitivity and glycemic control, preventing metabolic disorders that can impair arginase function and nitric oxide regulation.

Plant-Based Diet on Arginase-Related Health Outcomes

Cardiovascular Health

1. **Blood Pressure Regulation:** A plant-based diet rich in L-arginine, antioxidants, and anti-inflammatory compounds supports nitric oxide production and endothelial function, contributing to healthy blood pressure regulation.
2. **Atherosclerosis Prevention:** The anti-inflammatory and antioxidant properties of plant-based foods reduce the risk of

atherosclerosis by preventing oxidative damage to blood vessels and maintaining a healthy balance between arginase and nitric oxide synthase.

Immune Function

1. **Anti-Inflammatory Effects:** Plant-based diets reduce systemic inflammation, modulating immune responses and arginase activity. This balance supports optimal immune function and reduces the risk of chronic inflammatory diseases.
2. **Infection Resistance:** Enhanced immune function and reduced inflammation from plant-based nutrients improve the body's ability to resist infections and recover from illnesses, highlighting the role of arginase in immune regulation.

Metabolic Health

1. **Diabetes Management:** Improved insulin sensitivity and glycemic control from a plant-based diet prevent metabolic dysfunctions that can impair arginase activity and nitric oxide regulation, aiding in diabetes management.
2. **Weight Loss and Maintenance:** Healthy weight management through a plant-based diet reduces inflammation and metabolic stress, promoting optimal arginase function and overall metabolic health.

Wound Healing and Tissue Repair

1. **Collagen Synthesis:** Plant-based nutrients, including vitamins C and E, support collagen synthesis and tissue repair, enhancing the wound healing process mediated by arginase activity.

2. **Cell Proliferation:** Amino acids from plant sources, such as arginine and glutamine, promote cell proliferation and tissue regeneration, aiding in recovery from injuries and surgeries.

Neurological Health

1. **Neuroprotection:** Antioxidants and anti-inflammatory compounds in plant-based diets protect against neurodegenerative diseases by reducing oxidative stress and inflammation, supporting neurological function and arginase regulation.
2. **Cognitive Function:** Improved vascular health and reduced inflammation from a plant-based diet enhance cognitive function and prevent age-related cognitive decline, highlighting the interplay between arginase, nitric oxide, and brain health.

Anti-Aging Effects

1. **Oxidative Stress Reduction:** The antioxidant-rich nature of plant-based diets helps combat oxidative stress, a key factor in aging. Reduced oxidative damage and improved arginase regulation contribute to healthier aging and better maintenance of physiological functions.
2. **Hormonal Balance:** Plant-based diets support hormonal balance, reducing the risk of age-related hormonal imbalances that can affect arginase activity and overall health.

Arginase plays a pivotal role in various physiological processes, including the urea cycle, amino acid metabolism, and the regulation of nitric oxide levels. Its production and regulation are influenced by genetic, nutritional, hormonal, and environmental factors.

26

Amino Acid Metabolism Enzymes

Phenylalanine Hydroxylase (PAH)

Phenylalanine hydroxylase (PAH) is a critical enzyme in the human body that plays a central role in the metabolism of the amino acid phenylalanine.

Function of Phenylalanine Hydroxylase

PAH is responsible for converting the essential amino acid phenylalanine into tyrosine, another amino acid that is a precursor for several important neurotransmitters and hormones. This conversion is crucial for preventing the accumulation of phenylalanine, which can lead to severe metabolic disorders.

In the Metabolic Pathway

1. **Conversion to Tyrosine**: PAH catalyzes the hydroxylation of phenylalanine to tyrosine. This reaction requires tetrahydrobiopterin (BH4) as a cofactor and involves the incorporation of one atom of oxygen into phenylalanine.
2. **Neurotransmitter Synthesis**: Tyrosine produced by the action of PAH is further metabolized into important neurotransmitters such as dopamine, norepinephrine, and epinephrine. These

neurotransmitters are essential for brain function, mood regulation, and the body's stress response.

3. **Hormone Production**: Tyrosine is also a precursor for thyroid hormones, which are critical for regulating metabolism, growth, and development.

Production of Phenylalanine Hydroxylase

PAH is primarily produced in the liver, with smaller amounts found in the kidney and other tissues. Its production involves complex genetic and biochemical processes.

Synthesis

1. **Gene Encoding**: The PAH gene is located on chromosome 12 and encodes the enzyme's polypeptide chain. Mutations in this gene can lead to phenylketonuria (PKU), a metabolic disorder characterized by the inability to metabolize phenylalanine properly.
2. **Enzyme Structure**: PAH is a tetrameric enzyme, meaning it is composed of four subunits. Each subunit has a specific site for binding phenylalanine and the cofactor BH4, which is essential for the enzyme's activity.

Regulation by Cofactors and Substrates

1. **Tetrahydrobiopterin (BH4)**: BH4 is a critical cofactor for PAH. It is synthesized in the body from guanosine triphosphate (GTP) through a series of enzymatic reactions. BH4 not only activates PAH but also stabilizes its structure.
2. **Phenylalanine**: The substrate itself can regulate PAH activity. High levels of phenylalanine activate the enzyme, ensuring that excess phenylalanine is efficiently converted to tyrosine.

Regulation of Phenylalanine Hydroxylase

The regulation of PAH involves multiple feedback mechanisms and external factors that influence its activity and stability.

Feedback Mechanisms

1. **Negative Feedback**: Tyrosine, the product of the PAH-catalyzed reaction, can provide feedback inhibition. High levels of tyrosine decrease PAH activity, preventing excessive depletion of phenylalanine.
2. **Positive Feedback**: Conversely, low levels of tyrosine can relieve this inhibition, enhancing PAH activity to produce more tyrosine as needed.

External Factors

1. **Dietary Influence**: Diet plays a significant role in regulating PAH activity. A diet rich in phenylalanine (found in high-protein foods) increases the enzyme's activity. Conversely, a low-phenylalanine diet, often prescribed for individuals with PKU, reduces PAH activity.
2. **Plant-Based Diets**: Plant-based diets can influence PAH regulation through the availability of phenylalanine and other nutrients that support overall metabolic health. Plant-based sources of phenylalanine include soy products, legumes, nuts, seeds, and whole grains.
3. **Exercise and Stress**: Physical activity and stress levels can impact PAH regulation. Exercise increases the demand for neurotransmitter production, which can enhance PAH activity. Chronic stress, however, may disrupt this balance.

Plant-Based Diet and Phenylalanine Hydroxylase Regulation

A plant-based diet offers several benefits for the regulation of PAH and overall metabolic health. This section explores how plant-based nutrients and dietary patterns support PAH function and balance.

Nutrient Density

Plant-based diets provide a variety of essential nutrients that support enzyme function and metabolic health.

1. **Vitamins and Minerals**: Vitamins such as B6, B12, and folate, and minerals like iron and magnesium, play crucial roles in amino acid metabolism and enzyme function. These nutrients are abundant in plant-based foods like leafy greens, legumes, nuts, seeds, and fortified cereals.
2. **Antioxidants**: Fruits and vegetables are rich in antioxidants, which help reduce oxidative stress. Lower oxidative stress levels are associated with improved enzyme function, including PAH activity. Antioxidants like vitamins C and E found in citrus fruits, berries, nuts, and seeds can protect PAH from oxidative damage.

Amino Acids

Plant-based diets can provide adequate amounts of essential amino acids, including phenylalanine, through a diverse intake of protein-rich plants.

1. **Complete Proteins**: Certain plant foods, such as quinoa, soy, and buckwheat, are complete proteins, meaning they contain all essential amino acids. These foods ensure sufficient phenylalanine intake to support PAH activity.
2. **Amino Acid Synergy**: Combining different plant foods can provide a full spectrum of amino acids. For example, combining legumes with grains (e.g., beans and rice) can ensure balanced amino acid intake, supporting overall metabolic health.

Healthy Fats

Plant-based sources of fats, such as avocados, nuts, and seeds, provide essential fatty acids that support enzyme production and function.

1. **Omega-3 Fatty Acids**: Omega-3s, found in flaxseeds, chia seeds, and walnuts, have anti-inflammatory properties that can enhance metabolic function and support PAH activity.
2. **Monounsaturated Fats**: Sources like olive oil and avocados support overall health and provide energy for metabolic processes without the negative effects of saturated fats.

Fiber

High-fiber diets, common in plant-based eating, support gut health and metabolic regulation.

1. **Gut Microbiome**: A healthy gut microbiome can influence metabolic health and enzyme function through the production of short-chain fatty acids and other metabolites. Fiber-rich foods like fruits, vegetables, legumes, and whole grains support a diverse and healthy gut microbiome.
2. **Blood Sugar Regulation**: Fiber helps regulate blood sugar levels, preventing insulin resistance, which can negatively impact metabolic enzymes including PAH.

Plant-Based Diet on PAH-Related Health Outcomes

Metabolic Health

A plant-based diet supports metabolic health, reducing the risk of disorders related to PAH function.

1. **Phenylketonuria (PKU)**: For individuals with PKU, a plant-based diet can be tailored to manage phenylalanine intake while

ensuring adequate nutrition. Foods low in phenylalanine but rich in other essential nutrients help maintain metabolic balance.

2. **Obesity and Insulin Resistance**: Plant-based diets are effective for weight management and improving insulin sensitivity. Lower body fat and better glycemic control enhance overall metabolic health, supporting PAH function.

Brain Health

The role of PAH in neurotransmitter production links its activity to brain health and cognitive function.

1. **Cognitive Function**: Adequate production of tyrosine and its conversion to neurotransmitters like dopamine is crucial for cognitive health. A plant-based diet supports brain health through nutrient-rich foods that enhance enzyme function and neurotransmitter synthesis.
2. **Mental Health**: Emerging evidence suggests that plant-based diets may benefit mental health by reducing inflammation and oxidative stress, which are linked to mood disorders. Improved PAH function supports the production of neurotransmitters that regulate mood and mental well-being.

Cardiovascular Health

Tyrosine, produced by PAH, is a precursor for catecholamines like norepinephrine and epinephrine, which influence cardiovascular health.

1. **Blood Pressure Regulation**: Catecholamines play a role in regulating blood pressure. A plant-based diet, rich in nutrients and low in sodium, supports cardiovascular health and helps maintain healthy blood pressure levels.
2. **Cholesterol Levels**: Plant-based diets, particularly those low in saturated fats and high in fiber, can improve cholesterol levels.

Better lipid profiles support overall cardiovascular health and reduce the risk of related disorders.

Phenylalanine hydroxylase (PAH) plays a pivotal role in amino acid metabolism, neurotransmitter production, and overall metabolic health. Its function, production, and regulation are influenced by various factors, including diet, exercise, and stress.

Tyrosine Hydroxylase (TH)

Tyrosine Hydroxylase (TH) is a critical enzyme in the biosynthesis of catecholamines, including dopamine, norepinephrine, and epinephrine, which are essential neurotransmitters and hormones in the body.

Function of Tyrosine Hydroxylase

Tyrosine Hydroxylase plays a pivotal role in the synthesis of catecholamines, which are involved in various physiological processes, including mood regulation, stress response, and cardiovascular function.

In the Nervous System

1. **Dopamine Synthesis**: TH catalyzes the conversion of the amino acid tyrosine to L-DOPA, the precursor of dopamine. Dopamine is crucial for motor control, motivation, and reward mechanisms.
2. **Norepinephrine and Epinephrine Synthesis**: Following its conversion to dopamine, L-DOPA is further processed into norepinephrine and epinephrine. These neurotransmitters are vital for the fight-or-flight response, blood pressure regulation, and mood stabilization.

In the Adrenal Medulla

1. **Stress Response**: TH is active in the adrenal medulla, where it initiates the production of epinephrine and norepinephrine in response to stress, enhancing the body's ability to cope with immediate threats.

Additional Roles

1. **Metabolic Regulation**: Catecholamines synthesized through the action of TH influence metabolic processes, including glucose metabolism and energy expenditure.
2. **Cardiovascular Health**: Norepinephrine and epinephrine regulate heart rate and blood vessel constriction, playing a key role in maintaining cardiovascular stability.

Production of Tyrosine Hydroxylase

Tyrosine Hydroxylase is produced in various tissues, including the brain, adrenal medulla, and sympathetic nervous system, through a series of complex biochemical processes.

Synthesis

1. **Gene Encoding**: The TH gene is located on chromosome 11 and encodes the enzyme responsible for catalyzing the conversion of tyrosine to L-DOPA.
2. **Protein Structure**: TH is a tetrameric enzyme composed of four identical subunits, each containing a catalytic domain necessary for its function.

Regulation by Transcription Factors

1. **CREB (cAMP Response Element-Binding Protein)**: CREB is a transcription factor that binds to the promoter region of the TH gene, enhancing its transcription in response to increased cAMP levels.
2. **AP-1 (Activator Protein-1)**: AP-1 also regulates TH gene expression by responding to various extracellular signals, including stress and growth factors.

Influencing Factors

1. **Neuronal Activity**: Increased neuronal firing enhances TH expression to meet the heightened demand for catecholamine synthesis.
2. **Hormonal Influence**: Hormones such as glucocorticoids can upregulate TH expression, particularly in the adrenal medulla during stress responses.
3. **Environmental Stimuli**: External factors such as stress, drugs, and toxins can modulate TH production.

Regulation of Tyrosine Hydroxylase

The regulation of TH involves multiple mechanisms, including feedback inhibition, phosphorylation, and environmental factors.

Feedback Inhibition

1. **End-Product Inhibition**: High levels of catecholamines inhibit TH activity through feedback mechanisms, ensuring balanced neurotransmitter production.

Phosphorylation

1. **Protein Kinases**: Various kinases, including PKA (Protein Kinase A) and PKC (Protein Kinase C), phosphorylate TH at specific serine residues, enhancing its enzymatic activity.
2. **Stress-Induced Phosphorylation**: Acute stress increases TH phosphorylation, boosting catecholamine synthesis to prepare the body for the fight-or-flight response.

Environmental and Dietary Influences

1. **Dietary Tyrosine**: Tyrosine, obtained from dietary sources, is a precursor for TH activity. Plant-based foods rich in tyrosine, such as soy products, nuts, and seeds, support optimal TH function.
2. **Antioxidants**: Antioxidants found in plant-based diets reduce oxidative stress, preserving TH activity and enhancing catecholamine production.

Plant-Based Diet and Tyrosine Hydroxylase Regulation

A plant-based diet can positively influence TH regulation and catecholamine synthesis through various mechanisms.

Nutrient Density

1. **Amino Acids**: Plant-based sources of tyrosine, including legumes, nuts, and seeds, provide the necessary substrates for TH activity and catecholamine synthesis.
2. **Vitamins and Minerals**: Vitamins such as B6, found in whole grains and bananas, act as cofactors for TH, enhancing its enzymatic activity.

Antioxidants

1. **Oxidative Stress Reduction**: Fruits and vegetables are rich in antioxidants, which reduce oxidative stress and prevent damage to TH, ensuring efficient catecholamine production.

Healthy Fats

1. **Omega-3 Fatty Acids**: Plant-based sources of omega-3s, such as flaxseeds and chia seeds, have anti-inflammatory properties that support overall brain health and TH function.

Fiber

1. **Gut Health**: A high-fiber diet supports a healthy gut microbiome, which can influence brain health and neurotransmitter production, including catecholamines synthesized by TH.

Caloric Balance

1. **Weight Management**: Maintaining a healthy weight through a balanced plant-based diet prevents obesity-related hormonal imbalances that can affect TH activity.

Glycemic Control

1. **Stable Blood Glucose**: Plant-based diets help maintain stable blood glucose levels, preventing insulin resistance, which can negatively impact overall hormonal balance and TH function.

Plant-Based Diet on TH-Related Health Outcomes
Mental Health

1. **Mood Regulation**: A plant-based diet supports the production of dopamine and other catecholamines, improving mood and reducing symptoms of depression and anxiety.
2. **Cognitive Function**: Adequate catecholamine levels, supported by a nutrient-rich diet, enhance cognitive function and protect against neurodegenerative diseases.

Cardiovascular Health

1. **Blood Pressure Regulation**: Catecholamines synthesized through TH activity regulate blood pressure. A diet rich in plant-based nutrients supports cardiovascular health by maintaining balanced catecholamine levels.
2. **Stress Response**: Plant-based diets, which reduce overall stress levels, prevent the overproduction of catecholamines, reducing the risk of hypertension and other stress-related disorders.

Metabolic Health

1. **Glucose Metabolism**: Catecholamines play a role in glucose metabolism. A plant-based diet supports healthy glucose levels, enhancing metabolic function and reducing the risk of diabetes.
2. **Energy Expenditure**: Efficient catecholamine production, supported by a plant-based diet, enhances energy expenditure and weight management.

Anti-Aging Effects

1. **Oxidative Stress Reduction**: Antioxidants in plant-based diets combat oxidative stress, preserving TH activity and promoting healthy aging.
2. **Hormonal Balance**: Maintaining balanced catecholamine levels through a nutrient-rich diet supports overall hormonal balance and longevity.

This detailed analysis highlights the critical role of Tyrosine Hydroxylase in the synthesis of catecholamines and its regulation through various mechanisms, including dietary influences.

DOPA Decarboxylase (DDC)

DOPA decarboxylase (DDC), also known as aromatic L-amino acid decarboxylase (AADC), is a critical enzyme in the biosynthesis of several neurotransmitters. This enzyme is pivotal in the metabolic pathways that convert L-DOPA to dopamine, as well as L-5-hydroxytryptophan to serotonin.

Function of DOPA Decarboxylase

DOPA decarboxylase plays a crucial role in the central nervous system and peripheral tissues by catalyzing the decarboxylation of L-DOPA to dopamine and L-5-hydroxytryptophan to serotonin, which are vital neurotransmitters in the human body.

Neurotransmitter Synthesis

1. **Dopamine Production**: DDC converts L-DOPA into dopamine, a neurotransmitter essential for motor control, reward pathways, and various neuroendocrine functions.
2. **Serotonin Production**: DDC catalyzes the conversion of L-5-hydroxytryptophan to serotonin, which is involved in mood regulation, appetite control, and sleep.

Role in the Central Nervous System

1. **Motor Control**: Dopamine produced by DDC is critical for the coordination of smooth and voluntary movements.
2. **Mood and Behavior**: Serotonin synthesized by DDC influences mood, anxiety, and overall mental health.
3. **Cognitive Functions**: Both dopamine and serotonin are involved in learning, memory, and executive functions.

Peripheral Functions

1. **Cardiovascular Health**: Dopamine acts as a vasodilator, influencing blood flow and pressure.
2. **Gastrointestinal Function**: Serotonin regulates intestinal movements and secretion.
3. **Hormonal Regulation**: Dopamine and serotonin impact the release of various hormones, including prolactin and cortisol.

Production of DOPA Decarboxylase

The production of DOPA decarboxylase involves a series of genetic, transcriptional, and translational processes regulated by various factors.

Gene Encoding

1. **Gene Location**: The DDC gene is located on chromosome 7p12.2. It encodes the enzyme responsible for decarboxylating aromatic L-amino acids.
2. **Expression Patterns**: DDC is expressed in various tissues, including the brain, kidneys, liver, and intestines.

Synthesis and Structure

1. **Protein Structure**: DDC is a pyridoxal phosphate (PLP)-dependent enzyme, meaning it requires vitamin B6 as a cofactor for its activity.
2. **Isoforms**: Different isoforms of DDC exist, resulting from alternative splicing and post-translational modifications.

Regulation by Genetic and Epigenetic Factors

1. **Transcriptional Regulation**: The expression of the DDC gene is regulated by various transcription factors, including NF-κB and Sp1.
2. **Epigenetic Modifications:** DNA methylation and histone acetylation influence the expression levels of DDC.

Regulation of DOPA Decarboxylase

The regulation of DOPA decarboxylase is complex, involving feedback mechanisms, nutritional status, and external factors.

Feedback Mechanisms

1. **Dopamine and Serotonin Levels**: High levels of dopamine and serotonin provide negative feedback to regulate the activity and expression of DDC.

2. **Hormonal Influence**: Hormones such as glucocorticoids can modulate DDC expression and activity.

Nutritional Influence

1. **Vitamin B6**: As a cofactor, adequate levels of vitamin B6 are crucial for DDC activity. Plant-based sources rich in vitamin B6 include chickpeas, bananas, and potatoes.
2. **Amino Acids**: The availability of L-DOPA and L-5-hydroxytryptophan, derived from dietary amino acids like phenylalanine and tryptophan, directly affects DDC activity.

External Factors

1. **Stress and Exercise**: Chronic stress and intense physical activity can alter DDC activity through changes in neurotransmitter demand.
2. **Medications and Toxins**: Certain drugs and environmental toxins can inhibit or enhance DDC activity, impacting neurotransmitter levels.

Plant-Based Diet and DOPA Decarboxylase Regulation

A plant-based diet, rich in fruits, vegetables, whole grains, nuts, and seeds, can positively influence the regulation and activity of DOPA decarboxylase through various mechanisms.

Nutrient Density

1. **Vitamin B6-Rich Foods**: Plant-based sources such as sunflower seeds, pistachios, and avocados provide vitamin B6, essential for DDC activity.

2. **Amino Acid Sources**: Plant proteins from beans, lentils, and quinoa supply the necessary amino acids for the synthesis of L-DOPA and L-5-hydroxytryptophan.

Antioxidants

Fruits and vegetables are rich in antioxidants, which help reduce oxidative stress. Lower oxidative stress levels are associated with improved enzymatic function, including that of DDC.

Fiber

High-fiber diets, common in plant-based eating, support gut health and nutrient absorption, indirectly influencing the availability of cofactors and precursors needed for DDC activity.

Healthy Fats

Plant-based sources of fats, such as chia seeds, flaxseeds, and walnuts, provide essential fatty acids that support overall brain health and neurotransmitter function.

Plant-Based Diet on DDC-Related Health Outcomes

Neurological Health

1. **Mood and Mental Health**: A plant-based diet supports serotonin production, aiding in the management of mood disorders like depression and anxiety.
2. **Neurodegenerative Diseases**: Antioxidants and anti-inflammatory compounds in plant foods may protect against neurodegenerative diseases like Parkinson's, where dopamine production is compromised.

Cardiovascular Health

1. **Blood Pressure Regulation**: Dopamine's vasodilatory effects are supported by a plant-based diet, which can help maintain healthy blood pressure levels.

2. **Heart Health**: Nutrients in plant foods support overall cardiovascular function, indirectly influencing neurotransmitter-related cardiovascular health.

Digestive Health

A diet rich in plant-based fibers supports a healthy gut microbiome, which plays a role in serotonin production and overall digestive health.

DOPA decarboxylase is a pivotal enzyme in the production of key neurotransmitters such as dopamine and serotonin. Its function, production, and regulation are influenced by a variety of genetic, nutritional, and environmental factors.

Dopamine Beta-Hydroxylase (DBH)

Dopamine Beta-Hydroxylase (DBH) is a key enzyme in the biosynthesis of norepinephrine from dopamine, playing a crucial role in the functioning of the sympathetic nervous system.

Function of Dopamine Beta-Hydroxylase

DBH is vital for the conversion of dopamine to norepinephrine, which is essential for maintaining several physiological functions.

In the Nervous System

1. **Neurotransmitter Synthesis**: DBH catalyzes the conversion of dopamine to norepinephrine, an important neurotransmitter involved in arousal, alertness, and the fight-or-flight response.
2. **Sympathetic Nervous System**: Norepinephrine produced by DBH is critical for the function of the sympathetic nervous system, which regulates cardiovascular, respiratory, and metabolic responses to stress.

In the Adrenal Glands

1. **Catecholamine Production**: In the adrenal medulla, DBH facilitates the production of norepinephrine, which is further converted to epinephrine (adrenaline), playing a crucial role in stress response.
2. **Regulation of Blood Pressure**: Norepinephrine and epinephrine produced through the DBH pathway help regulate blood pressure by modulating heart rate and vascular tone.

Production of Dopamine Beta-Hydroxylase

DBH is produced through a series of complex biochemical processes and is regulated by genetic and environmental factors.

Synthesis

1. **Gene Encoding**: The DBH gene, located on chromosome 9q34, encodes the DBH enzyme. Variations in this gene can affect the enzyme's activity and stability.
2. **Protein Structure**: DBH is a copper-containing monooxygenase, requiring copper ions for its catalytic activity. It is synthesized as a pre-proenzyme that undergoes post-translational modifications to become active.

Cellular Localization

1. **Chromaffin Cells**: In the adrenal medulla, DBH is stored in chromaffin granules alongside dopamine and norepinephrine.
2. **Neurons**: Within the central and peripheral nervous systems, DBH is found in vesicles in noradrenergic neurons, where it converts dopamine to norepinephrine during neurotransmission.

Regulation of Dopamine Beta-Hydroxylase

The regulation of DBH involves a complex interplay of genetic, biochemical, and environmental factors.

Genetic Regulation

1. **Polymorphisms**: Genetic polymorphisms in the DBH gene can influence enzyme activity, impacting norepinephrine levels and associated physiological functions.
2. **Gene Expression**: Factors such as stress and dietary components can influence DBH gene expression, altering enzyme levels and activity.

Cofactor Availability

1. **Copper Ions**: DBH requires copper ions as a cofactor for its enzymatic activity. Copper deficiency can impair DBH function, reducing norepinephrine synthesis.
2. **Ascorbic Acid**: Vitamin C (ascorbic acid) is essential for DBH activity, acting as a cofactor in the hydroxylation process. Adequate dietary intake of vitamin C is crucial for optimal DBH function.

Environmental and Dietary Influences

1. **Stress**: Chronic stress can upregulate DBH expression and activity, leading to increased norepinephrine production.
2. **Diet**: Nutritional factors, particularly those found in plant-based diets, can influence DBH activity and overall norepinephrine levels.

Plant-Based Diet and Dopamine Beta-Hydroxylase Regulation

A plant-based diet, rich in essential nutrients and antioxidants, can positively influence DBH regulation through various mechanisms.

Nutrient Density

1. **Vitamin C**: Abundant in fruits and vegetables like citrus fruits, bell peppers, and broccoli, vitamin C is a crucial cofactor for DBH. Regular consumption ensures adequate enzyme activity.
2. **Copper**: Plant-based sources of copper, such as nuts, seeds, and whole grains, support DBH function by providing the necessary cofactor for its enzymatic activity.

Antioxidants

1. **Polyphenols**: Found in a variety of plant foods, polyphenols have antioxidant properties that protect DBH from oxidative damage, ensuring its proper function.
2. **Flavonoids**: These compounds, present in fruits, vegetables, and tea, can modulate enzyme activity and protect against oxidative stress.

Amino Acids

1. **Phenylalanine and Tyrosine**: Essential for dopamine synthesis, these amino acids are found in plant-based proteins like legumes, nuts, and seeds. Adequate intake supports the initial steps of norepinephrine synthesis.
2. **Tryptophan**: Though not directly involved in DBH function, tryptophan supports overall neurotransmitter balance and is found in plant foods like pumpkin seeds and tofu.

Dietary Patterns

1. **Low Saturated Fat**: Plant-based diets are typically low in saturated fats, which can support overall cardiovascular health and optimal enzyme function.
2. **High Fiber**: Dietary fiber from plant foods supports gut health, which in turn can influence overall metabolic and hormonal balance, including the regulation of DBH.

Plant-Based Diet on DBH-Related Health Outcomes

A plant-based diet can have several beneficial effects on health outcomes related to DBH and norepinephrine function.

Cardiovascular Health

1. **Blood Pressure Regulation**: By supporting optimal norepinephrine levels, a plant-based diet can help regulate blood pressure, reducing the risk of hypertension and related cardiovascular diseases.
2. **Heart Health**: Antioxidants and healthy fats in plant foods support cardiovascular health by reducing oxidative stress and inflammation, which can influence DBH activity and norepinephrine levels.

Mental Health

1. **Stress Response**: A plant-based diet rich in antioxidants and anti-inflammatory compounds can modulate the stress response, potentially reducing chronic stress and its impact on DBH activity.
2. **Mood Regulation**: Adequate intake of vitamins and minerals from plant foods supports neurotransmitter synthesis and function, contributing to better mood regulation and mental health.

Neuroprotection

1. **Cognitive Function**: Nutrients like vitamin C and polyphenols in plant foods support cognitive function by protecting neurons and maintaining neurotransmitter balance.
2. **Neurodegenerative Diseases**: A diet rich in antioxidants may protect against neurodegenerative diseases by reducing oxidative stress and inflammation, which can affect DBH activity and norepinephrine levels.

Dopamine Beta-Hydroxylase plays a pivotal role in the synthesis of norepinephrine, essential for various physiological functions, including cardiovascular regulation and stress response. Its production and regulation are influenced by genetic, environmental, and dietary factors.

Norepinephrine N-Methyltransferase (NNMT)

Norepinephrine N-Methyltransferase (NNMT) is an important enzyme in the human body, primarily involved in the metabolism of catecholamines. This enzyme is responsible for the methylation of norepinephrine to form epinephrine, playing a crucial role in the regulation of the fight-or-flight response, energy metabolism, and stress.

Function of Norepinephrine N-Methyltransferase

Norepinephrine N-Methyltransferase is integral to several physiological processes due to its role in catecholamine metabolism.

In Catecholamine Metabolism

1. **Methylation of Norepinephrine**: NNMT catalyzes the transfer of a methyl group from S-adenosylmethionine (SAM) to

norepinephrine, converting it into epinephrine. This process is crucial for the synthesis of epinephrine, which acts as a hormone and neurotransmitter.

2. **Stress Response**: Epinephrine, produced by the action of NNMT, is pivotal in the body's acute stress response, often referred to as the fight-or-flight response. It increases heart rate, blood pressure, and energy availability.
3. **Energy Metabolism**: By influencing the levels of epinephrine, NNMT indirectly affects glucose metabolism and lipolysis, providing energy during stress.
4. **Neurotransmission**: NNMT's activity ensures the proper balance of norepinephrine and epinephrine in the central nervous system, influencing mood, alertness, and cognitive function.

Additional Roles

1. **Detoxification**: NNMT also plays a role in detoxifying xenobiotics and drugs by methylation, aiding in their excretion.
2. **Regulation of Other Pathways**: Through its interaction with SAM, NNMT influences other methylation reactions and thus impacts numerous biological pathways beyond catecholamine metabolism.

Production of Norepinephrine N-Methyltransferase

NNMT production is regulated by various genetic and biochemical mechanisms.

Synthesis

1. **Gene Encoding**: The NNMT gene, located on chromosome 11, encodes the enzyme. The expression of this gene is tightly regulated by several transcription factors and environmental signals.

2. **Protein Structure**: NNMT is a cytosolic enzyme, and its active form consists of a single polypeptide chain. The enzyme's active site binds to norepinephrine and SAM, facilitating the transfer of the methyl group.

Regulation by the Nervous System

1. **Sympathetic Nervous System**: The activity of NNMT is influenced by the sympathetic nervous system. Increased sympathetic activity, often triggered by stress or exercise, enhances the enzyme's expression and activity.
2. **Feedback Mechanisms**: Levels of norepinephrine and epinephrine provide feedback to regulate NNMT activity. High levels of these catecholamines can inhibit further enzyme production to maintain homeostasis.

Regulation of Norepinephrine N-Methyltransferase

The regulation of NNMT involves a complex interplay of genetic, hormonal, and environmental factors.

Genetic Regulation

1. **Transcriptional Control**: Transcription factors such as NF-κB and AP-1 can bind to the promoter region of the NNMT gene, influencing its transcription in response to various stimuli.
2. **Epigenetic Modifications**: Methylation and acetylation of histones around the NNMT gene can alter its expression. For example, hypomethylation can lead to increased gene expression.

Hormonal Regulation

1. **Cortisol**: This stress hormone can upregulate NNMT expression, linking the enzyme's activity to the body's stress response.

2. **Insulin**: Insulin levels also impact NNMT activity, with hyperinsulinemia often leading to increased NNMT expression.

Nutritional and Environmental Factors

1. **Diet**: Certain dietary components, especially those found in plant-based diets, can modulate NNMT activity. For instance, flavonoids and polyphenols found in fruits and vegetables can influence enzyme expression and function.
2. **Exercise**: Physical activity has been shown to increase NNMT activity, contributing to improved stress resilience and energy metabolism.

Plant-Based Diet and Norepinephrine N-Methyltransferase Regulation

A plant-based diet, rich in diverse nutrients, can significantly influence NNMT activity and overall catecholamine balance.

Nutrient Density

Plant-based diets are high in vitamins, minerals, and phytonutrients that support overall health and enzymatic function.

1. **Vitamins and Minerals**: Vitamins such as B12 and folate, often found in fortified plant-based foods and supplements, are crucial for SAM synthesis, which is necessary for NNMT activity.
2. **Amino Acids**: Essential amino acids, such as methionine, found in legumes and seeds, are vital for the synthesis of SAM, impacting NNMT activity.

Antioxidants

Fruits and vegetables are rich in antioxidants, which can reduce oxidative stress and support the proper functioning of NNMT.

1. **Flavonoids and Polyphenols**: These compounds, abundant in plant foods, have been shown to modulate NNMT activity by influencing gene expression and protecting against oxidative damage.
2. **Vitamins C and E**: These antioxidants, found in various fruits and vegetables, help maintain cellular health and proper enzyme function.

Healthy Fats

Plant-based sources of fats, such as avocados, nuts, and seeds, provide essential fatty acids that support hormonal balance and enzymatic activity.

1. **Omega-3 Fatty Acids**: Found in flaxseeds, chia seeds, and walnuts, omega-3 fatty acids have anti-inflammatory properties that can enhance NNMT function and overall metabolic health.

Fiber

High-fiber diets, common in plant-based eating, support gut health and metabolic balance, indirectly affecting NNMT activity.

1. **Gut Microbiome**: A healthy gut microbiome, supported by dietary fiber, can influence systemic inflammation and metabolic pathways, impacting NNMT regulation.
2. **Metabolites**: Short-chain fatty acids produced by fiber fermentation in the gut can modulate systemic metabolic processes, including those involving NNMT.

Plant-Based Diet on NNMT-Related Health Outcomes
Stress Response and Mental Health

1. **Reduced Anxiety and Depression**: A plant-based diet, rich in antioxidants and essential nutrients, can help modulate the stress response and improve mood by supporting NNMT activity and catecholamine balance.
2. **Cognitive Function**: Improved NNMT activity can enhance cognitive function and reduce the risk of neurodegenerative diseases through better regulation of neurotransmitters.

Metabolic Health

1. **Energy Metabolism**: Plant-based diets support efficient energy metabolism by providing essential nutrients that enhance NNMT function, leading to improved glucose utilization and fat metabolism.
2. **Weight Management**: By supporting NNMT activity, a plant-based diet can aid in weight management and reduce the risk of obesity-related disorders.

Cardiovascular Health

1. **Blood Pressure Regulation**: NNMT activity influences catecholamine levels, which are critical for blood pressure regulation. A plant-based diet supports healthy NNMT function, contributing to better cardiovascular health.
2. **Reduced Risk of Hypertension**: The anti-inflammatory and antioxidant properties of plant-based foods help maintain vascular health and reduce the risk of hypertension by supporting balanced NNMT activity.

Detoxification and Disease Prevention

1. **Xenobiotic Metabolism**: Enhanced NNMT activity aids in the detoxification of harmful substances, reducing the risk of chronic diseases.
2. **Cancer Prevention**: By maintaining optimal NNMT function and catecholamine balance, a plant-based diet may lower the risk of certain cancers through improved detoxification and reduced oxidative stress.

Norepinephrine N-Methyltransferase plays a pivotal role in catecholamine metabolism, influencing the body's stress response, energy metabolism, and overall health. Its production and regulation are impacted by various factors, including genetic, hormonal, and environmental influences.

Nitric Oxide Synthase (NOS)

Nitric Oxide Synthase (NOS) is a pivotal enzyme in the human body responsible for the synthesis of nitric oxide (NO), a critical signaling molecule involved in various physiological processes.

Function of Nitric Oxide Synthase

Nitric oxide synthase exists in three isoforms: endothelial (eNOS), neuronal (nNOS), and inducible (iNOS), each with distinct functions in the body.

Endothelial NOS (eNOS):

- **Vasodilation**: eNOS produces NO in blood vessels, leading to vasodilation, which helps regulate blood pressure and ensures proper blood flow.
- **Cardiovascular Health**: eNOS-derived NO plays a crucial role in protecting the cardiovascular system by preventing platelet aggregation, reducing inflammation, and inhibiting the adhesion of white blood cells to the endothelium.

Neuronal NOS (nNOS):

- **Neurotransmission**: nNOS is involved in the production of NO in the nervous system, where it acts as a neurotransmitter and neuromodulator, influencing synaptic plasticity, memory, and learning.
- **Neuroprotection**: NO produced by nNOS also has neuroprotective effects, helping to mitigate neuronal damage and promoting neural repair mechanisms.

Inducible NOS (iNOS):

- **Immune Response**: iNOS is primarily expressed in immune cells such as macrophages and is induced during inflammatory responses. It produces large amounts of NO as a defense mechanism to destroy pathogens and tumor cells.
- **Inflammation**: While beneficial in pathogen defense, excessive NO production by iNOS can contribute to chronic inflammation and tissue damage in conditions like arthritis and inflammatory bowel disease.

Production of Nitric Oxide Synthase

NOS enzymes catalyze the production of NO from L-arginine, oxygen, and NADPH. This process involves several co-factors including tetrahydrobiopterin (BH4), flavin adenine dinucleotide (FAD), and flavin mononucleotide (FMN).

Gene Encoding:

- **eNOS:** Encoded by the NOS3 gene located on chromosome 7.
- **nNOS:** Encoded by the NOS1 gene on chromosome 12.
- **iNOS:** Encoded by the NOS2 gene on chromosome 17.

Isoform-Specific Regulation:

- **eNOS:** Regulated primarily by calcium/calmodulin and is localized in the endothelial cells of blood vessels.
- **nNOS:** Also regulated by calcium/calmodulin, nNOS is found in neuronal tissues and certain skeletal muscles.
- **iNOS:** Unlike eNOS and nNOS, iNOS is not regulated by calcium but is inducible by inflammatory cytokines like interferon-gamma (IFN-γ), tumor necrosis factor-alpha (TNF-α), and lipopolysaccharides (LPS).

Co-Factors and Enzyme Activation:

- **BH4, FAD, FMN:** These co-factors are essential for the catalytic activity of NOS enzymes. BH4, in particular, stabilizes the enzyme and facilitates the transfer of electrons required for NO production.

Regulation of Nitric Oxide Synthase

The regulation of NOS involves complex feedback mechanisms, external factors, and physiological states, influencing NO production and its subsequent effects on health.

Transcriptional Regulation:

- **Gene Expression**: The expression of NOS isoforms is tightly controlled at the transcriptional level. For instance, inflammatory cytokines upregulate iNOS expression, while factors like shear stress enhance eNOS expression.

Post-Translational Modifications:

- **Phosphorylation**: eNOS activity is modulated by phosphorylation. For example, phosphorylation at serine 1177 increases eNOS activity, enhancing NO production.
- **S-Nitrosylation**: This modification can alter the activity of NOS enzymes, often serving as a feedback mechanism to fine-tune NO levels.

Environmental and Lifestyle Factors:

- **Diet**: Nutritional status significantly impacts NOS activity. Diets rich in antioxidants, omega-3 fatty acids, and polyphenols from plant sources can enhance eNOS activity and NO production.
- **Exercise**: Regular physical activity upregulates eNOS expression and activity, contributing to improved cardiovascular health.
- **Stress**: Chronic stress can downregulate NOS activity, particularly eNOS, leading to impaired vascular function.

Plant-Based Diet and Nitric Oxide Synthase Regulation

A plant-based diet, rich in fruits, vegetables, whole grains, nuts, and seeds, can positively influence NOS regulation through various mechanisms.

Nutrient Density:

- **Arginine and Nitrate:** Plant foods like nuts, seeds, spinach, and beets are high in arginine and dietary nitrates, which are substrates for NO production. Dietary nitrates are converted to nitrites and subsequently to NO, enhancing NO bioavailability.
- **Antioxidants:** Vitamins C and E, polyphenols, and flavonoids in plant foods protect NOS enzymes from oxidative damage, ensuring optimal function.

Polyphenols and Flavonoids:

- **Enhancement of eNOS Activity:** Polyphenols from foods such as berries, green tea, and dark chocolate enhance eNOS expression and activity. These compounds increase the bioavailability of BH4, a critical co-factor for eNOS.
- **Anti-Inflammatory Effects:** Flavonoids and other anti-inflammatory compounds in plant-based diets reduce the expression of pro-inflammatory cytokines, thereby modulating iNOS activity and preventing chronic inflammation.

Healthy Fats:

- **Omega-3 Fatty Acids:** Found in flaxseeds, chia seeds, and walnuts, omega-3 fatty acids have been shown to upregulate eNOS expression and activity, improving endothelial function.
- **Reduction of Saturated Fats:** Plant-based diets are typically low in saturated fats, which can impair NOS activity. Reducing

saturated fat intake helps maintain NO production and vascular health.

Gut Microbiome:

- **Microbial Metabolites**: A high-fiber plant-based diet supports a healthy gut microbiome, which produces metabolites like short-chain fatty acids (SCFAs) that can influence NOS activity and NO production.
- **Gut-Heart Axis**: The interplay between gut microbiota and cardiovascular health is crucial. A healthy microbiome can enhance NO bioavailability and endothelial function through the gut-heart axis.

Plant-Based Diet on NOS-Related Health Outcomes
Cardiovascular Health:

- **Blood Pressure Regulation**: Plant-based diets are effective in lowering blood pressure by enhancing NO production through eNOS. Foods rich in nitrates like beets and leafy greens are particularly beneficial.
- **Atherosclerosis Prevention**: The anti-inflammatory and antioxidant properties of plant-based foods help prevent endothelial dysfunction and atherosclerosis by maintaining eNOS activity and reducing oxidative stress.

Neuroprotection:

- **Cognitive Function**: The neuroprotective effects of NO produced by nNOS are supported by plant-based diets rich in antioxidants and polyphenols. These compounds protect neurons from oxidative damage and support cognitive function.

- **Neurodegenerative Diseases**: Diets high in fruits, vegetables, and nuts may reduce the risk of neurodegenerative diseases by modulating NO levels and reducing neuroinflammation.

Immune Function:

- **Anti-Inflammatory Effects**: Plant-based diets help regulate iNOS activity by reducing the production of pro-inflammatory cytokines. This modulation prevents excessive NO production that can lead to chronic inflammation and tissue damage.
- **Infection Defense**: Adequate NO production by iNOS is essential for pathogen defense. Nutrients and phytochemicals in plant-based diets support immune function and the body's ability to fight infections.

Endothelial Function:

- **Improved Endothelial Health**: A plant-based diet enhances endothelial function by increasing eNOS activity and NO production. This improvement reduces the risk of cardiovascular diseases and promotes vascular health.
- **Exercise and Diet Synergy**: The combination of regular physical activity and a plant-based diet synergistically improves endothelial function and NO bioavailability, offering substantial cardiovascular benefits.

Metabolic Health:

- **Insulin Sensitivity**: NO plays a role in glucose uptake and insulin sensitivity. Plant-based diets, which are high in fiber and low in refined sugars, support healthy NO production and improve metabolic health.

- **Weight Management**: Maintaining a healthy weight through a plant-based diet reduces the risk of metabolic disorders. Reduced visceral fat and inflammation enhance NO production and vascular function.

Nitric Oxide Synthase plays a critical role in various physiological processes, including vasodilation, neurotransmission, and immune response. Its production and regulation are influenced by a range of factors, including diet, exercise, and stress.

27

Neurotransmitter Metabolism Enzymes

Choline Acetyltransferase (ChAT)

Choline Acetyltransferase (ChAT) is an essential enzyme in the nervous system, responsible for the synthesis of the neurotransmitter acetylcholine (ACh).

Function of Choline Acetyltransferase

Choline Acetyltransferase (ChAT) plays a critical role in the nervous system by synthesizing acetylcholine (ACh), a neurotransmitter vital for various physiological functions.

Role in Neurotransmission

1. **Acetylcholine Synthesis**: ChAT catalyzes the transfer of an acetyl group from acetyl-CoA to choline, producing acetylcholine. This reaction is fundamental for the cholinergic system, affecting both the central and peripheral nervous systems.
2. **Neuromuscular Junctions**: In the peripheral nervous system, ACh is essential for muscle contraction. ChAT activity in motor neurons ensures the availability of ACh at neuromuscular junctions, facilitating muscle movement.

3. **Cognitive Function**: In the central nervous system, ACh plays a pivotal role in cognitive processes such as learning, memory, and attention. ChAT activity in cholinergic neurons of the brain is crucial for maintaining these cognitive functions.
4. **Autonomic Nervous System**: ACh is involved in the autonomic nervous system, regulating involuntary bodily functions such as heart rate, digestion, and respiratory rate.

Additional Roles

1. **Neurodevelopment**: ChAT is crucial during neurodevelopment, influencing the growth and differentiation of cholinergic neurons.
2. **Neuroprotection**: ACh has neuroprotective properties, and adequate ChAT activity helps protect neurons from degenerative processes.
3. **Inflammation Modulation**: ACh has anti-inflammatory effects, and ChAT activity can influence immune responses by modulating acetylcholine levels.

Production of Choline Acetyltransferase

Choline Acetyltransferase is produced in cholinergic neurons through a well-orchestrated process involving gene expression, enzyme synthesis, and regulation.

Synthesis

1. **Gene Encoding**: The ChAT gene, located on chromosome 10q11.2, encodes the ChAT enzyme. This gene is highly expressed in cholinergic neurons.
2. **Protein Structure**: ChAT is a globular protein with an active site that binds acetyl-CoA and choline. The enzyme's structure is optimized for catalyzing the synthesis of acetylcholine efficiently.

Regulation by the Nervous System

1. **Neuronal Activity**: Neuronal activity regulates ChAT expression. Increased neuronal firing enhances ChAT synthesis to meet the demand for acetylcholine.
2. **Neurotrophic Factors**: Neurotrophic factors like nerve growth factor (NGF) and brain-derived neurotrophic factor (BDNF) influence ChAT expression by promoting the survival and growth of cholinergic neurons.
3. **Transcriptional Regulation**: Various transcription factors regulate ChAT gene expression, responding to neuronal activity and environmental cues.

Influencing Factors

1. **Age**: ChAT levels decline with age, contributing to decreased acetylcholine production and cognitive decline.
2. **Gender**: Hormonal differences between genders can influence ChAT activity, with estrogen shown to have a positive effect on ChAT expression.
3. **Exercise and Stress**: Physical activity can enhance ChAT activity by promoting neurotrophic factor release, while chronic stress may have a detrimental effect.

Regulation of Choline Acetyltransferase

The regulation of ChAT involves complex feedback mechanisms, environmental influences, and physiological states.

Feedback Mechanisms

1. **Acetylcholine Levels**: High levels of acetylcholine can provide feedback inhibition on ChAT activity, ensuring balanced neurotransmitter production.

2. **Acetylcholine Receptor Activity**: The activation of acetylcholine receptors can influence ChAT activity through intracellular signaling pathways.

Sleep

Sleep patterns significantly affect ChAT activity. Disrupted sleep can impair cholinergic function, leading to decreased acetylcholine synthesis.

Exercise

Regular physical activity supports ChAT activity by enhancing neuronal health and promoting the release of neurotrophic factors.

Nutritional Status

1. **Choline Intake**: Choline is a precursor for acetylcholine, and adequate dietary intake of choline is essential for optimal ChAT activity. Plant-based sources of choline include soybeans, quinoa, and cruciferous vegetables.
2. **Vitamins and Minerals**: Nutrients like vitamin B12, folate, and magnesium support ChAT activity and overall neuronal health. Plant-based diets can provide these nutrients through fortified foods and diverse plant sources.

Hormones

Hormones such as estrogen positively influence ChAT activity, enhancing acetylcholine production and cholinergic function.

Plant-Based Diet and Choline Acetyltransferase Regulation

A plant-based diet can positively influence ChAT regulation and cholinergic function through various mechanisms.

Nutrient Density

Plant-based diets offer a rich supply of essential nutrients, vitamins, and minerals that support overall health and ChAT activity. For instance, vitamin B12, found in fortified plant milk and nutritional yeast, is crucial for neuronal health.

Choline-Rich Foods

Certain plant foods are excellent sources of choline, such as soybeans, quinoa, and broccoli. These foods provide the necessary precursors for acetylcholine synthesis.

Antioxidants

Fruits and vegetables are rich in antioxidants, which reduce oxidative stress and support neuronal health. Lower oxidative stress levels are associated with improved ChAT activity.

Healthy Fats

Plant-based sources of fats, such as avocados, nuts, and seeds, provide essential fatty acids that support neuronal membrane integrity and function. Omega-3 fatty acids, in particular, have anti-inflammatory properties that enhance cholinergic function.

Fiber

High-fiber diets, common in plant-based eating, support gut health and can influence brain health through the gut-brain axis. A healthy gut microbiome can impact neurotransmitter production, including acetylcholine.

Caloric Balance

Maintaining a healthy weight through a balanced plant-based diet can prevent obesity-related neuronal imbalances. Excess body fat is linked to chronic inflammation, which can negatively impact ChAT activity.

Glycemic Control

Plant-based diets, which are low in refined sugars and high in complex carbohydrates, help maintain stable blood glucose levels. This stability supports overall brain health and ChAT activity.

Plant-Based Diet on ChAT-Related Health Outcomes
Cognitive Health

1. **Memory and Learning**: A plant-based diet supports cognitive health by providing essential nutrients and reducing oxidative stress. Improved ChAT activity enhances acetylcholine synthesis, which is crucial for memory and learning.
2. **Neuroprotection**: Antioxidants and anti-inflammatory compounds in plant foods protect neurons from degenerative processes, supporting long-term cognitive health.

Neuromuscular Health

1. **Muscle Function**: Adequate ChAT activity ensures optimal acetylcholine levels at neuromuscular junctions, facilitating muscle contraction and coordination. Plant-based diets provide nutrients like magnesium and potassium that support muscle health.
2. **Exercise Performance**: Plant-based diets rich in complex carbohydrates provide sustained energy for physical activity, supporting neuromuscular function and enhancing exercise performance.

Mental Health

Emerging evidence suggests that plant-based diets may benefit mental health by reducing inflammation and oxidative stress, which are linked to mood disorders. Improved ChAT activity and acetylcholine levels support cognitive function and emotional well-being.

Anti-Aging Effects

The antioxidant-rich nature of plant-based diets helps combat oxidative stress, a key factor in aging. Improved ChAT activity, coupled with reduced oxidative damage, contributes to healthier aging and better maintenance of cognitive health.

Neurodegenerative Diseases

1. **Alzheimer's Disease**: Adequate ChAT activity is crucial for acetylcholine synthesis, which is significantly impaired in Alzheimer's disease. A plant-based diet can support cognitive function and potentially slow the progression of neurodegenerative diseases by providing neuroprotective nutrients.
2. **Parkinson's Disease**: Plant-based diets rich in antioxidants and anti-inflammatory compounds may help reduce the risk of Parkinson's disease by protecting dopaminergic neurons and supporting overall brain health.

Choline Acetyltransferase plays a pivotal role in the nervous system, regulating acetylcholine synthesis and supporting various physiological functions, from muscle contraction to cognitive processes. Its production and regulation are influenced by factors such as age, sleep, exercise, and diet.

Acetylcholinesterase (AChE)

Acetylcholinesterase (AChE) is a critical enzyme in the nervous system, responsible for the breakdown of the neurotransmitter acetylcholine (ACh). It plays an essential role in terminating synaptic transmission, thus ensuring proper functioning of the neuromuscular junctions and other cholinergic synapses.

Function of Acetylcholinesterase

Acetylcholinesterase is vital for maintaining the balance of neurotransmission in cholinergic synapses.

Breakdown of Acetylcholine

AChE hydrolyzes acetylcholine into acetate and choline, terminating the neurotransmitter's action at the synaptic cleft. This process is crucial for the proper functioning of the nervous system as it:

1. **Prevents Continuous Stimulation:** By breaking down ACh, AChE prevents continuous stimulation of postsynaptic receptors, which could lead to muscle fatigue or paralysis.
2. **Maintains Synaptic Efficiency:** Rapid degradation of ACh ensures that synaptic transmission remains precise and timely, allowing for accurate communication between neurons.

Neuromuscular Junction

In the neuromuscular junction, AChE is essential for muscle contraction and relaxation:

1. **Muscle Contraction:** ACh is released from motor neurons and binds to receptors on muscle cells, causing contraction.
2. **Muscle Relaxation:** AChE breaks down ACh, leading to muscle relaxation and readiness for the next contraction cycle.

Central Nervous System

In the brain, AChE regulates cholinergic neurotransmission, which is involved in:

1. **Cognitive Functions:** ACh is critical for learning, memory, and attention.
2. **Autonomic Functions:** AChE ensures the proper functioning of the autonomic nervous system, which controls involuntary body functions such as heart rate and digestion.

Production of Acetylcholinesterase

Acetylcholinesterase is produced in various tissues, primarily in the nervous system.

Synthesis

1. **Gene Encoding:** The gene encoding AChE is located on chromosome 7 in humans. It produces multiple mRNA transcripts through alternative splicing, resulting in different isoforms of AChE.
2. **Enzyme Structure:** AChE is a hydrolase enzyme that breaks down acetylcholine. It exists in various molecular forms, including monomers, dimers, and tetramers, which determine its localization and function in different tissues.

Cellular Production

1. **Neurons:** In neurons, AChE is synthesized in the endoplasmic reticulum and transported to the synaptic cleft.
2. **Muscle Cells:** In muscle cells, AChE is anchored to the synaptic basal lamina, ensuring its proximity to released acetylcholine.

Regulation of Acetylcholinesterase

The regulation of AChE involves genetic, biochemical, and environmental factors.

Genetic Regulation

1. **Gene Expression:** The expression of the AChE gene is regulated by transcription factors and epigenetic modifications, which influence the amount of enzyme produced.

2. **Alternative Splicing:** Different isoforms of AChE are produced through alternative splicing of its pre-mRNA, allowing for tissue-specific expression and function.

Biochemical Regulation

1. **Feedback Mechanisms:** The levels of acetylcholine can regulate AChE activity through feedback mechanisms. High levels of acetylcholine can induce the synthesis of more AChE.
2. **Post-Translational Modifications:** AChE activity can be modulated by post-translational modifications such as phosphorylation and glycosylation, affecting its stability and function.

Environmental Influences

1. **Diet and Nutrition:** Nutritional factors, including those from a plant-based diet, can influence AChE activity.
2. **Stress and Toxins:** Exposure to stress and environmental toxins, such as pesticides and nerve agents, can affect AChE levels and activity.

Plant-Based Diet and Acetylcholinesterase Regulation

A plant-based diet, rich in fruits, vegetables, whole grains, nuts, and seeds, can positively influence AChE regulation through various mechanisms.

Antioxidants

Plant-based foods are rich in antioxidants, which can protect AChE from oxidative damage:

1. **Vitamin E and C:** Found in nuts, seeds, and citrus fruits, these vitamins can reduce oxidative stress and maintain AChE activity.

2. **Polyphenols:** Present in berries, green tea, and grapes, polyphenols have neuroprotective properties that can support AChE function.

Anti-Inflammatory Compounds

Chronic inflammation can impair AChE activity. Anti-inflammatory compounds in plant-based foods can mitigate this effect:

1. **Omega-3 Fatty Acids:** Found in flaxseeds, chia seeds, and walnuts, omega-3 fatty acids reduce inflammation and support neural health.
2. **Flavonoids:** Found in a variety of fruits and vegetables, flavonoids have potent anti-inflammatory effects.

Nutrient Density

Essential nutrients from a plant-based diet support overall health and enzymatic function:

1. **B Vitamins:** Crucial for brain health, B vitamins (such as folate and B12) support neurotransmitter synthesis and AChE activity. Sources include leafy greens, legumes, and fortified plant-based milks.
2. **Magnesium:** Found in whole grains, nuts, and seeds, magnesium is essential for nerve function and may influence AChE activity.

Fiber

High-fiber diets support gut health and can influence AChE activity through the gut-brain axis:

1. **Gut Microbiota:** A healthy gut microbiome, supported by dietary fiber, produces metabolites that can influence brain function and enzyme activity.

Plant-Based Diet on AChE-Related Health Outcomes

Adopting a plant-based diet can have several positive effects on health outcomes related to AChE activity.

Neuroprotection

1. **Cognitive Health:** Antioxidants and anti-inflammatory compounds in plant-based foods protect against neurodegenerative diseases like Alzheimer's, where AChE activity is often compromised.
2. **Memory and Learning:** Nutrients from plant-based foods support cognitive functions dependent on cholinergic neurotransmission.

Mental Health

1. **Mood Regulation:** A balanced plant-based diet can improve mood and reduce symptoms of depression and anxiety by supporting neurotransmitter balance, including acetylcholine.
2. **Stress Reduction:** Antioxidants and nutrients in plant-based foods help mitigate the effects of chronic stress on the nervous system.

Muscle Function

1. **Neuromuscular Health:** Proper AChE function is essential for muscle contraction and relaxation. A plant-based diet provides the nutrients necessary for maintaining neuromuscular health.
2. **Reduced Muscle Fatigue:** Nutrients like magnesium and antioxidants support muscle function and reduce fatigue.

Acetylcholinesterase plays a crucial role in the nervous system by regulating acetylcholine levels and ensuring proper neurotransmission. Its production and regulation are influenced by genetic, biochemical, and environmental factors, including diet.

Monoamine Oxidase (MAO)

Monoamine oxidase (MAO) is a critical enzyme in the human body that plays a significant role in the catabolism of monoamine neurotransmitters, such as dopamine, norepinephrine, and serotonin.

Function of Monoamine Oxidase

Monoamine oxidase is essential for maintaining the balance of neurotransmitters in the brain, which is crucial for mood regulation, cognitive function, and overall mental health.

In Neurotransmitter Catabolism

1. **Deamination**: MAO catalyzes the oxidative deamination of monoamines, converting them into their corresponding aldehydes, ammonia, and hydrogen peroxide. This reaction is vital for the breakdown and inactivation of neurotransmitters.
2. **Regulation of Neurotransmitter Levels**: By breaking down excess neurotransmitters, MAO helps maintain optimal levels, preventing conditions like anxiety, depression, and other mood disorders.
3. **Types of MAO**: There are two isoforms of MAO – MAO-A and MAO-B. MAO-A primarily degrades serotonin, norepinephrine, and dopamine, while MAO-B mainly metabolizes phenylethylamine and certain other trace amines.

Additional Roles

1. **Neuroprotection**: MAO helps protect neurons from oxidative stress by breaking down potentially toxic amines.
2. **Mood Regulation**: By modulating neurotransmitter levels, MAO plays a crucial role in mood regulation and emotional stability.
3. **Cognitive Function**: Proper MAO activity is essential for maintaining cognitive functions such as memory, learning, and attention.

Production of Monoamine Oxidase Monoamine oxidase is produced by various tissues in the body, particularly in the brain, liver, and gastrointestinal tract, through a complex interaction of genetic and biochemical pathways.

Synthesis

1. **Gene Encoding**: The MAO genes are located on the X chromosome. MAO-A and MAO-B are encoded by separate genes, MAOA and MAOB, respectively.
2. **Protein Structure**: MAO is a flavin adenine dinucleotide (FAD)-dependent enzyme, meaning it requires FAD as a cofactor to function effectively.

Regulation by Cellular Mechanisms

1. **Transcriptional Control**: The expression of MAO genes is regulated at the transcriptional level by various factors, including transcription factors and promoter regions.
2. **Post-Translational Modifications**: After synthesis, MAO enzymes undergo post-translational modifications, such as phosphorylation, which can affect their activity and stability.

3. **Cellular Localization**: MAO is located in the outer mitochondrial membrane, which positions it strategically to interact with monoamine neurotransmitters and other substrates.

Influencing Factors

1. **Age**: MAO levels and activity can change with age, typically increasing in the brain during the aging process.
2. **Gender**: Due to the X-linked nature of MAO genes, there may be gender-specific differences in MAO expression and activity.
3. **Environmental Factors**: External factors, such as diet, stress, and exposure to toxins, can influence MAO activity.

Regulation of Monoamine Oxidase The regulation of MAO involves a complex interplay of genetic, biochemical, and environmental factors.

Feedback Mechanisms

1. **Negative Feedback**: High levels of monoamine neurotransmitters can inhibit the activity of MAO through feedback mechanisms, ensuring a balance in neurotransmitter levels.
2. **Positive Feedback**: Certain conditions, such as prolonged stress or high intake of amines, can upregulate MAO expression to manage increased substrate levels.

Sleep

Sleep patterns significantly influence MAO activity. Disrupted sleep can alter neurotransmitter levels and, consequently, MAO activity, impacting mood and cognitive function.

Exercise

Regular physical activity, particularly moderate exercise, supports healthy MAO levels. Exercise can increase the turnover of neurotransmitters, necessitating balanced MAO activity to maintain homeostasis.

Nutritional Status

1. **Fasting and Malnutrition**: Low energy availability, as seen in fasting or malnutrition, can suppress MAO activity. This suppression can affect neurotransmitter balance and mood.
2. **Dietary Amine Intake**: Diets high in amines, such as those found in certain cheeses, wines, and fermented foods, can influence MAO activity by increasing substrate availability.
3. **Plant-Based Nutrients**: Nutrients found in plant-based diets can support MAO production and overall neurotransmitter balance.

Plant-Based Diet and Monoamine Oxidase Regulation

A plant-based diet, rich in fruits, vegetables, whole grains, nuts, and seeds, can positively influence MAO regulation through various mechanisms.

Nutrient Density

Plant-based diets provide a wealth of essential nutrients, vitamins, and minerals that support overall health and enzymatic activity. For example, vitamin B6, found in bananas, potatoes, and spinach, is crucial for the synthesis and function of MAO.

Amino Acids

Certain amino acids, such as tryptophan and tyrosine, found in plant foods like nuts, seeds, and legumes, are precursors to monoamine neurotransmitters. These amino acids support neurotransmitter synthesis and balance.

Antioxidants

Fruits and vegetables are rich in antioxidants, which help reduce oxidative stress. Lower oxidative stress levels are associated with improved MAO activity and overall neurotransmitter balance.

Healthy Fats

Plant-based sources of fats, such as avocados, nuts, and seeds, provide essential fatty acids that support brain health and neurotransmitter function. Omega-3 fatty acids, in particular, have anti-inflammatory properties that can enhance MAO function.

Fiber

High-fiber diets, common in plant-based eating, support gut health and neurotransmitter regulation. A healthy gut microbiome can influence neurotransmitter levels through the production of short-chain fatty acids and other metabolites.

Caloric Balance

Maintaining a healthy weight through a balanced plant-based diet can prevent obesity-related imbalances in MAO activity. Excess body fat, particularly visceral fat, is linked to increased oxidative stress and disrupted neurotransmitter balance.

Glycemic Control

Plant-based diets, which are low in refined sugars and high in complex carbohydrates, help maintain stable blood glucose levels. This stability prevents insulin resistance, which can negatively impact neurotransmitter function and MAO activity.

Plant-Based Diet on MAO-Related Health Outcomes

Mental Health

1. **Mood Regulation**: A plant-based diet can support mood regulation by providing essential nutrients that promote neurotransmitter balance. For example, the folate found in leafy greens is crucial for the synthesis of serotonin and other monoamines.
2. **Cognitive Function**: Adequate intake of nutrients like antioxidants and omega-3 fatty acids from plant sources supports cognitive function and protects against neurodegenerative diseases.

Reproductive Health

1. **Hormonal Balance**: Plant-based diets can support hormonal balance by providing phytoestrogens and other compounds that influence endocrine function. Balanced hormones can positively impact MAO activity and neurotransmitter regulation.
2. **Fertility**: Nutrients found in plant-based diets, such as zinc and selenium, support reproductive health and optimal neurotransmitter function, enhancing fertility.

Cardiovascular Health

Plant-based diets are known to reduce the risk of cardiovascular diseases by improving lipid profiles and reducing inflammation. This improved cardiovascular health supports overall brain function and MAO activity by ensuring adequate blood flow and nutrient delivery to the brain.

Anti-Aging Effects

The antioxidant-rich nature of plant-based diets helps combat oxidative stress, a key factor in aging. Improved MAO function, coupled with reduced oxidative damage, contributes to healthier aging and better maintenance of neurotransmitter balance.

Weight Management

Plant-based diets are effective for weight management, reducing body fat, and improving insulin sensitivity. Lower body fat and better glycemic control enhance overall enzymatic activity, including MAO function.

Gut Health

A high-fiber, plant-based diet promotes a healthy gut microbiome, which plays a crucial role in neurotransmitter synthesis and regulation. Short-chain fatty acids produced by gut bacteria can influence brain function and MAO activity.

Immune Function

Nutrients found in plant-based diets, such as vitamins C and E, support immune function. A strong immune system can protect against infections and inflammation that may disrupt neurotransmitter balance and MAO activity.

Monoamine oxidase plays a pivotal role in mental health and cognitive function by regulating neurotransmitter levels. Its production and regulation are influenced by various factors, including age, sleep, exercise, and diet.

Histone Acetyltransferase (HAT)

Histone acetyltransferases (HATs) are crucial enzymes in the regulation of gene expression through the modification of histones. These enzymes play a significant role in chromatin remodeling, influencing various cellular processes, including transcription, DNA repair, and replication.

Function of Histone Acetyltransferase

Histone acetyltransferases have a wide array of functions that are vital for maintaining cellular homeostasis and regulating gene expression.

Chromatin Remodeling

HATs catalyze the addition of acetyl groups to lysine residues on histone proteins, leading to a more relaxed chromatin structure. This process is essential for:

1. **Transcription Activation:** Acetylation of histones by HATs reduces the positive charge on histones, decreasing their affinity for the negatively charged DNA. This relaxed state allows

transcription factors easier access to the DNA, thereby promoting gene expression.

2. **DNA Repair:** HATs play a role in DNA damage response by acetylating histones and non-histone proteins involved in the repair processes. This modification facilitates the recruitment of repair proteins to sites of damage.
3. **Replication:** During DNA replication, HATs ensure that newly synthesized histones are acetylated, maintaining an open chromatin state that allows replication machinery access to the DNA.

Non-Histone Protein Acetylation

HATs also acetylate a variety of non-histone proteins, influencing numerous cellular functions:

1. **Protein Stability:** Acetylation can affect the stability and degradation of proteins, either marking them for degradation or protecting them from it.
2. **Protein-Protein Interactions:** Acetylation can modulate interactions between proteins, influencing signaling pathways and cellular responses.
3. **Enzyme Activity:** The acetylation of enzymes can either activate or inhibit their catalytic activity, thus regulating metabolic pathways and other cellular processes.

Production of Histone Acetyltransferase

The production and synthesis of HATs are tightly regulated at both the transcriptional and translational levels.

Gene Encoding

1. **HAT Families:** HATs are categorized into several families based on their sequence homology and functional similarities, including the GNAT (Gcn5-related N-acetyltransferase), MYST

(MOZ, Ybf2/Sas3, Sas2, and Tip60), and p300/CBP (CREB-binding protein) families.

2. **Gene Location:** The genes encoding HATs are located on various chromosomes and are subject to regulation by transcription factors and epigenetic modifications.

Synthesis

1. **Transcriptional Regulation:** The expression of HAT genes is regulated by multiple factors, including transcription factors that respond to cellular signals and environmental cues.
2. **Post-Transcriptional Modifications:** mRNA stability and translation efficiency of HATs can be influenced by microRNAs and RNA-binding proteins, which modulate their levels in response to cellular conditions.

Regulation of Histone Acetyltransferase

The activity of HATs is regulated through a complex interplay of mechanisms, ensuring precise control over gene expression and cellular functions.

Post-Translational Modifications

1. **Phosphorylation:** Phosphorylation of HATs can either activate or inhibit their enzymatic activity, allowing cells to rapidly respond to internal and external signals.
2. **Ubiquitination:** HATs can be tagged for degradation by ubiquitination, thus controlling their abundance and activity within the cell.

Protein-Protein Interactions

HATs often function as part of larger multi-protein complexes, where interactions with other proteins can modulate their activity and specificity. These interactions are crucial for targeting HATs to specific genomic loci and substrates.

Feedback Mechanisms

HAT activity is subject to feedback regulation, where the products of their enzymatic activity (e.g., acetylated histones) can influence the further activity of HATs. This ensures a balanced and self-regulating system.

Plant-Based Diet and Histone Acetyltransferase Regulation

A plant-based diet, rich in fruits, vegetables, whole grains, nuts, and seeds, can positively influence the regulation and activity of HATs through various mechanisms.

Nutrient Density

Plant-based diets provide a wealth of essential nutrients, vitamins, and minerals that support overall health and enzymatic functions:

1. **Vitamins and Minerals:** Nutrients such as vitamin E, found in nuts and seeds, and magnesium, found in leafy greens, are crucial for maintaining the enzymatic activity of HATs and other proteins.
2. **Phytonutrients:** Compounds like flavonoids and polyphenols found in fruits and vegetables can modulate HAT activity by influencing their expression and function.

Amino Acids

Certain amino acids found in plant foods support the synthesis and activity of HATs:

- **Lysine and Arginine:** These amino acids, abundant in legumes and nuts, are precursors for protein acetylation and are essential for the enzymatic function of HATs.

Antioxidants

Fruits and vegetables are rich in antioxidants, which help reduce oxidative stress and support cellular health:

- **Oxidative Stress Reduction:** Lower oxidative stress levels are associated with improved cellular functions, including the regulation of HAT activity.

Healthy Fats

Plant-based sources of fats, such as avocados, nuts, and seeds, provide essential fatty acids that support cellular health and enzyme function:

- **Omega-3 Fatty Acids:** These fatty acids have anti-inflammatory properties that can enhance the function of HATs and overall cellular health.

Fiber

High-fiber diets, common in plant-based eating, support gut health and hormone regulation:

- **Gut Microbiome:** A healthy gut microbiome can influence the regulation of HAT activity through the production of short-chain fatty acids and other metabolites.

Caloric Balance

Maintaining a healthy weight through a balanced plant-based diet can prevent obesity-related hormonal imbalances that affect HAT regulation:

- **Body Fat and Inflammation:** Excess body fat is linked to increased production of inflammatory markers, which can disrupt the regulation of HAT activity.

Glycemic Control

Plant-based diets, which are low in refined sugars and high in complex carbohydrates, help maintain stable blood glucose levels:

- **Insulin Sensitivity:** Stable blood glucose levels prevent insulin resistance, which can negatively impact the regulation of HATs and other enzymes.

Plant-Based Diet on HAT-Related Health Outcomes

Cancer Prevention

HATs play a critical role in regulating gene expression involved in cell proliferation and apoptosis. A plant-based diet can contribute to cancer prevention by:

1. **Antioxidant Properties:** Phytonutrients in plant foods protect cells from oxidative damage, reducing the risk of mutations and cancer development.
2. **Anti-Inflammatory Effects:** The anti-inflammatory properties of plant-based diets help maintain a balanced cellular environment, preventing the dysregulation of HAT activity associated with cancer.

Cardiovascular Health

HATs are involved in the regulation of genes that control lipid metabolism and inflammation. A plant-based diet can support cardiovascular health by:

1. **Cholesterol Regulation:** High-fiber diets help reduce cholesterol levels, promoting a healthy lipid profile and reducing the risk of cardiovascular disease.

2. **Blood Pressure Control:** Nutrients like potassium and magnesium, abundant in plant foods, help regulate blood pressure and support vascular health.

Neuroprotection

HATs play a role in the regulation of genes involved in neuronal function and plasticity. A plant-based diet can contribute to neuroprotection by:

1. **Cognitive Function:** Antioxidants and anti-inflammatory compounds in plant foods support brain health and protect against neurodegenerative diseases.
2. **Mood Regulation:** Nutrients like omega-3 fatty acids support the production of neurotransmitters and promote mental well-being.

Longevity and Healthy Aging

HATs are involved in the regulation of genes associated with aging and cellular senescence. A plant-based diet can promote longevity and healthy aging by:

1. **Anti-Aging Properties:** Antioxidants in plant foods combat oxidative stress, a key factor in aging, and support cellular health.
2. **Hormonal Balance:** Maintaining a healthy weight and stable blood glucose levels helps prevent age-related hormonal imbalances that can affect HAT regulation.

"The human body contains a vast array of enzymes, far too many to list comprehensively here. Therefore, I have chosen to focus on the top 50 most significant enzymes."

28

G-Protein-Coupled Receptors (GPCRs)

Human cell receptors play a pivotal role in the intricate network of communication within the body. These specialized proteins, located on the surface of cells, are responsible for receiving and transmitting signals that regulate various physiological processes. From hormone action to immune responses, cell receptors are essential for maintaining homeostasis and responding to environmental changes.

Types of Cell Receptors

There are several types of cell receptors, each with distinct functions and mechanisms. The major classes include:

1. **G Protein-Coupled Receptors (GPCRs)**
2. **Receptor Tyrosine Kinases (RTKs)**
3. **Ion Channel Receptors**
4. **Nuclear Receptors**
5. **Cytokine Receptors**

G Protein-Coupled Receptors (GPCRs)

GPCRs represent the largest family of cell receptors, involved in numerous physiological processes. These receptors respond to a variety of ligands, including hormones, neurotransmitters, and sensory stimuli.

Structure and Function: GPCRs are characterized by their seven transmembrane helices. Upon ligand binding, these receptors undergo a conformational change that activates an associated G protein. The G protein then interacts with various intracellular effectors, such as adenylyl cyclase or phospholipase C, leading to the generation of second messengers like cAMP or IP3.

Examples:

- **Adrenergic Receptors:** These receptors respond to adrenaline and noradrenaline, playing a critical role in the fight-or-flight response.
- **Rhodopsin:** A photoreceptor in the retina involved in vision.

Receptor Tyrosine Kinases (RTKs)

RTKs are key players in cellular growth, differentiation, and metabolism. These receptors have intrinsic kinase activity, meaning they can phosphorylate themselves and other proteins upon activation.

Structure and Function: RTKs are composed of an extracellular ligand-binding domain, a single transmembrane helix, and an intracellular tyrosine kinase domain. Ligand binding induces dimerization and autophosphorylation of the receptor, triggering a cascade of downstream signaling pathways, such as the MAPK and PI3K-Akt pathways.

Examples:

- **Epidermal Growth Factor Receptor (EGFR):** Involved in cell proliferation and differentiation.
- **Insulin Receptor:** Plays a crucial role in glucose homeostasis.

Ion Channel Receptors

Ion channel receptors, also known as ligand-gated ion channels, are critical for rapid signal transduction, particularly in the nervous system.

Structure and Function: These receptors consist of multiple subunits that form a pore in the cell membrane. Ligand binding causes a conformational change, opening the channel and allowing specific ions (such as Na+, K+, Ca2+, or Cl-) to flow across the membrane. This ion movement generates an electrical signal that can trigger various cellular responses.

Examples:

- **Nicotinic Acetylcholine Receptor:** Mediates synaptic transmission at neuromuscular junctions.
- **GABA_A Receptor:** Involved in inhibitory neurotransmission in the central nervous system.

Nuclear Receptors

Nuclear receptors are a unique class of receptors that function as transcription factors. They are involved in regulating gene expression in response to hormones and other ligands.

Structure and Function: Nuclear receptors have a modular structure with a ligand-binding domain, a DNA-binding domain, and a transcriptional activation domain. Upon ligand binding, these receptors translocate to the nucleus, where they bind to specific DNA sequences and modulate the transcription of target genes.

Examples:

- **Estrogen Receptor:** Regulates reproductive and other physiological processes.
- **Glucocorticoid Receptor:** Involved in stress response and metabolism.

Cytokine Receptors

Cytokine receptors are involved in immune responses, inflammation, and cell growth. They typically lack intrinsic enzymatic activity and rely on associated kinases for signal transduction.

Structure and Function: Cytokine receptors consist of extracellular ligand-binding domains, transmembrane domains, and intracellular domains that associate with Janus kinases (JAKs). Ligand binding induces receptor dimerization and activation of JAKs, which phosphorylate and activate STAT transcription factors, leading to gene expression changes.

Examples:

- **Interleukin-2 Receptor:** Important for T cell proliferation.
- **Tumor Necrosis Factor Receptor:** Mediates inflammatory responses.

Mechanisms of Signal Transduction

Cell receptors convert extracellular signals into intracellular responses through various mechanisms. These include:

1. **Ligand Binding and Conformational Change**
2. **Receptor Dimerization and Autophosphorylation**
3. **Second Messenger Generation**
4. **Activation of Intracellular Signaling Cascades**
5. **Regulation of Gene Expression**

Ligand Binding and Conformational Change

The initial step in receptor activation involves the binding of a specific ligand to the receptor's extracellular domain. This binding induces a conformational change in the receptor, which is crucial for the subsequent steps in signal transduction.

Example:

- In GPCRs, ligand binding causes a conformational change that allows the receptor to interact with and activate a G protein.

Receptor Dimerization and Autophosphorylation

For many receptors, particularly RTKs, ligand binding induces dimerization or oligomerization. This process brings the intracellular kinase domains of the receptors into close proximity, allowing them to phosphorylate each other on specific tyrosine residues.

Example:

- The activation of the EGFR involves dimerization and autophosphorylation, which then recruits and activates downstream signaling proteins.

Second Messenger Generation

Second messengers are small molecules that propagate the signal initiated by receptor activation. They amplify the signal and mediate various intracellular responses.

Example:

- In the case of GPCRs, activation of adenylyl cyclase leads to the production of cAMP, a second messenger that activates protein kinase A (PKA).

Activation of Intracellular Signaling Cascades

Receptor activation often triggers a cascade of intracellular signaling events, involving multiple proteins and pathways. These cascades amplify the signal and ensure a coordinated cellular response.

Example:

- The MAPK pathway, activated by RTKs, involves a series of phosphorylation events that ultimately lead to changes in gene expression and cell behavior.

Regulation of Gene Expression

Nuclear receptors and some cell surface receptors can influence gene expression by modulating the activity of transcription factors. This regulation is critical for long-term cellular responses, such as differentiation, proliferation, and apoptosis.

Example:

- The binding of cortisol to the glucocorticoid receptor leads to its translocation to the nucleus, where it regulates the expression of genes involved in stress response and metabolism.

Physiological Roles of Cell Receptors

Cell receptors are involved in virtually every physiological process in the body. Some key roles include:

1. **Regulation of Metabolism**
2. **Immune Response and Inflammation**
3. **Neurotransmission and Synaptic Plasticity**
4. **Cell Growth and Differentiation**
5. **Sensory Perception**

Regulation of Metabolism

Receptors such as the insulin receptor and nuclear receptors like the thyroid hormone receptor play crucial roles in regulating metabolism.

They ensure that cells respond appropriately to changes in nutrient availability and energy demands.

Example:

- The insulin receptor facilitates glucose uptake into cells, thereby lowering blood glucose levels and providing energy for cellular processes.

Immune Response and Inflammation

Cytokine receptors and other immune receptors are essential for coordinating immune responses and inflammation. They enable immune cells to recognize and respond to pathogens, as well as to regulate the intensity and duration of inflammatory responses.

Example:

- The interleukin-1 receptor is involved in the inflammatory response, mediating the effects of IL-1, a key pro-inflammatory cytokine.

Neurotransmission and Synaptic Plasticity

Ion channel receptors and GPCRs are vital for neurotransmission in the nervous system. They mediate rapid communication between neurons and are involved in synaptic plasticity, which underlies learning and memory.

Example:

- The NMDA receptor, an ion channel receptor, is crucial for synaptic plasticity and memory formation.

Cell Growth and Differentiation

RTKs and other growth factor receptors regulate cell growth, differentiation, and survival. These receptors are critical for development, tissue repair, and maintaining tissue homeostasis.

Example:

- The fibroblast growth factor receptor (FGFR) regulates cell proliferation and differentiation during development and wound healing.

Sensory Perception

Receptors such as rhodopsin in the retina and olfactory receptors in the nasal epithelium are involved in sensory perception. They enable organisms to detect and respond to environmental stimuli.

Example:

- Rhodopsin is a GPCR involved in the detection of light, essential for vision.

Dysfunction and Disease

Dysfunction in cell receptors can lead to a variety of diseases and disorders. Mutations, overexpression, or aberrant signaling can disrupt normal cellular function and contribute to pathogenesis.

Cancer

Aberrant activation of RTKs and other growth factor receptors is a common feature in many cancers. Mutations that lead to constitutive activation of these receptors can drive uncontrolled cell proliferation and survival.

Example:

- Mutations in the EGFR gene are associated with several types of cancer, including non-small cell lung cancer.

Diabetes

Impaired insulin receptor signaling is a hallmark of diabetes mellitus. Insulin resistance, a condition where cells fail to respond properly to insulin, leads to elevated blood glucose levels and associated complications.

Example:

- Type 2 diabetes is characterized by insulin resistance and often involves defects in insulin receptor function and downstream signaling pathways.

Neurodegenerative Diseases

Dysfunction in neurotransmitter receptors, such as the NMDA receptor and dopamine receptors, is implicated in neurodegenerative diseases like Alzheimer's disease and Parkinson's disease.

Example:

- Altered NMDA receptor function is associated with synaptic dysfunction and cognitive deficits in Alzheimer's disease.

Autoimmune Diseases

Abnormal signaling through cytokine receptors can contribute to autoimmune diseases, where the immune system attacks the body's own tissues.

Example:

- Overactivation of the interleukin-6 receptor is implicated in rheumatoid arthritis, leading to chronic inflammation and joint damage.

Cardiovascular Diseases

Dysregulation of receptors involved in cardiovascular function, such as adrenergic receptors and angiotensin receptors, can lead to hypertension, heart failure, and other cardiovascular diseases.

Example:

- Overactivation of beta-adrenergic receptors can contribute to heart failure by increasing cardiac workload and promoting maladaptive remodeling.

Therapeutic Targeting of Cell Receptors

Given their roles in various physiological processes and diseases, cell receptors are important targets for therapeutic interventions. Many drugs are designed to modulate receptor function, either by activating or inhibiting their activity.

Agonists and Antagonists

Agonists are compounds that bind to and activate receptors, mimicking the effect of natural ligands. Antagonists, on the other hand, bind to receptors and block their activation, inhibiting the effect of natural ligands.

Examples:

- **Beta-Blockers:** These antagonists of beta-adrenergic receptors are used to treat hypertension and heart conditions by reducing heart rate and contractility.
- **Glucocorticoids:** These agonists of the glucocorticoid receptor are used to reduce inflammation in conditions like asthma and rheumatoid arthritis.

Monoclonal Antibodies

Monoclonal antibodies are engineered proteins that can specifically bind to cell receptors, either blocking their activation or targeting them for destruction by the immune system.

Examples:

- **Trastuzumab (Herceptin):** A monoclonal antibody that targets the HER2 receptor, used in the treatment of HER2-positive breast cancer.
- **Infliximab (Remicade):** A monoclonal antibody that targets TNF-alpha, used in the treatment of autoimmune diseases like Crohn's disease and rheumatoid arthritis.

Small Molecule Inhibitors

Small molecule inhibitors are compounds that can enter cells and inhibit the activity of intracellular receptor domains or downstream signaling proteins.

Examples:

- **Imatinib (Gleevec):** A tyrosine kinase inhibitor that targets the BCR-ABL fusion protein in chronic myeloid leukemia.

- **Erlotinib (Tarceva):** An EGFR inhibitor used in the treatment of non-small cell lung cancer.

Gene Therapy

Gene therapy approaches aim to correct genetic defects in receptors or their signaling pathways. This can involve delivering functional copies of genes, using RNA interference to silence defective genes, or employing CRISPR-Cas9 technology for gene editing.

Example:

- Gene therapy for severe combined immunodeficiency (SCID) involves introducing a functional copy of the defective gene into the patient's immune cells, restoring immune function.

Human cell receptors are fundamental to the proper functioning of the body's physiological processes. They mediate communication between cells and their environment, ensuring appropriate responses to a wide range of stimuli. Dysfunction in these receptors can lead to various diseases, making them critical targets for therapeutic interventions.

Beta-adrenergic Receptors (β-adrenergic receptors)

Beta-adrenergic receptors (β-adrenergic receptors) are a class of G protein-coupled receptors that are targets of the catecholamines, especially norepinephrine (noradrenaline) and epinephrine (adrenaline). These receptors play crucial roles in the regulation of heart rate, smooth muscle relaxation, and metabolic processes. There are three main subtypes of beta-adrenergic receptors: β1, β2, and β3, each with distinct functions and tissue distributions.

Function of Beta-Adrenergic Receptors

β1-Adrenergic Receptors

β1-adrenergic receptors are primarily located in the heart. Their activation leads to an increase in heart rate (chronotropy) and force of contraction (inotropy). This response is part of the body's 'fight or flight' mechanism, preparing the body for rapid action in response to stress. Additionally, β1 receptors are found in the kidneys, where they stimulate the release of renin, a key enzyme in the regulation of blood pressure.

β2-Adrenergic Receptors

β2-adrenergic receptors are found predominantly in the smooth muscles of the airways, blood vessels, and uterus. Their activation results in smooth muscle relaxation, leading to bronchodilation, vasodilation, and uterine relaxation. This makes β2 receptors important in managing conditions like asthma, where bronchodilation is beneficial. These receptors also influence metabolic processes, such as glycogenolysis and gluconeogenesis, aiding in the mobilization of energy reserves during stress.

β3-Adrenergic Receptors

β3-adrenergic receptors are mainly found in adipose tissue. Their primary role is in the regulation of lipolysis, the breakdown of fat stores into free fatty acids and glycerol. This process is essential for energy homeostasis, especially during periods of fasting or increased energy demand. β3 receptors also contribute to thermogenesis in brown adipose tissue, a process important for maintaining body temperature in cold environments.

Production of Beta-Adrenergic Receptors

The production of beta-adrenergic receptors is a complex process regulated at multiple levels, including gene expression, receptor synthesis, and post-translational modifications. The genes encoding β1, β2, and β3 receptors are ADRB1, ADRB2, and ADRB3, respectively.

Gene Expression

Gene expression of beta-adrenergic receptors is controlled by various transcription factors and regulatory elements. These include promoter regions upstream of the ADRB genes that bind specific proteins to initiate transcription. The expression of these genes can be influenced by several factors, including hormones, stress, and dietary components.

Receptor Synthesis

Once transcribed, the mRNA of beta-adrenergic receptors is translated into protein in the endoplasmic reticulum. These proteins undergo folding and glycosylation, essential for their proper function and stability. The receptors are then transported to the cell membrane, where they become functional.

Post-Translational Modifications

Beta-adrenergic receptors undergo various post-translational modifications, such as phosphorylation, which regulate their activity, desensitization, and internalization. Phosphorylation of these receptors by kinases, such as PKA and GRKs, can lead to receptor desensitization, reducing their responsiveness to agonists like norepinephrine and epinephrine.

Regulation of Beta-Adrenergic Receptors

The regulation of beta-adrenergic receptors involves multiple mechanisms to ensure appropriate cellular responses to catecholamines.

Desensitization and Downregulation

Prolonged exposure to agonists can lead to receptor desensitization, where the receptor's responsiveness is diminished. This is often followed by downregulation, where the number of receptors on the cell surface is reduced. These processes are crucial in preventing overstimulation and maintaining homeostasis. Desensitization involves receptor phosphorylation by kinases such as GRKs, leading to the binding of β-arrestins, which uncouple the receptors from G proteins and target them for internalization.

Receptor Recycling and Degradation

Internalized receptors can either be recycled back to the cell membrane or degraded in lysosomes. The balance between these processes determines the overall number of functional receptors on the cell surface. Recycling allows the cell to quickly restore receptor sensitivity, while degradation reduces the receptor density, providing long-term regulation.

Role of Plant-Based Compounds in Regulation

Plant-based diets can influence the regulation of beta-adrenergic receptors through various bioactive compounds. Phytochemicals, such as flavonoids, have been shown to modulate receptor activity and expression.

Flavonoids

Flavonoids are a group of polyphenolic compounds found in fruits, vegetables, tea, and other plant-based foods. They have been reported to influence the beta-adrenergic signaling pathway by inhibiting catecholamine-induced responses. For instance, quercetin, a flavonoid found in apples, onions, and berries, can inhibit β2-adrenergic receptor-mediated lipolysis in adipocytes.

Dietary Fiber

High-fiber diets, typical of plant-based nutrition, can improve insulin sensitivity and reduce sympathetic nervous system activity. This, in turn, may modulate the activity of beta-adrenergic receptors, as insulin and sympathetic activity are linked to receptor regulation.

Omega-3 Fatty Acids

Plant sources of omega-3 fatty acids, such as flaxseeds and chia seeds, have anti-inflammatory properties and can influence adrenergic receptor function. Omega-3 fatty acids have been shown to decrease the expression of β-adrenergic receptors in adipose tissue, potentially affecting lipolysis and energy metabolism.

Plant-Based Diets and Beta-Adrenergic Receptors

Adopting a plant-based diet can have significant impacts on the regulation and function of beta-adrenergic receptors. The intake of various nutrients and bioactive compounds from plants can modulate the adrenergic system, contributing to overall health benefits.

Cardiovascular Health

Plant-based diets are rich in antioxidants, dietary fiber, and healthy fats, which are beneficial for cardiovascular health. The regulation of β1-adrenergic receptors in the heart can be positively influenced by these dietary components. For example, antioxidants can reduce oxidative stress, which is known to impair β1 receptor function. Additionally, dietary fiber helps in managing blood pressure by improving endothelial function and reducing systemic inflammation.

Metabolic Health

The influence of plant-based diets on β2-adrenergic receptors can enhance metabolic health. Foods rich in flavonoids and omega-3 fatty acids can improve insulin sensitivity and reduce the risk of metabolic disorders such as type 2 diabetes. By modulating β2 receptor activity, these diets can enhance glucose uptake and utilization, contributing to better glycemic control.

Weight Management

β3-adrenergic receptors play a crucial role in fat metabolism and thermogenesis. Plant-based diets, which are typically lower in calories and higher in fiber, can support weight management by enhancing the function of β3 receptors. The presence of bioactive compounds in plant foods can stimulate β3 receptor-mediated lipolysis, aiding in the reduction of fat stores and promoting healthy weight loss.

Beta-adrenergic receptors are essential for various physiological processes, including cardiovascular function, smooth muscle relaxation, and metabolic regulation. The production and regulation of these receptors involve complex mechanisms influenced by genetic and environmental factors.

Alpha-Adrenergic Receptors (α-adrenergic receptors)

Alpha-adrenergic receptors (α-adrenergic receptors) are a class of G protein-coupled receptors that respond to catecholamines, particularly norepinephrine (noradrenaline) and epinephrine (adrenaline). These receptors play pivotal roles in various physiological processes, including vascular tone regulation, smooth muscle contraction, and neurotransmitter release inhibition. The two main subtypes of alpha-adrenergic receptors are α1 and α2, each with distinct functions and tissue distributions.

Function of Alpha-Adrenergic Receptors

α1-Adrenergic Receptors

Vascular Smooth Muscle Contraction: α1-adrenergic receptors are predominantly located in the smooth muscles of blood vessels. Their activation causes vasoconstriction, which increases peripheral resistance and blood pressure. This mechanism is vital in maintaining vascular tone and ensuring adequate blood flow to vital organs during stress or hemorrhage.

Genitourinary Smooth Muscle Contraction: In the genitourinary system, α1 receptors facilitate the contraction of the bladder sphincter, and prostate, which helps in controlling urine flow and maintaining continence. They also play a role in ejaculation by inducing the contraction of the vas deferens and seminal vesicles.

Hepatic Glycogenolysis: Activation of α1 receptors in the liver stimulates glycogenolysis, the breakdown of glycogen to glucose, which provides an immediate energy source during stress.

α2-Adrenergic Receptors

Inhibition of Neurotransmitter Release: α2-adrenergic receptors are located on presynaptic nerve terminals, where they inhibit the release of norepinephrine. This negative feedback mechanism helps regulate neurotransmitter levels, preventing overstimulation and maintaining homeostasis.

Platelet Aggregation: These receptors also promote platelet aggregation, which is crucial for blood clotting and wound healing. Their activation helps in the formation of a platelet plug during vascular injury.

Insulin Secretion Inhibition: In the pancreas, α2 receptors inhibit insulin secretion from beta cells. This modulation helps in balancing blood glucose levels, especially during stress when energy needs are high.

Production of Alpha-Adrenergic Receptors

The production of alpha-adrenergic receptors involves intricate processes regulated at the genetic, transcriptional, and post-translational levels. The genes encoding α1 and α2 receptors are ADRA1 and ADRA2, respectively.

Gene Expression

Regulatory Elements: The expression of alpha-adrenergic receptor genes is controlled by various regulatory elements and transcription factors. Promoter regions upstream of ADRA1 and ADRA2 genes bind specific proteins that initiate transcription. Hormones, stress, and dietary factors can influence this gene expression.

Transcription Factors: Key transcription factors, such as cAMP response element-binding protein (CREB) and nuclear factor-kappa B (NF-κB), play crucial roles in the regulation of alpha-adrenergic receptor genes. These factors respond to various intracellular signals, including stress and inflammatory cytokines.

Receptor Synthesis

Protein Translation: The mRNA transcribed from ADRA1 and ADRA2 genes is translated into receptor proteins in the endoplasmic reticulum. These proteins undergo proper folding and glycosylation, essential for their stability and function.

Membrane Trafficking: After synthesis, alpha-adrenergic receptors are transported to the cell membrane, where they become functional. Proper trafficking ensures that receptors are correctly positioned to respond to catecholamines.

Post-Translational Modifications

Phosphorylation: Alpha-adrenergic receptors undergo post-translational modifications, such as phosphorylation, which regulate their activity. Kinases like PKA and GRKs phosphorylate these receptors, leading to changes in their responsiveness and desensitization.

Glycosylation: Glycosylation of alpha-adrenergic receptors is crucial for their stability and membrane localization. This modification helps protect the receptors from degradation and ensures their proper function.

Regulation of Alpha-Adrenergic Receptors

The regulation of alpha-adrenergic receptors involves multiple mechanisms to maintain appropriate cellular responses to catecholamines.

Desensitization and Downregulation

Prolonged Agonist Exposure: Continuous exposure to agonists can lead to receptor desensitization, reducing their responsiveness. This is followed by downregulation, where receptor numbers on the cell surface decrease. These processes prevent overstimulation and maintain cellular homeostasis.

Receptor Phosphorylation: Desensitization involves receptor phosphorylation by kinases such as GRKs, which facilitate the binding of β-arrestins. β-arrestins uncouple receptors from G proteins, leading to receptor internalization and decreased signaling.

Receptor Recycling and Degradation

Internalization: Internalized receptors can be recycled back to the cell membrane or degraded in lysosomes. The balance between recycling and degradation determines the number of functional receptors available for signaling.

Recycling: Recycling allows rapid restoration of receptor sensitivity, enabling cells to respond to new stimuli. This mechanism is essential for maintaining receptor functionality during fluctuating catecholamine levels.

Degradation: Degradation reduces receptor density on the cell surface, providing long-term regulation. This process helps in preventing excessive receptor activity and maintaining cellular equilibrium.

Role of Plant-Based Compounds in Regulation

Plant-based diets can influence the regulation of alpha-adrenergic receptors through various bioactive compounds. Phytochemicals, dietary fiber, and omega-3 fatty acids have been shown to modulate receptor activity and expression.

Phytochemicals

Flavonoids: Flavonoids are polyphenolic compounds found in fruits, vegetables, tea, and other plant-based foods. They can modulate adrenergic receptor activity by inhibiting catecholamine-induced responses. For instance, quercetin, a flavonoid in apples, onions, and berries, can inhibit α1-adrenergic receptor-mediated vasoconstriction.

Catechins: Catechins, present in green tea, can influence alpha-adrenergic receptors by enhancing vasodilation and reducing oxidative stress. These effects contribute to cardiovascular health by improving blood flow and reducing arterial stiffness.

Dietary Fiber

Insulin Sensitivity: High-fiber diets, typical of plant-based nutrition, can improve insulin sensitivity and reduce sympathetic nervous system activity. Improved insulin sensitivity can modulate the activity of α2-adrenergic receptors, as insulin and sympathetic activity are linked to receptor regulation.

Gut Microbiota: Dietary fiber influences gut microbiota composition, which can affect adrenergic receptor regulation. A healthy gut microbiome can produce metabolites that modulate inflammation and adrenergic signaling.

Omega-3 Fatty Acids

Anti-Inflammatory Properties: Plant sources of omega-3 fatty acids, such as flaxseeds and chia seeds, possess anti-inflammatory properties and can influence adrenergic receptor function. Omega-3 fatty acids have been shown to decrease the expression of α-adrenergic receptors in adipose tissue, potentially affecting lipid metabolism and energy homeostasis.

Cardiovascular Health: Omega-3 fatty acids contribute to cardiovascular health by modulating adrenergic receptor-mediated vasoconstriction. They can enhance endothelial function, reduce arterial stiffness, and improve blood pressure regulation.

Plant-Based Diets and Alpha-Adrenergic Receptors

Adopting a plant-based diet can have significant impacts on the regulation and function of alpha-adrenergic receptors. The intake of various nutrients and bioactive compounds from plants can modulate the adrenergic system, contributing to overall health benefits.

Cardiovascular Health

Antioxidants: Plant-based diets are rich in antioxidants, which protect against oxidative stress. Oxidative stress can impair α1-adrenergic receptor function, leading to vascular dysfunction. Antioxidants from fruits and vegetables help maintain receptor functionality and improve vascular health.

Dietary Fiber: Dietary fiber from plant-based foods can lower blood pressure by improving endothelial function and reducing systemic inflammation. This, in turn, positively influences α1-adrenergic receptor-mediated vasoconstriction.

Metabolic Health

Flavonoids: Flavonoid-rich foods can enhance metabolic health by modulating α2-adrenergic receptors. Improved insulin sensitivity and reduced inflammation contribute to better glucose uptake and utilization, aiding in the management of metabolic disorders like type 2 diabetes.

Omega-3 Fatty Acids: Omega-3 fatty acids from plant sources can improve lipid metabolism and energy homeostasis by influencing α-adrenergic receptor activity. These fatty acids can enhance thermogenesis and fat oxidation, supporting weight management and metabolic health.

Weight Management

Thermogenesis: α-adrenergic receptors play a crucial role in thermogenesis and fat metabolism. Plant-based diets, which are typically lower in calories and higher in fiber, can support weight management by enhancing α-adrenergic receptor-mediated lipolysis. The presence of bioactive compounds in plant foods stimulates fat breakdown and promotes healthy weight loss.

Appetite Regulation: High-fiber diets increase satiety and reduce calorie intake, aiding in weight management. The modulation of adrenergic receptors by dietary components helps in maintaining energy balance and preventing obesity.

Plant-Based Diets and Disease Prevention

Hypertension: A plant-based diet can reduce the risk of hypertension by modulating α1-adrenergic receptor-mediated vasoconstriction. Nutrients such as potassium, magnesium, and antioxidants from plant foods help in lowering blood pressure and improving vascular health.

Diabetes: Improved insulin sensitivity from a plant-based diet positively influences α2-adrenergic receptor activity, aiding in glucose regulation. The anti-inflammatory properties of plant-based foods further contribute to diabetes prevention and management.

Cardiovascular Diseases: By enhancing α-adrenergic receptor function and reducing oxidative stress, plant-based diets lower the risk of cardiovascular diseases. The regulation of adrenergic receptors through diet plays a vital role in maintaining heart health and preventing atherosclerosis.

Alpha-adrenergic receptors are essential for various physiological processes, including vascular tone regulation, smooth muscle contraction, and neurotransmitter release inhibition. The production and regulation of these receptors involve complex mechanisms influenced by genetic and environmental factors.

Dopamine Receptors (D1, D2, D3, D4, D5)

Dopamine receptors are a class of G protein-coupled receptors (GPCRs) that play critical roles in various neurological processes, including motivation, pleasure, cognition, memory, learning, and fine motor control. There are five known subtypes of dopamine receptors: D1, D2, D3, D4, and D5, each with distinct functions and tissue distributions. These receptors are essential for the normal functioning of the central nervous system (CNS) and are implicated in a range of neuropsychiatric disorders.

Function of Dopamine Receptors

D1 Dopamine Receptors

D1 receptors are primarily located in the striatum, cerebral cortex, and limbic system. They are involved in modulating cognitive functions, emotional regulation, and motor control. Activation of D1 receptors stimulates the production of cyclic adenosine monophosphate (cAMP), which enhances the signaling pathways responsible for learning and memory. In the basal ganglia, D1 receptors play a pivotal role in facilitating voluntary movement.

D2 Dopamine Receptors

D2 receptors are widely distributed in the brain, particularly in the striatum, substantia nigra, and pituitary gland. They are crucial for motor control, reward, and neuroendocrine regulation. D2 receptors exist in two forms: pre-synaptic and post-synaptic. Pre-synaptic D2 receptors act as autoreceptors that inhibit dopamine release, whereas post-synaptic D2 receptors modulate the postsynaptic neuron's excitability. This dual role is vital for maintaining dopamine homeostasis and modulating behaviors related to reward and addiction.

D3 Dopamine Receptors

D3 receptors are predominantly found in the limbic areas of the brain, such as the nucleus accumbens, olfactory tubercle, and islands of Calleja. They are involved in regulating emotional responses, motivation, and reward-related behaviors. D3 receptors have a high affinity for dopamine and are believed to play a role in the pathophysiology of psychiatric disorders like schizophrenia and bipolar disorder.

D4 Dopamine Receptors

D4 receptors are expressed in the frontal cortex, amygdala, hypothalamus, and the mesolimbic pathway. They are implicated in cognitive and emotional processes, including attention and impulse control. Variations in the D4 receptor gene (DRD4) have been associated with personality traits and susceptibility to neuropsychiatric conditions, such as attention deficit hyperactivity disorder (ADHD) and schizophrenia.

D5 Dopamine Receptors

D5 receptors are primarily located in the hippocampus, hypothalamus, and limbic system. They share a high degree of structural similarity with D1 receptors but have a higher affinity for dopamine. D5 receptors are involved in modulating synaptic plasticity, memory formation, and neuroendocrine functions. They also play a role in the regulation of blood pressure and renal function.

Production of Dopamine Receptors

The production of dopamine receptors involves gene expression, receptor synthesis, and post-translational modifications. The genes encoding the D1, D2, D3, D4, and D5 receptors are DRD1, DRD2, DRD3, DRD4, and DRD5, respectively.

Gene Expression

Gene expression of dopamine receptors is regulated by transcription factors and promoter regions that initiate the transcription process. Various intracellular and extracellular signals, including hormonal changes, stress, and dietary factors, can influence the expression of these genes. For instance, stress hormones like glucocorticoids can alter dopamine receptor gene expression, impacting receptor density and function.

Receptor Synthesis

Once the dopamine receptor genes are transcribed, the mRNA is translated into protein in the endoplasmic reticulum. These proteins undergo folding and glycosylation, which are crucial for their stability and proper functioning. The receptors are then transported to the cell membrane, where they become functional.

Post-Translational Modifications

Dopamine receptors undergo several post-translational modifications, such as phosphorylation, palmitoylation, and ubiquitination. These modifications regulate receptor activity, desensitization, and internalization. For example, phosphorylation of dopamine receptors by kinases can lead to receptor desensitization, reducing their responsiveness to dopamine.

Regulation of Dopamine Receptors

The regulation of dopamine receptors involves multiple mechanisms to ensure appropriate cellular responses to dopamine.

Desensitization and Downregulation

Prolonged exposure to dopamine can lead to receptor desensitization, where the receptor's responsiveness is diminished. This is often followed by downregulation, where the number of receptors on the cell surface is reduced. Desensitization involves receptor phosphorylation by kinases, such as GRKs, leading to the binding of β-arrestins, which uncouple the receptors from G proteins and target them for internalization.

Receptor Recycling and Degradation

Internalized receptors can either be recycled back to the cell membrane or degraded in lysosomes. The balance between these processes determines the overall number of functional receptors on the cell surface. Recycling allows the cell to quickly restore receptor sensitivity, while degradation reduces receptor density, providing long-term regulation.

Role of Plant-Based Compounds in Regulation

Plant-based diets can influence the regulation of dopamine receptors through various bioactive compounds. Phytochemicals, such as flavonoids, have been shown to modulate receptor activity and expression.

Flavonoids

Flavonoids are a group of polyphenolic compounds found in fruits, vegetables, tea, and other plant-based foods. They have been reported to influence dopamine signaling pathways by modulating receptor activity and expression. For instance, quercetin, a flavonoid found in apples, onions, and berries, can enhance D1 receptor-mediated signaling and protect dopaminergic neurons from oxidative stress.

Polyphenols

Polyphenols, found in foods like grapes, berries, and green tea, have neuroprotective properties and can modulate dopamine receptor function. Resveratrol, a polyphenol in red grapes, has been shown to enhance dopamine D2 receptor signaling and improve cognitive function in animal models of neurodegenerative diseases.

Omega-3 Fatty Acids

Plant sources of omega-3 fatty acids, such as flaxseeds and chia seeds, have anti-inflammatory properties and can influence dopaminergic signaling. Omega-3 fatty acids have been shown to increase the expression of D2 receptors and improve dopamine-related behaviors, potentially benefiting conditions like ADHD and depression.

Plant-Based Diets and Dopamine Receptors

Adopting a plant-based diet can significantly impact the regulation and function of dopamine receptors. The intake of various nutrients and bioactive compounds from plants can modulate the dopaminergic system, contributing to overall mental and neurological health.

Cognitive Health

Plant-based diets are rich in antioxidants, dietary fiber, and healthy fats, which are beneficial for cognitive health. The regulation of D1 receptors in the brain can be positively influenced by these dietary components. For example, antioxidants can reduce oxidative stress, which is known to impair D1 receptor function. Additionally, dietary fiber helps in managing blood sugar levels, which can influence dopamine metabolism and cognitive functions.

Emotional and Behavioral Health

The influence of plant-based diets on D2 and D3 dopamine receptors can enhance emotional and behavioral health. Foods rich in flavonoids and omega-3 fatty acids can improve mood and reduce the risk of psychiatric disorders such as depression and anxiety. By modulating D2 and D3 receptor activity, these diets can enhance reward-related behaviors and emotional regulation.

Neuroprotection

Dopamine receptors, particularly D4 and D5, play a role in neuroprotection. Plant-based diets, which are typically high in antioxidants and polyphenols, can support the neuroprotective functions of these receptors. The presence of bioactive compounds in plant foods can protect dopaminergic neurons from oxidative stress and inflammation, aiding in the prevention of neurodegenerative diseases like Parkinson's and Alzheimer's.

Dopamine receptors are essential for various neurological processes, including cognitive functions, emotional regulation, and motor control. The production and regulation of these receptors involve complex mechanisms influenced by genetic and environmental factors.

Serotonin Receptors (5-HT1, 5-HT2, 5-HT3, 5-HT4)

Serotonin receptors (5-HT receptors) are a class of G protein-coupled receptors and ligand-gated ion channels found in the central and peripheral nervous systems. These receptors mediate the effects of serotonin (5-hydroxytryptamine, 5-HT), a key neurotransmitter involved in regulating mood, cognition, reward, learning, memory, and numerous physiological processes. There are several subtypes of serotonin receptors, including 5-HT1, 5-HT2, 5-HT3, and 5-HT4, each with distinct functions and tissue distributions.

Function of Serotonin Receptors

5-HT1 Receptors

5-HT1 receptors are primarily inhibitory and are found in both the central and peripheral nervous systems. The 5-HT1 receptor family includes several subtypes, such as 5-HT1A, 5-HT1B, 5-HT1D, 5-HT1E, and 5-HT1F. These receptors play crucial roles in regulating mood, anxiety, and thermoregulation.

- **5-HT1A Receptors**: These are located in brain regions like the hippocampus, cortex, and raphe nuclei. Activation of 5-HT1A receptors leads to inhibition of adenylate cyclase, resulting in reduced cAMP levels and neuronal hyperpolarization. This receptor is implicated in the anxiolytic and antidepressant effects of serotonin, as well as in thermoregulation and feeding behavior.
- **5-HT1B and 5-HT1D Receptors**: These receptors are involved in vasoconstriction and are targets for triptans, a class of drugs

used to treat migraines. They also play a role in the modulation of neurotransmitter release, particularly in the basal ganglia and other areas associated with movement and reward.

5-HT2 Receptors

5-HT2 receptors are excitatory and are found in various tissues, including the brain, cardiovascular system, and gastrointestinal tract. The 5-HT2 receptor family includes 5-HT2A, 5-HT2B, and 5-HT2C receptors.

- **5-HT2A Receptors**: These are widely distributed in the cortex, and their activation leads to an increase in intracellular calcium levels and protein kinase C activity. 5-HT2A receptors are involved in the regulation of mood, perception, and cognition. They are the primary targets for many psychedelic substances, such as LSD and psilocybin.
- **5-HT2B Receptors**: Found in the heart, gut, and brain, 5-HT2B receptors play roles in cardiovascular function, smooth muscle contraction, and gut motility. Overactivation of 5-HT2B receptors has been associated with valvular heart disease.
- **5-HT2C Receptors**: These receptors are primarily located in the choroid plexus and the brain. Activation of 5-HT2C receptors influences appetite, mood, and endocrine secretion. They are targets for drugs used in the treatment of obesity and mood disorders.

5-HT3 Receptors

5-HT3 receptors are unique among serotonin receptors because they are ligand-gated ion channels rather than G protein-coupled receptors. These receptors are found in the central and peripheral nervous systems, particularly in the brainstem and gastrointestinal tract.

- **Function**: Activation of 5-HT3 receptors results in rapid depolarization of neurons by allowing the influx of cations such as sodium and calcium. They play a critical role in nausea and vomiting, particularly in response to chemotherapy. 5-HT3 receptor antagonists, such as ondansetron, are used to prevent chemotherapy-induced nausea and vomiting.

5-HT4 Receptors

5-HT4 receptors are G protein-coupled receptors found in the brain, heart, and gastrointestinal tract.

- **Function**: Activation of 5-HT4 receptors stimulates adenylate cyclase, increasing cAMP levels and promoting smooth muscle relaxation and enhanced gastrointestinal motility. These receptors are involved in cognitive processes and have been investigated for their potential role in treating Alzheimer's disease and other cognitive disorders.

Production of Serotonin Receptors

The production of serotonin receptors involves gene expression, receptor synthesis, and post-translational modifications. Each subtype of the serotonin receptor is encoded by distinct genes, and their expression is regulated by various factors, including developmental cues, hormonal influences, and environmental factors.

Gene Expression

- **5-HT1 Receptors**: The genes encoding the 5-HT1 receptor subtypes are HTR1A, HTR1B, HTR1D, HTR1E, and HTR1F. Their expression is regulated by transcription factors and promoter regions specific to each gene. For example, the HTR1A gene is influenced by factors such as stress and glucocorticoids, which can affect its expression levels.

- **5-HT2 Receptors**: The genes for the 5-HT2 receptors are HTR2A, HTR2B, and HTR2C. The expression of these genes can be modulated by various factors, including neurotransmitter levels, hormonal changes, and pharmacological agents. For instance, antipsychotic drugs can upregulate HTR2A expression, influencing the density of 5-HT2A receptors in the brain.
- **5-HT3 Receptors**: The 5-HT3 receptor is encoded by the HTR3A and HTR3B genes. The regulation of these genes involves multiple promoter elements and transcription factors that respond to neural activity and environmental cues.
- **5-HT4 Receptors**: The HTR4 gene encodes the 5-HT4 receptor, and its expression is regulated by factors such as neuronal activity, hormonal status, and developmental signals.

Receptor Synthesis

Once transcribed, the mRNA of serotonin receptors is translated into protein in the endoplasmic reticulum. These proteins undergo folding and glycosylation, essential for their proper function and stability. The receptors are then transported to the cell membrane, where they become functional.

Post-Translational Modifications

Serotonin receptors undergo various post-translational modifications that regulate their activity, desensitization, and internalization. These modifications include phosphorylation, palmitoylation, and glycosylation.

- **Phosphorylation**: This modification involves the addition of phosphate groups by kinases such as PKA and PKC, which can influence receptor activity and signaling. For example, phosphorylation of 5-HT1A receptors can modulate their coupling to G proteins and downstream signaling pathways.
- **Palmitoylation**: This lipid modification enhances the receptor's membrane association and stability. Palmitoylation of 5-HT1A

receptors is crucial for their localization and function in the neuronal membrane.

- **Glycosylation**: The addition of carbohydrate groups to the receptor protein can affect its folding, stability, and cell surface expression. Glycosylation is essential for the proper function of receptors like 5-HT3, which require this modification for efficient ion channel activity.

Regulation of Serotonin Receptors

The regulation of serotonin receptors involves mechanisms to ensure appropriate cellular responses to serotonin.

Desensitization and Downregulation

Prolonged exposure to agonists can lead to receptor desensitization, where the receptor's responsiveness is diminished. This is often followed by downregulation, where the number of receptors on the cell surface is reduced. These processes are crucial in preventing overstimulation and maintaining homeostasis.

- **Desensitization**: Involves receptor phosphorylation by kinases such as GRKs, leading to the binding of β-arrestins, which uncouple the receptors from G proteins and target them for internalization. For example, chronic activation of 5-HT2A receptors can lead to desensitization and reduced receptor density.
- **Downregulation**: Involves the internalization and degradation of receptors in lysosomes. The balance between receptor recycling and degradation determines the overall number of functional receptors on the cell surface.

Receptor Recycling and Degradation

Internalized receptors can either be recycled back to the cell membrane or degraded in lysosomes. The balance between these processes determines the overall number of functional receptors on the cell surface. Recycling allows the cell to quickly restore receptor sensitivity, while degradation reduces the receptor density, providing long-term regulation.

Role of Plant-Based Compounds in Regulation

Plant-based diets can influence the regulation of serotonin receptors through various bioactive compounds. Phytochemicals, such as flavonoids, have been shown to modulate receptor activity and expression.

- **Flavonoids**: These are polyphenolic compounds found in fruits, vegetables, tea, and other plant-based foods. They have been reported to influence serotonin receptor signaling pathways. For instance, quercetin, a flavonoid found in apples, onions, and berries, can modulate 5-HT receptor activity and has potential anxiolytic and antidepressant effects.
- **Dietary Fiber**: High-fiber diets typical of plant-based nutrition can improve gut health and influence serotonin levels. The gut microbiota can metabolize dietary fiber into short-chain fatty acids, which can modulate the gut-brain axis and serotonin signaling.
- **Omega-3 Fatty Acids**: Plant sources of omega-3 fatty acids, such as flaxseeds and chia seeds, have anti-inflammatory properties and can influence serotonin receptor function. Omega-3 fatty acids have been shown to modulate the expression and activity of serotonin receptors, potentially impacting mood and cognitive functions.

Plant-Based Diets and Serotonin Receptors

Adopting a plant-based diet can have significant impacts on the regulation and function of serotonin receptors. The intake of various nutrients and bioactive compounds from plants can modulate the serotonergic system, contributing to overall health benefits.

Mood and Mental Health

Plant-based diets are rich in antioxidants, dietary fiber, and healthy fats, which are beneficial for mental health. The regulation of 5-HT1A and 5-HT2A receptors in the brain can be positively influenced by these dietary components. For example, antioxidants can reduce oxidative stress, which is known to impair receptor function. Additionally, dietary fiber helps in managing gut health, which is linked to serotonin production and mental well-being.

Cardiovascular Health

The influence of plant-based diets on 5-HT2B receptors can enhance cardiovascular health. Foods rich in flavonoids and omega-3 fatty acids can improve endothelial function and reduce the risk of cardiovascular diseases. By modulating 5-HT2B receptor activity, these diets can promote vascular health and reduce the incidence of hypertension and atherosclerosis.

Gastrointestinal Health

5-HT3 and 5-HT4 receptors play crucial roles in gut motility and function. Plant-based diets, which are typically high in fiber, can support gastrointestinal health by enhancing the function of these receptors. The presence of bioactive compounds in plant foods can stimulate receptor-mediated gut motility, aiding in the prevention of constipation and other gastrointestinal disorders.

Cognitive Health

Plant-based diets can benefit cognitive health through the regulation of 5-HT4 receptors. The intake of antioxidants and omega-3 fatty acids from plant sources can support cognitive functions and reduce the risk of neurodegenerative diseases. By modulating 5-HT4 receptor activity, these diets can enhance memory, learning, and overall brain health.

Weight Management

Serotonin receptors, particularly 5-HT2C, play a role in appetite regulation and energy balance. Plant-based diets, which are typically lower in calories and higher in fiber, can support weight management by enhancing the function of these receptors. The presence of bioactive compounds in plant foods can modulate serotonin signaling pathways, aiding in appetite control and promoting healthy weight loss.

Serotonin receptors are essential for various physiological processes, including mood regulation, cardiovascular function, gut motility, and cognitive health. The production and regulation of these receptors involve complex mechanisms influenced by genetic and environmental factors.

Histamine Receptors (H1, H2, H3, H4)

Histamine receptors are a class of G protein-coupled receptors (GPCRs) that mediate the effects of histamine, a biogenic amine involved in local immune responses, regulating physiological function in the gut, and acting as a neurotransmitter. These receptors are divided into four main subtypes: H1, H2, H3, and H4, each with distinct functions, tissue distributions, and regulatory mechanisms.

Function of Histamine Receptors

H1 Receptors

H1 receptors are primarily found in smooth muscles, endothelial cells, and the central nervous system (CNS). Their activation is involved in allergic reactions, promoting symptoms such as vasodilation, increased vascular permeability, and bronchoconstriction. In the CNS, H1 receptors play a role in regulating wakefulness and cognitive functions.

Allergic Reactions

H1 receptors are key mediators of allergic responses. Upon activation by histamine, these receptors cause vasodilation and increased permeability of blood vessels, leading to symptoms such as redness, swelling, and itchiness. This is a protective mechanism that facilitates the arrival of immune cells to the site of injury or infection.

CNS Functions

In the brain, H1 receptors are involved in the regulation of sleep-wake cycles and cognitive processes. Histamine, acting through H1 receptors, promotes wakefulness and alertness. Antihistamines that block H1 receptors can cause drowsiness, highlighting the role of these receptors in maintaining wakefulness.

H2 Receptors

H2 receptors are predominantly located in the stomach, heart, and various other tissues. Their primary function is to regulate gastric acid secretion, but they also play roles in modulating heart rate and immune responses.

Gastric Acid Secretion

H2 receptors in the stomach are found on the parietal cells, where their activation by histamine stimulates the production and release of gastric acid. This process is crucial for digestion and maintaining the acidic environment of the stomach, which helps in the breakdown of food and the elimination of pathogens.

Cardiovascular Functions

H2 receptors also influence cardiovascular function by modulating heart rate and the force of cardiac contractions. They can cause vasodilation and are involved in regulating blood pressure.

H3 Receptors

H3 receptors are primarily located in the central and peripheral nervous systems. They act as auto-receptors, modulating the release of histamine and other neurotransmitters.

Neurotransmitter Regulation

H3 receptors regulate the release of histamine and other neurotransmitters, including dopamine, serotonin, and acetylcholine. This modulation is essential for maintaining neurotransmitter balance and proper functioning of the nervous system.

Cognitive and Behavioral Functions

H3 receptors play a role in cognitive and behavioral functions, including learning, memory, and attention. Their regulation of neurotransmitter release influences various neural circuits involved in these processes.

H4 Receptors

H4 receptors are predominantly expressed in bone marrow and white blood cells, such as eosinophils, mast cells, and dendritic cells. They are involved in immune response modulation and inflammatory processes.

Immune Response

H4 receptors are involved in the chemotaxis of immune cells to sites of inflammation. They play a role in the regulation of immune cell migration and the release of pro-inflammatory cytokines, contributing to the body's defense mechanisms.

Inflammatory Processes

By modulating the activity of immune cells, H4 receptors influence the inflammatory response. This makes them potential targets for the treatment of inflammatory and autoimmune diseases.

Production of Histamine Receptors

The production of histamine receptors is a complex process regulated at the genetic and molecular levels. The genes encoding these receptors are HRH1, HRH2, HRH3, and HRH4.

Gene Expression

Gene expression of histamine receptors is controlled by various transcription factors and regulatory elements. These include promoter regions upstream of the HRH genes that bind specific proteins to initiate transcription. The expression of these genes can be influenced by several factors, including hormones, stress, and dietary components.

HRH1 Gene

The HRH1 gene encodes the H1 receptor. Its expression is regulated by factors such as inflammatory cytokines and hormones, which can increase or decrease receptor levels in response to physiological needs.

HRH2 Gene

The HRH2 gene encodes the H2 receptor. Gastric hormones such as gastrin and somatostatin regulate the expression of this gene, influencing gastric acid secretion.

HRH3 Gene

The HRH3 gene encodes the H3 receptor. Its expression is primarily regulated by neural activity and various neurotransmitters, reflecting its role in the nervous system.

HRH4 Gene

The HRH4 gene encodes the H4 receptor. The expression of this gene is regulated by immune signals and cytokines, aligning with its role in immune response modulation.

Receptor Synthesis

Once transcribed, the mRNA of histamine receptors is translated into protein in the endoplasmic reticulum. These proteins undergo folding and glycosylation, essential for their proper function and stability. The receptors are then transported to the cell membrane, where they become functional.

Post-Translational Modifications

Histamine receptors undergo various post-translational modifications, such as phosphorylation and glycosylation, which regulate their activity, desensitization, and internalization. Phosphorylation of these receptors by kinases can lead to receptor desensitization, reducing their responsiveness to histamine.

Regulation of Histamine Receptors

The regulation of histamine receptors involves multiple mechanisms to ensure appropriate cellular responses to histamine.

Desensitization and Downregulation

Prolonged exposure to histamine can lead to receptor desensitization, where the receptor's responsiveness is diminished. This is often followed by downregulation, where the number of receptors on the cell surface is reduced. These processes are crucial in preventing overstimulation and maintaining homeostasis.

H1 Receptors

Desensitization of H1 receptors involves phosphorylation by specific kinases, leading to receptor internalization and reduced cell surface expression. This prevents excessive allergic reactions and maintains balance.

H2 Receptors

H2 receptor regulation involves mechanisms such as receptor phosphorylation and interaction with regulatory proteins. This modulation ensures appropriate gastric acid secretion and cardiovascular responses.

Receptor Recycling and Degradation

Internalized receptors can either be recycled back to the cell membrane or degraded in lysosomes. The balance between these processes determines the overall number of functional receptors on the cell surface.

H3 Receptors

H3 receptors undergo recycling and degradation processes that regulate their availability and function in the nervous system. This modulation is essential for maintaining neurotransmitter balance.

H4 Receptors

The regulation of H4 receptors involves similar mechanisms, ensuring appropriate immune responses and preventing excessive inflammation.

Role of Plant-Based Compounds in Regulation

Plant-based diets can influence the regulation of histamine receptors through various bioactive compounds. Phytochemicals, such as flavonoids, have been shown to modulate receptor activity and expression.

Flavonoids

Flavonoids are a group of polyphenolic compounds found in fruits, vegetables, tea, and other plant-based foods. They have been reported to influence histamine receptor signaling pathways.

Quercetin

Quercetin, a flavonoid found in apples, onions, and berries, can inhibit histamine release from mast cells and reduce H1 receptor-mediated allergic responses.

Resveratrol

Resveratrol, found in grapes and red wine, has anti-inflammatory properties and can modulate H2 receptor activity, reducing gastric acid secretion and protecting against ulcers.

Curcumin

Curcumin, the active compound in turmeric, has been shown to inhibit histamine release and H1 receptor activity, contributing to its anti-inflammatory and anti-allergic effects.

Dietary Fiber

High-fiber diets, typical of plant-based nutrition, can improve gut health and reduce inflammation, indirectly influencing histamine receptor activity. Fiber can modulate the gut microbiota, leading to the production of short-chain fatty acids (SCFAs) that have anti-inflammatory effects.

Omega-3 Fatty Acids

Plant sources of omega-3 fatty acids, such as flaxseeds and chia seeds, have anti-inflammatory properties and can influence histamine receptor function. Omega-3 fatty acids can reduce the expression of histamine receptors in immune cells, potentially affecting allergic and inflammatory responses.

Plant-Based Diets and Histamine Receptors

Adopting a plant-based diet can have significant impacts on the regulation and function of histamine receptors. The intake of various nutrients and bioactive compounds from plants can modulate the histaminergic system, contributing to overall health benefits.

Cardiovascular Health

Plant-based diets are rich in antioxidants, dietary fiber, and healthy fats, which are beneficial for cardiovascular health. The regulation of H2 receptors in the heart can be positively influenced by these dietary components. For example, antioxidants can reduce oxidative stress, which is known to impair H2 receptor function.

Allergic and Inflammatory Conditions

The influence of plant-based diets on H1 and H4 receptors can help manage allergic and inflammatory conditions. Foods rich in flavonoids and omega-3 fatty acids can reduce histamine release and receptor activity, alleviating symptoms of allergies and inflammation.

Gastrointestinal Health

H2 receptors play a crucial role in gastric acid secretion and gastrointestinal health. Plant-based diets, which are typically lower in fat and higher in fiber, can support digestive health by modulating H2 receptor activity and reducing the risk of acid-related disorders.

Neurological Health

H3 receptors are involved in cognitive and behavioral functions. Plant-based diets rich in antioxidants and anti-inflammatory compounds can protect neural tissues and support healthy brain function by modulating H3 receptor activity.

Histamine receptors are essential for various physiological processes, including immune responses, gastric acid secretion, and neurotransmitter regulation.

Muscarinic Acetylcholine Receptors (M1, M2, M3, M4, M5)

Muscarinic acetylcholine receptors (mAChRs) are a class of G protein-coupled receptors (GPCRs) that are activated by the neurotransmitter acetylcholine. These receptors play vital roles in various physiological processes, including modulation of neurotransmission, smooth muscle contraction, and glandular secretion. There are five distinct subtypes of muscarinic receptors: M1, M2, M3, M4, and M5, each with specific functions and tissue distributions.

Function of Muscarinic Acetylcholine Receptors

M1 Muscarinic Receptors

M1 receptors are primarily located in the central nervous system (CNS), including the cerebral cortex, hippocampus, and striatum. They are involved in cognitive functions such as learning and memory. Activation of M1 receptors enhances synaptic plasticity and neuronal excitability, contributing to the processes underlying memory formation and retention. Additionally, M1 receptors play a role in the modulation of pain perception and are implicated in various neuropsychiatric disorders, including schizophrenia and Alzheimer's disease.

M2 Muscarinic Receptors

M2 receptors are predominantly found in the heart, where they mediate parasympathetic control of cardiac function. Activation of M2 receptors results in a decrease in heart rate (negative chronotropy) and reduction of the force of contraction (negative inotropy), primarily through inhibition of adenylate cyclase and subsequent reduction in cyclic AMP levels. M2 receptors are also present in the CNS and play a role in regulating neurotransmitter release and synaptic transmission.

M3 Muscarinic Receptors

M3 receptors are widely distributed in smooth muscles and glandular tissues. Their activation leads to smooth muscle contraction and glandular secretion. In the gastrointestinal tract, M3 receptors facilitate peristalsis and secretion of digestive enzymes. In the respiratory system, they induce bronchoconstriction, while in the urinary system, they promote bladder contraction. M3 receptors also stimulate secretion from exocrine glands, such as salivary and sweat glands.

M4 Muscarinic Receptors

M4 receptors are primarily expressed in the CNS, particularly in the striatum and cerebral cortex. They play a role in modulating dopaminergic neurotransmission and are involved in motor control and cognitive processes. M4 receptors are also implicated in the pathophysiology of various neurological disorders, including Parkinson's disease and addiction. Activation of M4 receptors can inhibit the release of certain neurotransmitters, thus modulating synaptic activity and neuronal signaling.

M5 Muscarinic Receptors

M5 receptors are the least understood of the muscarinic receptor subtypes, with limited expression in the CNS and peripheral tissues. They are found in the substantia nigra and ventral tegmental area, regions associated with dopaminergic signaling. M5 receptors are believed to play a role in regulating cerebral blood flow and modulating dopamine release. Emerging evidence suggests that M5 receptors may be involved in addiction and reward mechanisms.

Production of Muscarinic Acetylcholine Receptors

The production of muscarinic acetylcholine receptors involves several steps, including gene expression, receptor synthesis, and post-translational modifications.

Gene Expression

The genes encoding muscarinic receptors are CHRM1, CHRM2, CHRM3, CHRM4, and CHRM5. The expression of these genes is regulated by various transcription factors and promoter regions. Factors such as neuronal activity, hormonal changes, and dietary components can influence the transcription of muscarinic receptor genes. For example, certain plant-derived compounds, such as polyphenols, have been shown to modulate gene expression by interacting with transcription factors.

Receptor Synthesis

Once transcribed, the mRNA of muscarinic receptors is translated into protein in the endoplasmic reticulum. These proteins undergo folding and glycosylation, processes essential for their proper function and stability. Chaperone proteins assist in the correct folding of the receptors, ensuring they attain their functional conformation. The synthesized receptors are then transported to the Golgi apparatus for further processing and eventual delivery to the cell membrane.

Post-Translational Modifications

Muscarinic receptors undergo various post-translational modifications, such as phosphorylation, which regulate their activity and localization. Phosphorylation by kinases can modulate receptor sensitivity, desensitization, and internalization. Additionally, glycosylation and palmitoylation of muscarinic receptors play critical roles in their stability and membrane localization. These modifications ensure that the receptors are correctly positioned and functional on the cell surface.

Regulation of Muscarinic Acetylcholine Receptors

The regulation of muscarinic acetylcholine receptors involves multiple mechanisms to ensure appropriate cellular responses to acetylcholine.

Desensitization and Downregulation

Prolonged exposure to agonists can lead to receptor desensitization, where the receptor's responsiveness diminishes. This is often followed by downregulation, where the number of receptors on the cell surface is reduced. These processes are crucial in preventing overstimulation and maintaining homeostasis. Desensitization involves receptor phosphorylation by kinases such as GRKs, leading to the binding of β-arrestins, which uncouple the receptors from G proteins and target them for internalization.

Receptor Recycling and Degradation

Internalized receptors can either be recycled back to the cell membrane or degraded in lysosomes. The balance between these processes determines the overall number of functional receptors on the cell surface. Recycling allows the cell to quickly restore receptor sensitivity, while degradation reduces the receptor density, providing long-term regulation.

Role of Plant-Based Compounds in Regulation

Plant-based diets can influence the regulation of muscarinic receptors through various bioactive compounds. Phytochemicals, such as flavonoids and polyphenols, have been shown to modulate receptor activity and expression.

Flavonoids

Flavonoids are a group of polyphenolic compounds found in fruits, vegetables, tea, and other plant-based foods. They have been reported to influence the muscarinic signaling pathway by modulating receptor activity and gene expression. For instance, quercetin, a flavonoid found in apples, onions, and berries, can enhance M1 receptor-mediated cognitive functions and reduce oxidative stress in neuronal cells.

Polyphenols

Polyphenols, abundant in plant-based foods, can interact with muscarinic receptors and influence their regulation. Resveratrol, a polyphenol found in grapes and red wine, has been shown to enhance M2 receptor-mediated cardioprotective effects by reducing oxidative stress and inflammation in cardiac tissues. Additionally, polyphenols can modulate the expression of muscarinic receptors through their antioxidant properties, protecting cells from oxidative damage and maintaining receptor function.

Omega-3 Fatty Acids

Plant sources of omega-3 fatty acids, such as flaxseeds and chia seeds, have anti-inflammatory properties and can influence muscarinic receptor function. Omega-3 fatty acids have been shown to modulate M3 receptor activity in smooth muscle cells, potentially affecting gastrointestinal motility and secretion. These fatty acids can also reduce inflammation in glandular tissues, enhancing M3 receptor-mediated secretory functions.

Plant-Based Diets and Muscarinic Acetylcholine Receptors

Adopting a plant-based diet can have significant impacts on the regulation and function of muscarinic acetylcholine receptors. The intake of various nutrients and bioactive compounds from plants can modulate the muscarinic system, contributing to overall health benefits.

Cognitive Health

Plant-based diets rich in antioxidants, polyphenols, and flavonoids can support cognitive health by modulating M1 receptor activity. These compounds can enhance synaptic plasticity, protect neuronal cells from oxidative stress, and improve memory and learning functions. For example, a diet high in berries, rich in flavonoids, has been associated with improved cognitive performance and a reduced risk of neurodegenerative diseases.

Cardiovascular Health

The regulation of M2 receptors in the heart can be positively influenced by plant-based dietary components. Antioxidants from plant foods can reduce oxidative stress, which is known to impair M2 receptor function. Additionally, dietary polyphenols can enhance the cardioprotective effects of M2 receptors by reducing inflammation and improving endothelial function. Consuming a diet rich in fruits, vegetables, and whole grains can support cardiovascular health by modulating M2 receptor activity and maintaining heart function.

Gastrointestinal Health

M3 receptors play a crucial role in gastrointestinal motility and secretion. A plant-based diet, high in fiber and plant-derived bioactive compounds, can support gastrointestinal health by modulating M3 receptor activity. Dietary fiber improves gut motility and facilitates the secretion of digestive enzymes, while polyphenols can reduce inflammation and oxidative stress in the gastrointestinal tract. This combination promotes healthy digestion and prevents gastrointestinal disorders.

Respiratory Health

Plant-based diets can benefit respiratory health by modulating M3 receptor activity in the airways. Flavonoids and polyphenols from plant foods can reduce bronchoconstriction and inflammation, enhancing M3 receptor-mediated bronchodilation. For individuals with respiratory conditions such as asthma, a diet rich in plant-based antioxidants can improve lung function and reduce the frequency and severity of asthma attacks.

Metabolic Health

M4 receptors are involved in the regulation of metabolic processes, including insulin secretion and glucose homeostasis. Plant-based diets, rich in fiber, antioxidants, and anti-inflammatory compounds, can enhance M4 receptor function and improve metabolic health. For instance, dietary fiber improves insulin sensitivity, while polyphenols reduce oxidative stress and inflammation, supporting overall metabolic function. This can reduce the risk of metabolic disorders such as type 2 diabetes.

Neurological Health

M5 receptors, though less understood, are believed to play a role in dopaminergic signaling and neurological health. Plant-based diets, which provide a variety of bioactive compounds, can support the function of M5 receptors and protect against neurodegenerative diseases. Antioxidants and polyphenols from plant foods can reduce oxidative stress and inflammation in the brain, promoting healthy dopaminergic signaling and reducing the risk of neurological disorders.

Muscarinic acetylcholine receptors are essential for various physiological processes, including cognitive function, cardiovascular health, gastrointestinal motility, respiratory function, and metabolic regulation. The production and regulation of these receptors involve complex mechanisms influenced by genetic and environmental factors. Adopting a plant-based diet can significantly impact the regulation and function of muscarinic receptors, providing overall health benefits. Bioactive compounds from plant foods, such as flavonoids, polyphenols, and omega-3 fatty acids, can modulate receptor activity and expression, enhancing the body's ability to maintain homeostasis and prevent disease.

Opioid Receptors (Mu, Delta, Kappa)

Opioid receptors are a class of G protein-coupled receptors (GPCRs) that are primarily involved in the modulation of pain and analgesia, but also play roles in mood regulation, immune response, and gastrointestinal function. There are three main subtypes of opioid receptors: Mu (μ), Delta (δ), and Kappa (κ), each with distinct functions and tissue distributions.

Function of Opioid Receptors

Mu (μ) Opioid Receptors

Mu opioid receptors (MOR) are predominantly found in the brain, spinal cord, and digestive tract. Their activation is primarily associated with analgesic effects, making them critical targets for pain management. Activation of MOR leads to:

- **Analgesia**: MORs are highly effective in reducing both acute and chronic pain by inhibiting pain signals in the central and peripheral nervous systems.
- **Euphoria**: Stimulation of MORs in the brain's reward centers can produce feelings of euphoria, which is why opioids can be addictive.
- **Respiratory Depression**: MOR activation can depress respiratory function, which is a major risk factor in opioid overdose.

- **Gastrointestinal Effects**: MORs in the digestive tract slow down gastrointestinal motility, often leading to constipation.

Delta (δ) Opioid Receptors

Delta opioid receptors (DOR) are found in the brain and peripheral nervous system. They play a role in modulating mood and emotional responses. Key functions include:

- **Analgesia**: DORs contribute to pain relief, although to a lesser extent than MORs.
- **Antidepressant Effects**: Activation of DORs has been shown to produce antidepressant-like effects, potentially making them targets for mood disorder treatments.
- **Neuroprotection**: DOR activation has neuroprotective effects and may protect against neurodegenerative diseases.

Kappa (κ) Opioid Receptors

Kappa opioid receptors (KOR) are located in the brain, spinal cord, and some peripheral tissues. Their activation produces effects that are often opposite to those of MORs. These include:

- **Analgesia**: KORs are involved in pain relief, particularly in spinal-level analgesia.
- **Dysphoria**: Activation of KORs can lead to feelings of dysphoria and anxiety, which limits their use in pain management.
- **Diuresis**: KOR activation can increase urine production by influencing kidney function.
- **Antipruritic Effects**: KORs can reduce itching, making them useful in treating pruritus.

Production of Opioid Receptors

The production of opioid receptors is regulated at multiple levels, including gene expression, receptor synthesis, and post-translational modifications. The genes encoding μ, δ, and κ receptors are OPRM1, OPRD1, and OPRK1, respectively.

Gene Expression

Gene expression of opioid receptors is controlled by various transcription factors and regulatory elements. These include promoter regions upstream of the OPR genes that bind specific proteins to initiate transcription. Factors influencing their expression include stress, hormones, and dietary components.

Receptor Synthesis

Once transcribed, the mRNA of opioid receptors is translated into protein in the endoplasmic reticulum. These proteins undergo folding and glycosylation, which are essential for their proper function and stability. The receptors are then transported to the cell membrane, where they become functional.

Post-Translational Modifications

Opioid receptors undergo various post-translational modifications, such as phosphorylation, which regulate their activity, desensitization, and internalization. Phosphorylation of these receptors by kinases can lead to receptor desensitization, reducing their responsiveness to agonists.

Regulation of Opioid Receptors

The regulation of opioid receptors involves multiple mechanisms to ensure appropriate cellular responses to endogenous and exogenous opioids.

Desensitization and Downregulation

Prolonged exposure to agonists can lead to receptor desensitization, where the receptor's responsiveness is diminished. This is often followed by downregulation, where the number of receptors on the cell surface is reduced. These processes are crucial in preventing overstimulation and maintaining homeostasis. Desensitization involves receptor phosphorylation by kinases, leading to the binding of β-arrestins, which uncouple the receptors from G proteins and target them for internalization.

Receptor Recycling and Degradation

Internalized receptors can either be recycled back to the cell membrane or degraded in lysosomes. The balance between these processes determines the overall number of functional receptors on the cell surface. Recycling allows the cell to quickly restore receptor sensitivity, while degradation reduces the receptor density, providing long-term regulation.

Role of Plant-Based Compounds in Regulation

Plant-based diets can influence the regulation of opioid receptors through various bioactive compounds. Phytochemicals, such as flavonoids, alkaloids, and terpenes, have been shown to modulate receptor activity and expression.

Flavonoids

Flavonoids are a group of polyphenolic compounds found in fruits, vegetables, tea, and other plant-based foods. They have been reported to influence the opioid signaling pathway by inhibiting receptor-mediated responses. For instance, quercetin, a flavonoid found in apples, onions, and berries, can modulate opioid receptor activity and enhance analgesic effects.

Alkaloids

Certain plant alkaloids, such as those found in Kratom (Mitragyna speciosa), can interact with opioid receptors. Mitragynine and 7-hydroxymitragynine, the primary active compounds in Kratom, have been shown to act on opioid receptors, providing pain relief and mood enhancement.

Terpenes

Terpenes, such as those found in cannabis (e.g., beta-caryophyllene), can interact with opioid receptors and modulate their effects. These compounds can enhance the analgesic properties of endogenous opioids and reduce inflammation.

Plant-Based Diets and Opioid Receptors

Adopting a plant-based diet can have significant impacts on the regulation and function of opioid receptors. The intake of various nutrients and bioactive compounds from plants can modulate the opioid system, contributing to overall health benefits.

Pain Management

Plant-based diets rich in anti-inflammatory compounds, such as flavonoids and omega-3 fatty acids, can enhance the body's natural pain relief mechanisms. By modulating opioid receptor activity, these diets can provide effective pain management without the risks associated with opioid medications.

Mood Regulation

The influence of plant-based diets on DORs can improve mood and reduce the risk of mood disorders. Foods rich in phytochemicals, such as berries, nuts, and seeds, can enhance the production and function of neurotransmitters that interact with opioid receptors, promoting emotional well-being.

Immune Function

Opioid receptors play a role in modulating immune responses. Plant-based diets, which are high in antioxidants and anti-inflammatory compounds, can support immune function by regulating opioid receptor activity in immune cells. This can help in reducing chronic inflammation and enhancing immune defense.

Gastrointestinal Health

A diet rich in fiber and plant-based compounds can support gastrointestinal health by modulating the activity of opioid receptors in the digestive tract. This can help in managing conditions like irritable bowel syndrome (IBS) and promoting overall gut health.

Angiotensin Receptors (AT1, AT2)

Angiotensin receptors, specifically the subtypes AT1 and AT2, are critical components of the renin-angiotensin system (RAS), playing essential roles in the regulation of blood pressure, fluid balance, and cardiovascular health. These receptors are G protein-coupled receptors activated by the peptide hormone angiotensin II.

Function of Angiotensin Receptors

AT1 Receptors

AT1 receptors are the primary mediators of the classical actions of angiotensin II. These receptors are widely distributed in various tissues, including the heart, blood vessels, kidneys, and adrenal glands. Activation of AT1 receptors leads to several physiological responses:

1. **Vasoconstriction**: Angiotensin II binding to AT1 receptors on vascular smooth muscle cells causes vasoconstriction, leading to an increase in blood pressure.
2. **Aldosterone Secretion**: In the adrenal cortex, AT1 receptor activation stimulates the release of aldosterone, a hormone that promotes sodium and water reabsorption in the kidneys, further contributing to blood pressure regulation.
3. **Cardiac Effects**: AT1 receptors in the heart mediate cardiac hypertrophy and fibrosis, which can be detrimental in conditions of chronic high blood pressure.
4. **Renal Effects**: In the kidneys, AT1 receptor activation enhances sodium reabsorption, contributing to the regulation of fluid and electrolyte balance.

5. **Sympathetic Nervous System**: AT1 receptors also influence the sympathetic nervous system, enhancing norepinephrine release and increasing sympathetic tone.

AT2 Receptors

AT2 receptors, although less understood than AT1 receptors, counterbalance many of the effects mediated by AT1 receptors. They are expressed in various tissues, particularly during fetal development, and are involved in:

1. **Vasodilation**: Activation of AT2 receptors induces vasodilation, opposing the vasoconstrictive effects of AT1 receptors.
2. **Anti-proliferative Effects**: AT2 receptors inhibit cell growth and proliferation, contributing to tissue repair and anti-fibrotic effects.
3. **Apoptosis**: These receptors promote apoptosis in certain cell types, aiding in the removal of damaged cells and tissue remodeling.
4. **Neuromodulation**: AT2 receptors modulate neuronal function and can influence pain perception and neuroprotection.

Production of Angiotensin Receptors

Gene Expression

The genes encoding AT1 and AT2 receptors are AGTR1 and AGTR2, respectively. The expression of these genes is regulated by various transcription factors and can be influenced by physiological and pathological conditions.

1. **Transcriptional Regulation**: Specific promoter regions upstream of AGTR1 and AGTR2 bind transcription factors that initiate gene transcription. Factors such as hypoxia, oxidative

stress, and inflammatory cytokines can modulate the expression of these genes.

2. **Epigenetic Modifications**: DNA methylation and histone modifications also play a role in the regulation of angiotensin receptor gene expression. These epigenetic changes can be influenced by environmental factors, including diet and lifestyle.

Receptor Synthesis

Once transcribed, the mRNA for AT1 and AT2 receptors is translated into proteins in the endoplasmic reticulum. These proteins undergo folding and post-translational modifications essential for their proper function and stability.

1. **Protein Folding**: Proper folding of the receptor proteins is facilitated by molecular chaperones within the endoplasmic reticulum.
2. **Glycosylation**: The receptors undergo glycosylation, which is crucial for their stability, trafficking, and function.
3. **Transport to Membrane**: After folding and modification, the receptors are transported to the cell membrane, where they become functional.

Post-Translational Modifications

Angiotensin receptors undergo various post-translational modifications that regulate their activity, desensitization, and internalization.

1. **Phosphorylation**: Kinases such as GRKs phosphorylate the receptors, leading to desensitization and reduced responsiveness to angiotensin II.
2. **Ubiquitination**: This modification targets the receptors for degradation, regulating the number of receptors on the cell surface.

Regulation of Angiotensin Receptors

Desensitization and Downregulation

Prolonged exposure to angiotensin II can lead to receptor desensitization and downregulation, essential mechanisms to prevent overstimulation and maintain homeostasis.

1. **Desensitization**: Phosphorylation by GRKs and subsequent binding of β-arrestins uncouples the receptors from G proteins, reducing their activity.
2. **Downregulation**: Internalized receptors can be degraded in lysosomes, reducing receptor density on the cell surface.

Receptor Recycling and Degradation

Internalized receptors can be either recycled back to the membrane or degraded, balancing receptor availability and responsiveness.

1. **Recycling**: This process allows the cell to quickly restore receptor sensitivity after desensitization.
2. **Degradation**: Reduces receptor density, providing long-term regulation and preventing overstimulation.

Role of Plant-Based Compounds in Regulation

Plant-based diets can influence the regulation of angiotensin receptors through various bioactive compounds, such as flavonoids, polyphenols, and dietary fibers.

1. **Flavonoids**: Compounds like quercetin and kaempferol, found in many fruits and vegetables, have been shown to modulate angiotensin receptor activity. Quercetin, for example, can inhibit the expression of AT1 receptors, reducing angiotensin II-mediated vasoconstriction.

2. **Polyphenols**: Polyphenols, such as resveratrol found in grapes, have antioxidant properties that can protect against oxidative stress, a factor known to upregulate AT1 receptor expression.
3. **Dietary Fiber**: High-fiber diets, typical of plant-based nutrition, can improve overall cardiovascular health by modulating the activity of angiotensin receptors. Improved gut health and reduced systemic inflammation from high fiber intake can influence receptor expression and function.

Plant-Based Diets and Angiotensin Receptors
Cardiovascular Health

Plant-based diets, rich in antioxidants, dietary fiber, and healthy fats, have significant benefits for cardiovascular health. These diets can positively influence the regulation of angiotensin receptors, contributing to better blood pressure control and reduced risk of cardiovascular diseases.

1. **Antioxidants**: Antioxidant-rich foods, such as berries and leafy greens, can reduce oxidative stress, which is known to impair the function of angiotensin receptors. Reducing oxidative stress helps maintain receptor balance and function, preventing hypertension and cardiovascular damage.
2. **Dietary Fiber**: Fiber helps manage blood pressure by improving endothelial function and reducing systemic inflammation. Whole grains, legumes, and vegetables are excellent sources of dietary fiber, which supports cardiovascular health through modulation of the RAS.
3. **Healthy Fats**: Plant-based sources of healthy fats, like nuts and seeds, provide omega-3 fatty acids that have anti-inflammatory properties. These fatty acids can decrease the expression of AT1 receptors, potentially reducing vasoconstriction and blood pressure.

Metabolic Health

Plant-based diets can also enhance metabolic health by modulating angiotensin receptor activity, improving insulin sensitivity, and reducing the risk of metabolic disorders such as type 2 diabetes.

1. **Insulin Sensitivity**: Foods rich in flavonoids and polyphenols, such as berries and green tea, can improve insulin sensitivity. Enhanced insulin sensitivity helps regulate blood sugar levels and may influence the activity of AT1 receptors, contributing to better metabolic control.
2. **Anti-inflammatory Effects**: Plant-based diets are known for their anti-inflammatory properties, which can mitigate the chronic inflammation associated with metabolic disorders. This reduction in inflammation can modulate the RAS and improve overall metabolic health.

Weight Management

Angiotensin receptors, particularly AT1 receptors, play a crucial role in fat metabolism and energy balance. Plant-based diets, typically lower in calories and higher in fiber, can support weight management by influencing these receptors.

1. **Caloric Density**: Plant-based diets tend to be lower in calories but high in nutrients, promoting healthy weight management without excessive caloric intake. This helps in maintaining a healthy balance of angiotensin receptor activity.
2. **Bioactive Compounds**: The presence of bioactive compounds in plant foods can inhibit AT1 receptor-mediated adipogenesis, aiding in the reduction of fat stores and promoting healthy weight loss.

Immune Function

The regulation of angiotensin receptors is also linked to immune function. Plant-based diets, rich in vitamins, minerals, and antioxidants, can enhance immune health and influence receptor activity.

1. **Anti-inflammatory Properties**: Plant-based diets reduce systemic inflammation, which can positively affect immune function. This reduction in inflammation helps maintain the proper regulation of angiotensin receptors, contributing to overall immune health.
2. **Nutrient Density**: The high nutrient density of plant-based diets ensures adequate intake of essential vitamins and minerals necessary for optimal immune function. Proper nutrition supports the balanced regulation of angiotensin receptors, aiding in immune response and protection.

Angiotensin receptors, specifically AT1 and AT2, are vital components of the renin-angiotensin system, playing crucial roles in regulating blood pressure, fluid balance, and cardiovascular health. The production and regulation of these receptors involve complex mechanisms influenced by genetic, environmental, and dietary factors.

Plant-based diets offer significant benefits in the regulation and function of angiotensin receptors. The intake of various nutrients and bioactive compounds from plants can modulate the angiotensin system, contributing to improved cardiovascular, metabolic, and immune health. Incorporating antioxidant-rich foods, dietary fiber, and healthy fats from plant sources can enhance the balance and activity of angiotensin receptors, promoting overall well-being and reducing the risk of chronic diseases.

Vasopressin Receptors (V1a, V1b, V2)

Vasopressin receptors, including V1a, V1b, and V2 subtypes, are crucial components of the body's physiological regulation systems. These receptors, primarily activated by the hormone vasopressin (also known as antidiuretic hormone, ADH), play significant roles in maintaining water balance, blood pressure, and various neuroendocrine functions.

Function of Vasopressin Receptors

V1a Receptors

V1a receptors are located in various tissues, including vascular smooth muscle, liver, and the brain. Their activation leads to several physiological responses:

1. **Vasoconstriction**: Vasopressin binding to V1a receptors on vascular smooth muscle cells causes vasoconstriction, leading to an increase in blood pressure.
2. **Glycogenolysis**: In the liver, V1a receptor activation stimulates glycogenolysis, the breakdown of glycogen into glucose, which can be critical during stress or hypoglycemia.
3. **Platelet Aggregation**: V1a receptors are involved in promoting platelet aggregation, which is essential for blood clotting and wound healing.
4. **Behavioral and Neurological Effects**: In the brain, V1a receptors influence social behavior, stress response, and memory formation.

V1b Receptors

V1b receptors, also known as V3 receptors, are primarily found in the anterior pituitary gland but also in the brain and pancreas. They are involved in:

1. **ACTH Secretion**: Activation of V1b receptors in the pituitary gland stimulates the release of adrenocorticotropic hormone

(ACTH), which in turn stimulates cortisol production by the adrenal glands, playing a vital role in the stress response.

2. **Insulin Secretion**: V1b receptors in the pancreas can influence insulin secretion, although their role in this process is less well-defined compared to their role in ACTH release.

V2 Receptors

V2 receptors are primarily located in the kidney's collecting ducts and play a key role in regulating water balance:

1. **Antidiuretic Effect**: Vasopressin binding to V2 receptors increases the permeability of the collecting ducts to water, leading to water reabsorption and concentrated urine production, thus conserving body water.
2. **Release of Coagulation Factors**: V2 receptors also stimulate the release of coagulation factors such as von Willebrand factor and factor VIII, which are important for blood clotting.

Production of Vasopressin Receptors

Gene Expression

The genes encoding V1a, V1b, and V2 receptors are AVPR1A, AVPR1B, and AVPR2, respectively. The expression of these genes is tightly regulated and can be influenced by various physiological and environmental factors.

1. **Transcriptional Regulation**: Specific promoter regions upstream of AVPR1A, AVPR1B, and AVPR2 bind transcription factors that initiate gene transcription. These transcription factors can be influenced by stress, hormonal levels, and other signaling molecules.
2. **Epigenetic Modifications**: DNA methylation and histone modifications also play a role in the regulation of vasopressin receptor

gene expression. These epigenetic changes can be influenced by environmental factors, including diet and lifestyle.

Receptor Synthesis

Once transcribed, the mRNA for V1a, V1b, and V2 receptors is translated into proteins in the endoplasmic reticulum. These proteins undergo folding and post-translational modifications essential for their proper function and stability.

1. **Protein Folding**: Proper folding of the receptor proteins is facilitated by molecular chaperones within the endoplasmic reticulum.
2. **Glycosylation**: The receptors undergo glycosylation, which is crucial for their stability, trafficking, and function.
3. **Transport to Membrane**: After folding and modification, the receptors are transported to the cell membrane, where they become functional.

Post-Translational Modifications

Vasopressin receptors undergo various post-translational modifications that regulate their activity, desensitization, and internalization.

1. **Phosphorylation**: Kinases such as GRKs phosphorylate the receptors, leading to desensitization and reduced responsiveness to vasopressin.
2. **Ubiquitination**: This modification targets the receptors for degradation, regulating the number of receptors on the cell surface.

Regulation of Vasopressin Receptors

Desensitization and Downregulation

Prolonged exposure to vasopressin can lead to receptor desensitization and downregulation, essential mechanisms to prevent overstimulation and maintain homeostasis.

1. **Desensitization**: Phosphorylation by GRKs and subsequent binding of β-arrestins uncouples the receptors from G proteins, reducing their activity.
2. **Downregulation**: Internalized receptors can be degraded in lysosomes, reducing receptor density on the cell surface.

Receptor Recycling and Degradation

Internalized receptors can be either recycled back to the membrane or degraded, balancing receptor availability and responsiveness.

1. **Recycling**: This process allows the cell to quickly restore receptor sensitivity after desensitization.
2. **Degradation**: Reduces receptor density, providing long-term regulation and preventing overstimulation.

Role of Plant-Based Compounds in Regulation

Plant-based diets can influence the regulation of vasopressin receptors through various bioactive compounds, such as flavonoids, polyphenols, and dietary fibers.

1. **Flavonoids**: Compounds like quercetin and kaempferol, found in many fruits and vegetables, have been shown to modulate vasopressin receptor activity. Quercetin, for example, can inhibit the expression of V1a receptors, reducing vasopressin-mediated vasoconstriction.

2. **Polyphenols**: Polyphenols, such as resveratrol found in grapes, have antioxidant properties that can protect against oxidative stress, a factor known to upregulate V1 receptor expression.
3. **Dietary Fiber**: High-fiber diets, typical of plant-based nutrition, can improve overall cardiovascular health by modulating the activity of vasopressin receptors. Improved gut health and reduced systemic inflammation from high fiber intake can influence receptor expression and function.

Plant-Based Diets and Vasopressin Receptors
Cardiovascular Health

Plant-based diets, rich in antioxidants, dietary fiber, and healthy fats, have significant benefits for cardiovascular health. These diets can positively influence the regulation of vasopressin receptors, contributing to better blood pressure control and reduced risk of cardiovascular diseases.

1. **Antioxidants**: Antioxidant-rich foods, such as berries and leafy greens, can reduce oxidative stress, which is known to impair the function of vasopressin receptors. Reducing oxidative stress helps maintain receptor balance and function, preventing hypertension and cardiovascular damage.
2. **Dietary Fiber**: Fiber helps manage blood pressure by improving endothelial function and reducing systemic inflammation. Whole grains, legumes, and vegetables are excellent sources of dietary fiber, which supports cardiovascular health through modulation of the vasopressin system.
3. **Healthy Fats**: Plant-based sources of healthy fats, like nuts and seeds, provide omega-3 fatty acids that have anti-inflammatory properties. These fatty acids can decrease the expression of V1a receptors, potentially reducing vasoconstriction and blood pressure.

Metabolic Health

Plant-based diets can also enhance metabolic health by modulating vasopressin receptor activity, improving insulin sensitivity, and reducing the risk of metabolic disorders such as type 2 diabetes.

1. **Insulin Sensitivity**: Foods rich in flavonoids and polyphenols, such as berries and green tea, can improve insulin sensitivity. Enhanced insulin sensitivity helps regulate blood sugar levels and may influence the activity of vasopressin receptors, contributing to better metabolic control.
2. **Anti-inflammatory Effects**: Plant-based diets are known for their anti-inflammatory properties, which can mitigate the chronic inflammation associated with metabolic disorders. This reduction in inflammation can modulate the vasopressin system and improve overall metabolic health.

Weight Management

Vasopressin receptors, particularly V1a receptors, play a crucial role in fat metabolism and energy balance. Plant-based diets, typically lower in calories and higher in fiber, can support weight management by influencing these receptors.

1. **Caloric Density**: Plant-based diets tend to be lower in calories but high in nutrients, promoting healthy weight management without excessive caloric intake. This helps in maintaining a healthy balance of vasopressin receptor activity.
2. **Bioactive Compounds**: The presence of bioactive compounds in plant foods can inhibit V1a receptor-mediated adipogenesis, aiding in the reduction of fat stores and promoting healthy weight loss.

Immune Function

The regulation of vasopressin receptors is also linked to immune function. Plant-based diets, rich in vitamins, minerals, and antioxidants, can enhance immune health and influence receptor activity.

1. **Anti-inflammatory Properties**: Plant-based diets reduce systemic inflammation, which can positively affect immune function. This reduction in inflammation helps maintain the proper regulation of vasopressin receptors, contributing to overall immune health.
2. **Nutrient Density**: The high nutrient density of plant-based diets ensures adequate intake of essential vitamins and minerals necessary for optimal immune function. Proper nutrition supports the balanced regulation of vasopressin receptors, aiding in immune response and protection.

Vasopressin receptors, specifically V1a, V1b, and V2, are vital components of the body's physiological regulation systems, playing crucial roles in maintaining water balance, blood pressure, and various neuroendocrine functions. The production and regulation of these receptors involve complex mechanisms influenced by genetic, environmental, and dietary factors.

Glucagon Receptors

Glucagon receptors are integral to the regulation of glucose metabolism and play a critical role in maintaining glucose homeostasis. These receptors, which belong to the G protein-coupled receptor (GPCR) family, are primarily activated by glucagon, a hormone produced by the alpha cells of the pancreas. Understanding the function, production, and regulation of glucagon receptors, especially from a plant-based viewpoint, provides valuable insights into how diet can influence metabolic health.

Function of Glucagon Receptors

Glucagon receptors are predominantly found in the liver, where they mediate the effects of glucagon on glucose metabolism. However, they are also present in other tissues, including the kidneys, adipose tissue, heart, and brain.

Liver

In the liver, glucagon receptors play a vital role in the regulation of glycogenolysis and gluconeogenesis, processes crucial for maintaining blood glucose levels during fasting or between meals. Activation of glucagon receptors in hepatocytes leads to the conversion of glycogen to glucose and the production of glucose from non-carbohydrate sources, ensuring a continuous supply of glucose to the body.

Kidneys

In the kidneys, glucagon receptors help in the regulation of renal gluconeogenesis, contributing to overall glucose homeostasis. This process becomes particularly important during prolonged fasting or starvation when glucose availability is limited.

Adipose Tissue

In adipose tissue, glucagon receptors facilitate lipolysis, the breakdown of stored fats into free fatty acids and glycerol. This process provides substrates for gluconeogenesis and energy production during periods of low glucose availability.

Heart and Brain

Although less is known about the precise roles of glucagon receptors in the heart and brain, they are believed to contribute to overall metabolic regulation and energy balance in these tissues.

Production of Glucagon Receptors

The production of glucagon receptors is a complex process regulated at multiple levels, including gene expression, receptor synthesis, and post-translational modifications. The gene encoding the glucagon receptor is GCG.

Gene Expression

The expression of the glucagon receptor gene (GCG) is regulated by various transcription factors and signaling pathways. Nutritional status, hormonal signals, and other environmental factors can influence the transcription of the GCG gene. For example, fasting and low insulin levels tend to upregulate GCG expression, increasing the number of glucagon receptors available for activation.

Receptor Synthesis

Following transcription, the mRNA for the glucagon receptor is translated into protein in the endoplasmic reticulum. The receptor protein undergoes folding and glycosylation, which are crucial for its proper function and stability. These modifications ensure that the receptor maintains its structural integrity and functional capacity.

Post-Translational Modifications

Post-translational modifications, such as phosphorylation, further regulate the activity and responsiveness of glucagon receptors. Phosphorylation can affect receptor sensitivity, desensitization, and internalization, fine-tuning the receptor's ability to respond to glucagon.

Regulation of Glucagon Receptors

The regulation of glucagon receptors involves intricate mechanisms to ensure appropriate cellular responses to glucagon.

Desensitization and Downregulation

Prolonged exposure to high levels of glucagon can lead to receptor desensitization, reducing the receptor's responsiveness. This is followed by downregulation, where the number of receptors on the cell surface is decreased. These processes prevent overstimulation and help maintain metabolic balance. Desensitization involves receptor phosphorylation by specific kinases, which uncouple the receptors from G proteins and target them for internalization.

Receptor Recycling and Degradation

Internalized receptors can either be recycled back to the cell membrane or degraded in lysosomes. The balance between these processes determines the overall number of functional receptors available. Recycling allows the cell to quickly restore receptor sensitivity, while degradation reduces receptor density, providing long-term regulation.

Role of Plant-Based Compounds in Regulation

Plant-based diets can significantly influence the regulation of glucagon receptors through various bioactive compounds. Phytochemicals, dietary fiber, and healthy fats found in plant-based foods can modulate receptor activity and expression.

Phytochemicals

Phytochemicals, such as flavonoids, have been shown to influence glucagon receptor signaling pathways. For instance, quercetin, a flavonoid found in apples, onions, and berries, has been reported to modulate glucose metabolism by affecting glucagon receptor-mediated pathways. Studies suggest that quercetin can enhance insulin sensitivity and reduce hepatic glucose production, thereby influencing glucagon receptor activity.

Dietary Fiber

High-fiber diets typical of plant-based nutrition can improve insulin sensitivity and modulate glucagon receptor activity. Dietary fiber helps maintain stable blood glucose levels by slowing down glucose absorption and enhancing satiety, which reduces the need for glucagon-induced glucose production. This, in turn, can modulate the activity of glucagon receptors, contributing to better glucose homeostasis.

Omega-3 Fatty Acids

Plant sources of omega-3 fatty acids, such as flaxseeds and chia seeds, have anti-inflammatory properties and can influence glucagon receptor function. Omega-3 fatty acids have been shown to improve metabolic health by modulating the expression of glucagon receptors and enhancing the body's response to glucagon. This can lead to improved regulation of glucose and lipid metabolism.

Plant-Based Diets and Glucagon Receptors

Adopting a plant-based diet can have significant impacts on the regulation and function of glucagon receptors. The intake of various nutrients and bioactive compounds from plants can modulate the glucagon signaling system, contributing to overall health benefits.

Cardiovascular Health

Plant-based diets are rich in antioxidants, dietary fiber, and healthy fats, which are beneficial for cardiovascular health. The regulation of glucagon receptors in the liver and other tissues can be positively influenced by these dietary components. For example, antioxidants can reduce oxidative stress, which is known to impair glucagon receptor function. Additionally, dietary fiber helps in managing blood lipid levels and reducing systemic inflammation, which can improve overall metabolic health.

Metabolic Health

The influence of plant-based diets on glucagon receptors can enhance metabolic health. Foods rich in flavonoids and omega-3 fatty acids can improve insulin sensitivity and reduce the risk of metabolic disorders such as type 2 diabetes. By modulating glucagon receptor activity, these diets can enhance glucose uptake and utilization, contributing to better glycemic control and overall metabolic balance.

Weight Management

Glucagon receptors play a crucial role in fat metabolism and energy balance. Plant-based diets, which are typically lower in calories and higher in fiber, can support weight management by enhancing the function of glucagon receptors. The presence of bioactive compounds in plant foods can stimulate glucagon receptor-mediated lipolysis, aiding in the reduction of fat stores and promoting healthy weight loss.

Glucagon receptors are essential for various physiological processes, including glucose metabolism, lipid metabolism, and overall energy balance. The production and regulation of these receptors involve complex mechanisms influenced by genetic and environmental factors.

Chemokine Receptors

Chemokine receptors, particularly CCR5 and CXCR4, are integral components of the immune system, playing crucial roles in immune cell trafficking, and inflammation. These receptors, belonging to the G protein-coupled receptor (GPCR) family, respond to chemokines—small signaling proteins—that direct the movement of immune cells to sites of infection or injury.

Function of Chemokine Receptors

CCR5

CCR5 is primarily expressed on the surface of T cells, macrophages, dendritic cells, and some other immune cells. It binds to chemokines such as CCL3, CCL4, and CCL5 (RANTES), which are involved in the recruitment of immune cells to inflammatory sites.

Role in Immune Response: CCR5 is crucial for the immune system's ability to respond to infections and injuries. By binding to its ligands, CCR5 triggers intracellular signaling pathways that result in the migration of immune cells to sites where they are needed, enhancing the body's defense mechanisms.

CXCR4

CXCR4 is widely expressed on various cells, including hematopoietic stem cells, progenitor cells, and many types of leukocytes. Its primary ligand is CXCL12 (SDF-1).

Stem Cell Homing: CXCR4 plays a pivotal role in the homing and retention of hematopoietic stem cells within the bone marrow. The CXCR4-CXCL12 axis is essential for maintaining stem cell niches and facilitating the regeneration of blood cells.

Cancer Metastasis: CXCR4 is implicated in cancer metastasis. Many tumors express high levels of CXCR4, which allows them to migrate toward organs that produce CXCL12, thus promoting the spread of cancer cells to distant sites.

Production of Chemokine Receptors

The production of chemokine receptors involves gene expression, protein synthesis, and post-translational modifications.

Gene Expression

The genes encoding CCR5 and CXCR4 are regulated by various transcription factors and signaling pathways.

Transcriptional Regulation: For CCR5, transcription factors such as NF-κB and AP-1 play significant roles in its expression, especially during inflammatory responses. Similarly, CXCR4 gene expression is regulated by transcription factors like HIF-1α, which can induce CXCR4 expression under hypoxic conditions, commonly found in tumor microenvironments.

Protein Synthesis

Once the genes are transcribed, the resulting mRNA is translated into protein in the endoplasmic reticulum. The nascent receptors undergo folding and glycosylation, which are crucial for their stability and function. Properly folded receptors are then transported to the cell membrane.

Glycosylation: Glycosylation is particularly important for chemokine receptors as it affects their ligand-binding affinity and receptor signaling. Aberrant glycosylation can lead to dysfunctional receptors and impaired immune responses.

Regulation of Chemokine Receptors

Regulation of chemokine receptors is complex and involves various mechanisms to ensure appropriate responses to chemokines.

Desensitization and Internalization

Similar to other GPCRs, chemokine receptors undergo desensitization and internalization upon prolonged exposure to their ligands.

Desensitization: Phosphorylation of the receptor by GPCR kinases (GRKs) leads to the recruitment of β-arrestins, which uncouple the receptor from G proteins, thereby terminating the signal. This process prevents overstimulation and maintains cellular homeostasis.

Internalization and Recycling: Internalized receptors can either be recycled back to the cell surface or targeted for degradation in lysosomes. The balance between recycling and degradation determines the overall receptor density on the cell surface, influencing the cell's responsiveness to chemokines.

Role of Plant-Based Compounds in Regulation

Plant-based diets, rich in various bioactive compounds, can modulate the activity and expression of chemokine receptors, thereby influencing immune function and disease outcomes.

Polyphenols: Polyphenols, abundant in fruits, vegetables, and other plant-based foods, have been shown to affect chemokine receptor signaling. For example, resveratrol, a polyphenol found in grapes, can inhibit the expression of CCR5 and CXCR4, thereby reducing the migration of immune cells and potentially inhibiting cancer metastasis.

Dietary Fiber: High-fiber diets can influence immune responses by modulating gut microbiota and their metabolic products. Short-chain fatty acids (SCFAs), produced by the fermentation of dietary fiber, have anti-inflammatory properties and can downregulate the expression of chemokine receptors, including CCR5 and CXCR4.

Omega-3 Fatty Acids: Plant sources of omega-3 fatty acids, such as flaxseeds and chia seeds, exhibit anti-inflammatory effects. These fatty acids can modulate the expression of chemokine receptors and reduce the migration of inflammatory cells, which is beneficial in conditions like atherosclerosis and autoimmune diseases.

Plant-Based Diets and Chemokine Receptors

Adopting a plant-based diet can have significant impacts on the regulation and function of chemokine receptors, contributing to improved immune function and reduced risk of chronic diseases.

Immune Health: A plant-based diet rich in antioxidants, polyphenols, and dietary fiber supports a balanced immune response. By modulating chemokine receptor activity, such diets can enhance the body's ability to respond to infections while preventing excessive inflammation that can lead to chronic diseases.

Cancer Prevention: The anti-cancer properties of plant-based diets are partly due to their effects on chemokine receptors. Polyphenols like epigallocatechin gallate (EGCG) from green tea and curcumin from turmeric have been shown to inhibit CXCR4-mediated cancer cell migration and invasion, thereby reducing the risk of metastasis.

Cardiovascular Health: Omega-3 fatty acids and other bioactive compounds in plant-based diets can reduce the expression of chemokine receptors involved in atherosclerosis, such as CCR5. This results in decreased recruitment of inflammatory cells to the arterial wall, lowering the risk of plaque formation and cardiovascular events.

Chemokine receptors CCR5 and CXCR4 are critical for immune cell trafficking, inflammation, and the pathogenesis of various diseases, and cancer. Their function, production, and regulation are influenced by complex genetic and environmental factors.

29

Receptor Tyrosine Kinases (RTKs)

Epidermal Growth Factor Receptor (EGFR)

The Epidermal Growth Factor Receptor (EGFR) is a transmembrane protein that functions as a receptor for members of the epidermal growth factor family (EGF family) of extracellular protein ligands. It is also known as HER1 or ERBB1. This receptor plays a crucial role in regulating cell growth, survival, proliferation, and differentiation. EGFR is implicated in various cellular processes and has been extensively studied for its role in cancer development and progression.

Function of EGFR

- **Mechanism of Action**

EGFR is a member of the ErbB family of receptors, which includes HER2/neu (ErbB2), HER3 (ErbB3), and HER4 (ErbB4). Upon binding with its ligands, such as EGF or transforming growth factor-alpha (TGF-α), EGFR undergoes a conformational change that facilitates dimerization with another EGFR molecule or other members of the ErbB family. This dimerization activates the intrinsic tyrosine kinase activity of EGFR, leading to autophosphorylation of specific tyrosine residues in its cytoplasmic domain. These phosphorylated residues serve as docking sites for various signaling molecules, initiating a cascade of downstream signaling pathways, including the RAS-RAF-MEK-ERK pathway, the PI3K-AKT pathway, and the JAK-STAT pathway.

Cellular Processes

• Cell Proliferation

One of the primary roles of EGFR is to promote cell proliferation. The activation of the RAS-RAF-MEK-ERK pathway leads to the phosphorylation of ERK1/2, which translocates to the nucleus and activates transcription factors involved in cell cycle progression, such as c-Myc and cyclin D1. This promotes the transition from the G1 phase to the S phase of the cell cycle, leading to DNA synthesis and cell division.

• Cell Survival

EGFR also plays a critical role in promoting cell survival. The PI3K-AKT pathway, activated by EGFR signaling, leads to the phosphorylation and activation of AKT, a serine/threonine kinase. AKT phosphorylates and inhibits pro-apoptotic factors such as BAD and promotes the activity of anti-apoptotic proteins like Bcl-2 and Bcl-XL. This helps in preventing programmed cell death and supports cell survival under various stress conditions.

• Differentiation

EGFR signaling is involved in the differentiation of various cell types. For instance, in the skin, EGFR regulates the balance between proliferation and differentiation of keratinocytes, which is essential for maintaining skin homeostasis and repair. Abnormal EGFR signaling can disrupt this balance, leading to skin disorders and contributing to the pathogenesis of skin cancers.

Production of EGFR

• Gene Expression

The gene encoding EGFR is located on chromosome 7p11.2 and is composed of 28 exons. The regulation of EGFR gene expression involves various transcription factors and regulatory elements. Promoter regions upstream of the EGFR gene bind specific transcription factors, such as Sp1 and AP-2, to initiate transcription. Epigenetic modifications, including DNA methylation and histone acetylation, also play a significant role in regulating EGFR expression.

- **mRNA Processing**

After transcription, the pre-mRNA undergoes splicing to remove introns and join exons, resulting in a mature mRNA transcript. This mRNA is then transported from the nucleus to the cytoplasm, where it is translated into the EGFR protein in the endoplasmic reticulum.

- **Protein Synthesis and Post-Translational Modifications**

The newly synthesized EGFR protein undergoes folding and glycosylation in the endoplasmic reticulum, which is essential for its stability and function. Properly folded and glycosylated EGFR is then transported to the Golgi apparatus for further processing before being delivered to the cell membrane. Post-translational modifications, such as phosphorylation, ubiquitination, and acetylation, regulate EGFR activity, localization, and degradation.

Regulation of EGFR

- **Ligand Binding and Receptor Activation**

The primary mechanism of EGFR regulation is through ligand binding. Ligands such as EGF, TGF-α, amphiregulin, and heparin-binding EGF-like growth factor (HB-EGF) bind to the extracellular domain of EGFR, inducing receptor dimerization and activation. The availability of these ligands is tightly regulated by various mechanisms, including proteolytic cleavage of membrane-bound precursors and secretion of soluble ligands.

- **Receptor Endocytosis and Degradation**

Following activation, EGFR undergoes endocytosis, a process where the receptor-ligand complex is internalized into the cell. This can lead to receptor recycling back to the cell membrane or degradation in lysosomes. The balance between recycling and degradation determines the overall level of EGFR on the cell surface and its responsiveness to ligands. Ubiquitination of EGFR by E3 ubiquitin ligases, such as CBL, targets the receptor for degradation, thereby attenuating the signal.

- **Feedback Inhibition**

Several feedback mechanisms negatively regulate EGFR signaling to prevent overactivation. For example, the activation of ERK1/2 can induce the expression of negative regulators like Sprouty and LRIG1, which inhibit EGFR signaling. Additionally, activated AKT can phosphorylate and inhibit TSC2, a component of the TSC1/TSC2 complex, which negatively regulates mTOR signaling downstream of EGFR.

Role of Plant-Based Compounds in Regulation

- **Phytochemicals**

Phytochemicals, found in various plant-based foods, can modulate EGFR signaling. Flavonoids, polyphenols, and other bioactive compounds have been shown to influence EGFR activity and expression. For instance, curcumin, a polyphenol from turmeric, can inhibit EGFR activation and downstream signaling pathways, thereby exerting anti-proliferative and pro-apoptotic effects in cancer cells.

- **Dietary Fiber**

High-fiber diets, typical of plant-based nutrition, can influence EGFR signaling. Fiber fermentation by gut microbiota produces short-chain fatty acids (SCFAs), such as butyrate, which have been reported to inhibit histone deacetylases (HDACs). This inhibition can lead to increased acetylation of histones associated with the EGFR gene, affecting its expression and potentially reducing the overactivation of EGFR signaling in cancer cells.

- **Omega-3 Fatty Acids**

Plant sources of omega-3 fatty acids, such as flaxseeds and chia seeds, have anti-inflammatory properties and can influence EGFR function. Omega-3 fatty acids can modulate lipid rafts in the cell membrane, affecting the localization and signaling of EGFR. Additionally, omega-3 fatty acids have been shown to inhibit the expression of pro-inflammatory cytokines that can activate EGFR signaling pathways.

Plant-Based Diets and EGFR Regulation

- **Cancer Prevention**

Plant-based diets rich in fruits, vegetables, and whole grains provide a variety of phytochemicals and nutrients that can modulate EGFR signaling and reduce the risk of cancer. For example, sulforaphane, a compound found in cruciferous vegetables like broccoli and Brussels sprouts, can inhibit HDACs and modulate EGFR signaling, leading to reduced proliferation and increased apoptosis of cancer cells.

- **Skin Health**

EGFR plays a critical role in skin health, regulating keratinocyte proliferation and differentiation. Plant-based diets can provide essential vitamins, minerals, and antioxidants that support skin health and modulate EGFR activity. For instance, vitamins C and E, abundant in fruits and vegetables, can protect against oxidative stress and support the integrity of the skin barrier, potentially influencing EGFR-mediated processes.

- **Cardiovascular Health**

EGFR signaling is also involved in cardiovascular health, influencing processes such as vascular remodeling and endothelial function. Plant-based diets, which are rich in antioxidants and anti-inflammatory compounds, can positively impact cardiovascular health by modulating EGFR signaling pathways. For example, resveratrol, a polyphenol found in grapes and red wine, can inhibit EGFR activation and reduce the risk of atherosclerosis and other cardiovascular diseases.

- **Metabolic Health**

EGFR signaling is implicated in metabolic health, influencing processes such as insulin sensitivity and lipid metabolism. Plant-based diets can enhance metabolic health by providing nutrients and bioactive compounds that modulate EGFR signaling. For instance, dietary polyphenols can improve insulin sensitivity and reduce the risk of metabolic disorders by inhibiting EGFR activation and downstream signaling pathways.

The Epidermal Growth Factor Receptor (EGFR) is a critical regulator of cell growth, survival, proliferation, and differentiation. Its function, production, and regulation are complex processes influenced by various genetic and environmental factors. Plant-based diets, rich in phytochemicals, dietary fiber, and omega-3 fatty acids, can modulate EGFR signaling and provide numerous health benefits, including cancer prevention, improved skin health, cardiovascular health, and metabolic health.

Insulin Receptor

The insulin receptor (IR) is a transmembrane receptor that is activated by insulin, a hormone essential for regulating glucose homeostasis. The insulin receptor plays a critical role in metabolic processes, including the uptake of glucose into cells, the synthesis of glycogen, and the regulation of fat metabolism. It is fundamental in maintaining energy balance and has significant implications for conditions such as diabetes mellitus.

Function of Insulin Receptors

• Glucose Uptake

The primary function of the insulin receptor is to mediate the effects of insulin on cells, particularly in muscle and adipose tissues. When insulin binds to the insulin receptor on the cell surface, it triggers a cascade of intracellular events leading to the translocation of glucose transporter type 4 (GLUT4) to the cell membrane. This process enhances the uptake of glucose from the bloodstream into the cells, thus lowering blood glucose levels.

- **Glycogen Synthesis**

In the liver and muscle tissues, the activation of the insulin receptor promotes glycogen synthesis. Insulin stimulates the activity of enzymes such as glycogen synthase, which catalyzes the conversion of glucose to glycogen, the stored form of glucose. This function is crucial for energy storage and maintaining blood glucose levels during fasting.

- **Lipid Metabolism**

The insulin receptor also regulates lipid metabolism. Insulin signaling inhibits lipolysis, the breakdown of fat stores, by reducing the activity of hormone-sensitive lipase in adipose tissue. Concurrently, it promotes lipogenesis, the synthesis of fatty acids, through the activation of acetyl-CoA carboxylase and fatty acid synthase. This dual role helps to manage the body's fat stores and energy utilization.

- **Protein Synthesis**

Insulin signaling through its receptor promotes protein synthesis by stimulating the activity of the mammalian target of rapamycin (mTOR) pathway. This pathway increases the translation of mRNA into proteins, supporting muscle growth and repair, as well as overall cellular function.

- **Cellular Growth and Differentiation**

Beyond its metabolic functions, the insulin receptor is involved in cellular growth, differentiation, and survival. Insulin signaling can activate the mitogen-activated protein kinase (MAPK) pathway, which regulates gene expression related to cell growth and division. This function is particularly important in development and tissue regeneration.

Production of Insulin Receptors

- **Gene Expression**

The gene encoding the insulin receptor is INSR, located on chromosome 19 in humans. The expression of this gene is tightly regulated by various factors, including hormones, nutrients, and cellular energy status. Transcription factors such as FoxO1 and PGC-1α can modulate INSR expression in response to metabolic demands.

- **Receptor Synthesis**

The synthesis of the insulin receptor begins with the transcription of the INSR gene into mRNA, which is then translated into a polypeptide chain in the endoplasmic reticulum. The nascent receptor undergoes glycosylation, a post-translational modification essential for its proper folding and stability. After glycosylation, the receptor is transported to the Golgi apparatus for further processing and then to the cell membrane.

- **Post-Translational Modifications**

The insulin receptor is subject to various post-translational modifications that regulate its function. These include phosphorylation, ubiquitination, and glycosylation. Phosphorylation of tyrosine residues on the receptor is a key step in activating downstream signaling pathways. Ubiquitination can target the receptor for degradation, modulating its levels on the cell surface.

Regulation of Insulin Receptors

- **Insulin Sensitivity**

Insulin sensitivity refers to how effectively cells respond to insulin. Several factors influence insulin sensitivity, including diet, physical activity, and genetic predisposition. High insulin sensitivity allows for effective glucose uptake and metabolism, while low sensitivity, or insulin resistance, is a hallmark of type 2 diabetes.

- **Desensitization and Downregulation**

Chronic exposure to high levels of insulin can lead to desensitization of the insulin receptor, reducing its responsiveness. This is often followed by downregulation, where the number of receptors on the cell surface is decreased. These processes help to prevent overstimulation and maintain metabolic balance.

• **Receptor Recycling and Degradation**

After internalization, insulin receptors can be recycled back to the cell membrane or targeted for degradation in lysosomes. The balance between recycling and degradation determines the number of functional receptors available on the cell surface. Recycling allows for rapid resensitization to insulin, while degradation reduces receptor density, providing long-term regulation.

Role of Plant-Based Compounds in Regulation

• **Phytochemicals**

Plant-based diets are rich in phytochemicals, which can positively influence insulin receptor function and insulin sensitivity. These bioactive compounds include flavonoids, polyphenols, and carotenoids.

• **Flavonoids**

Flavonoids, found in fruits, vegetables, tea, and other plant-based foods, have been shown to enhance insulin sensitivity. Quercetin, a flavonoid present in apples and onions, can activate AMP-activated protein kinase (AMPK), which enhances insulin receptor signaling and glucose uptake in muscle cells.

• **Polyphenols**

Polyphenols, abundant in foods like berries, grapes, and nuts, exhibit anti-inflammatory and antioxidant properties that protect insulin receptors from oxidative stress. Resveratrol, a polyphenol in red grapes, has been shown to improve insulin sensitivity by enhancing the activity of the insulin receptor and downstream signaling pathways.

• **Dietary Fiber**

Dietary fiber, found in whole grains, legumes, fruits, and vegetables, can improve insulin sensitivity and reduce the risk of insulin resistance. High-fiber diets slow the absorption of glucose, leading to more stable blood glucose levels and reduced insulin demand. This can enhance the function and regulation of insulin receptors over time.

• Omega-3 Fatty Acids

Plant sources of omega-3 fatty acids, such as flaxseeds and chia seeds, have anti-inflammatory properties that can improve insulin sensitivity. Omega-3 fatty acids reduce inflammation and oxidative stress, protecting insulin receptors from damage and supporting their optimal function.

Plant-Based Diets and Insulin Receptors

Adopting a plant-based diet can significantly impact the regulation and function of insulin receptors. The intake of various nutrients and bioactive compounds from plants can modulate insulin signaling pathways, contributing to overall health benefits.

• Cardiovascular Health

Plant-based diets are rich in antioxidants, dietary fiber, and healthy fats, which are beneficial for cardiovascular health. The regulation of insulin receptors in endothelial cells can be positively influenced by these dietary components. For example, antioxidants can reduce oxidative stress, which impairs insulin receptor function. Additionally, dietary fiber helps in managing blood pressure and improving endothelial function.

• Metabolic Health

The influence of plant-based diets on insulin receptors can enhance metabolic health. Foods rich in flavonoids and omega-3 fatty acids can improve insulin sensitivity and reduce the risk of metabolic disorders such as type 2 diabetes. By modulating insulin receptor activity, these diets can enhance glucose uptake and utilization, contributing to better glycemic control.

• Weight Management

Plant-based diets, typically lower in calories and higher in fiber, support weight management by enhancing insulin receptor function. The presence of bioactive compounds in plant foods can improve insulin sensitivity, aiding in the reduction of fat stores and promoting healthy weight loss.

- **Inflammation and Oxidative Stress**

Chronic inflammation and oxidative stress are key factors in the development of insulin resistance. Plant-based diets, rich in anti-inflammatory and antioxidant compounds, can mitigate these factors, thus protecting insulin receptors and maintaining their function.

- **Gut Microbiota**

The gut microbiota plays a crucial role in metabolic health and insulin sensitivity. Plant-based diets promote a healthy gut microbiota composition, which can enhance the production of short-chain fatty acids (SCFAs) like butyrate. SCFAs have been shown to improve insulin sensitivity and protect insulin receptors from inflammation and oxidative stress.

- **Exercise and Insulin Sensitivity**

Physical activity is a well-known modulator of insulin sensitivity. Combining a plant-based diet with regular exercise can synergistically improve insulin receptor function. Exercise increases the translocation of GLUT4 to the cell membrane, enhancing glucose uptake and improving overall metabolic health.

Insulin receptors are pivotal in maintaining glucose homeostasis and regulating various metabolic processes. Their function, production, and regulation are influenced by numerous factors, including diet, physical activity, and genetic predisposition. Plant-based diets, rich in phytochemicals, dietary fiber, and omega-3 fatty acids, offer significant benefits for the regulation of insulin receptors. By enhancing insulin sensitivity, reducing inflammation, and protecting against oxidative stress, plant-based nutrition supports the optimal function of insulin receptors, contributing to improved metabolic health and reduced risk of conditions like type 2 diabetes.

Platelet-Derived Growth Factor Receptor (PDGFR)

Platelet-Derived Growth Factor Receptors (PDGFRs) are cell surface tyrosine kinase receptors critical for various cellular processes, including proliferation, differentiation, and survival. They are primarily activated by the binding of Platelet-Derived Growth Factors (PDGFs), which trigger a cascade of downstream signaling pathways. There are two main types of PDGFRs: PDGFR-α and PDGFR-β, each having unique and overlapping roles in cellular functions.

Function of Platelet-Derived Growth Factor Receptors

- **PDGFR-α**

PDGFR-α is primarily involved in embryonic development and the regulation of cell growth and differentiation. This receptor is crucial for the development of organs such as the lungs, kidneys, and central nervous system. Activation of PDGFR-α leads to autophosphorylation of the receptor, which then activates various intracellular signaling pathways, including the PI3K/Akt, Ras/MAPK, and PLCγ pathways. These pathways collectively contribute to cell survival, proliferation, and migration.

- **PDGFR-β**

PDGFR-β is predominantly expressed in mesenchymal cells and is essential for the regulation of blood vessel formation (angiogenesis) and the stability of blood vessels. It plays a significant role in wound healing and the response to injury by promoting the proliferation and migration of fibroblasts and smooth muscle cells. PDGFR-β activation also stimulates the production of extracellular matrix components, contributing to tissue repair and fibrosis.

- **Overlapping Functions**

Both PDGFR-α and PDGFR-β have overlapping roles in certain cellular processes, such as the regulation of cell proliferation and migration. They can form homo- or heterodimers upon ligand binding, which allows for diverse and context-specific signaling outcomes. This redundancy ensures that critical functions like tissue repair and development are robustly regulated.

Production of Platelet-Derived Growth Factor Receptors

• Gene Expression

The genes encoding PDGFR-α and PDGFR-β are PDGFRA and PDGFRB, respectively. Their expression is tightly regulated by various transcription factors and regulatory elements. Promoter regions upstream of these genes contain binding sites for proteins that initiate and control transcription. Factors such as growth factors, cytokines, and stress signals can modulate the expression of PDGFR genes. For example, hypoxia-inducible factor 1 (HIF-1) can upregulate PDGFR expression under low oxygen conditions, promoting angiogenesis.

• Receptor Synthesis

After transcription, PDGFR mRNA is translated into protein in the endoplasmic reticulum. The nascent receptors undergo folding and glycosylation, which are critical for their stability and function. Properly folded and modified PDGFRs are then transported to the Golgi apparatus for further processing before being delivered to the cell membrane.

• Post-Translational Modifications

PDGFRs undergo various post-translational modifications, including phosphorylation, ubiquitination, and glycosylation. These modifications regulate receptor activity, stability, and cellular localization. Phosphorylation of PDGFRs at specific tyrosine residues is crucial for activating downstream signaling pathways. Ubiquitination often marks the receptors for degradation, thus controlling their levels on the cell surface and preventing overactivation.

Regulation of Platelet-Derived Growth Factor Receptors

• Desensitization and Downregulation

Prolonged activation of PDGFRs can lead to receptor desensitization, where the receptors become less responsive to their ligands. This is often followed by downregulation, where the number of receptors on the cell surface is reduced. Desensitization involves receptor phosphorylation by kinases, leading to the recruitment of proteins such as c-Cbl that mediate receptor internalization and degradation. This process is crucial for preventing excessive signaling and maintaining cellular homeostasis.

- **Receptor Recycling and Degradation**

Internalized PDGFRs can either be recycled back to the cell membrane or targeted for degradation in lysosomes. The balance between these processes determines the overall number of functional receptors on the cell surface. Recycling allows for the rapid restoration of receptor sensitivity, while degradation reduces receptor density, providing long-term regulation.

Role of Plant-Based Compounds in Regulation

Plant-based diets can influence the regulation of PDGFRs through various bioactive compounds. Phytochemicals, such as flavonoids and polyphenols, have been shown to modulate receptor activity and expression.

- **Flavonoids**

Flavonoids are a group of polyphenolic compounds found in fruits, vegetables, tea, and other plant-based foods. They have been reported to influence PDGFR signaling pathways by inhibiting receptor activation. For instance, quercetin, a flavonoid found in apples, onions, and berries, can inhibit PDGFR-mediated cell proliferation and migration in vascular smooth muscle cells, which is beneficial in preventing pathological conditions such as atherosclerosis and restenosis.

- **Dietary Fiber**

High-fiber diets, typical of plant-based nutrition, can improve insulin sensitivity and reduce inflammatory responses. This, in turn, may modulate the activity of PDGFRs, as insulin and inflammatory cytokines are linked to receptor regulation. For example, dietary fibers from fruits and vegetables can reduce the levels of pro-inflammatory cytokines like TNF-α and IL-6, which are known to upregulate PDGFR expression.

• **Omega-3 Fatty Acids**

Plant sources of omega-3 fatty acids, such as flaxseeds and chia seeds, have anti-inflammatory properties and can influence PDGFR function. Omega-3 fatty acids can decrease the expression of PDGFRs in various cell types, potentially affecting processes like cell proliferation and migration. This regulation is particularly important in preventing chronic inflammatory conditions and promoting vascular health.

Plant-Based Diets and Platelet-Derived Growth Factor Receptors

• **Cardiovascular Health**

Plant-based diets are rich in antioxidants, dietary fiber, and healthy fats, which are beneficial for cardiovascular health. The regulation of PDGFRs in vascular smooth muscle cells and endothelial cells can be positively influenced by these dietary components. For example, antioxidants can reduce oxidative stress, which is known to impair PDGFR function. Additionally, dietary fiber helps in managing blood pressure and reducing systemic inflammation, which can influence PDGFR-mediated vascular responses.

• **Metabolic Health**

The influence of plant-based diets on PDGFRs can enhance metabolic health. Foods rich in flavonoids and omega-3 fatty acids can improve insulin sensitivity and reduce the risk of metabolic disorders such as type 2 diabetes. By modulating PDGFR activity, these diets can enhance glucose uptake and utilization, contributing to better glycemic control. Additionally, the anti-inflammatory properties of plant-based diets can mitigate the chronic inflammation associated with metabolic syndrome, further benefiting metabolic health.

• **Cancer Prevention**

PDGFRs are implicated in the progression of various cancers, including glioblastoma, breast cancer, and colorectal cancer. Plant-based diets, which are high in antioxidants and anti-inflammatory compounds, can help modulate PDGFR signaling pathways involved in cancer development. For example, curcumin, a polyphenol found in turmeric, has been shown to inhibit PDGFR-mediated cell proliferation and induce apoptosis in cancer cells. This suggests that a plant-based diet could play a role in cancer prevention and management by targeting PDGFR-related pathways.

- **Inflammatory and Autoimmune Diseases**

PDGFRs play a role in the pathogenesis of inflammatory and autoimmune diseases such as rheumatoid arthritis and multiple sclerosis. Plant-based diets, which are known to reduce inflammation and oxidative stress, can modulate PDGFR activity in immune cells and fibroblasts. For instance, resveratrol, a polyphenol found in grapes and berries, has been shown to inhibit PDGFR signaling in fibroblast-like synoviocytes, reducing inflammation and joint damage in rheumatoid arthritis models. This highlights the potential of plant-based diets in managing inflammatory and autoimmune diseases by targeting PDGFR pathways.

- **Tissue Repair and Regeneration**

PDGFRs are crucial for tissue repair and regeneration processes. A plant-based diet, rich in vitamins, minerals, and bioactive compounds, can support these processes by modulating PDGFR activity. For example, vitamin C, found abundantly in fruits and vegetables, is essential for collagen synthesis and tissue repair. It also modulates PDGFR signaling in fibroblasts, promoting wound healing and tissue regeneration. Furthermore, plant-derived omega-3 fatty acids can reduce inflammation and support tissue repair by modulating PDGFR activity in various cell types.

- **Neuroprotection**

PDGFRs are expressed in the central nervous system and play a role in neuroprotection and neural development. Plant-based diets, which are high in antioxidants and anti-inflammatory compounds, can support brain health by modulating PDGFR signaling pathways. For example, polyphenols such as quercetin and resveratrol have neuroprotective effects by inhibiting PDGFR-mediated neuroinflammation and oxidative stress in neuronal cells. This suggests that a plant-based diet could contribute to the prevention and management of neurodegenerative diseases by targeting PDGFR pathways.

Platelet-Derived Growth Factor Receptors (PDGFRs) are essential for various physiological processes, including cell proliferation, differentiation, migration, and survival. The production and regulation of these receptors involve complex mechanisms influenced by genetic and environmental factors. Plant-based diets, rich in antioxidants, dietary fiber, and healthy fats, can positively influence PDGFR activity and expression. Bioactive compounds found in plant foods, such as flavonoids and omega-3 fatty acids, have been shown to modulate PDGFR signaling pathways, contributing to the prevention and management of chronic diseases such as cardiovascular disease, cancer, and inflammatory conditions.

Vascular Endothelial Growth Factor Receptors (VEGFRs)

Vascular Endothelial Growth Factor Receptors (VEGFRs) are tyrosine kinase receptors that play a vital role in the regulation of angiogenesis, the process through which new blood vessels form from pre-existing ones. These receptors are essential for both physiological and pathological vascular formation, making them critical targets in the treatment of various diseases, including cancer and age-related macular degeneration. There are three primary types of VEGFRs: VEGFR-1 (Flt-1), VEGFR-2 (KDR/Flk-1), and VEGFR-3 (Flt-4), each with distinct roles and tissue distributions.

Function of VEGFR

• **VEGFR-1 (Flt-1)**

VEGFR-1 is predominantly involved in the regulation of angiogenesis during embryonic development and in adult physiology. It acts mainly as a decoy receptor to modulate the availability of VEGF-A, the primary ligand, preventing excessive angiogenic signaling. While its kinase activity is relatively low, VEGFR-1's role in controlling VEGF-A availability is crucial for maintaining vascular homeostasis.

• **VEGFR-2 (KDR/Flk-1)**

VEGFR-2 is the principal mediator of the angiogenic effects of VEGF-A. It is primarily expressed in endothelial cells and, upon binding to VEGF-A, undergoes dimerization and autophosphorylation, leading to the activation of several downstream signaling pathways. These pathways promote endothelial cell proliferation, migration, survival, and increased vascular permeability, all of which are essential for new blood vessel formation.

• **VEGFR-3 (Flt-4)**

VEGFR-3 is mainly expressed in lymphatic endothelial cells and is crucial for the development and maintenance of the lymphatic system. Its primary ligands are VEGF-C and VEGF-D. VEGFR-3 activation leads to lymphangiogenesis, the formation of lymphatic vessels, which is important for maintaining fluid balance and immune function.

Production of VEGFR

The production of VEGFRs is a complex process regulated at multiple levels, including gene expression, receptor synthesis, and post-translational modifications. The genes encoding VEGFR-1, VEGFR-2, and VEGFR-3 are FLT1, KDR, and FLT4, respectively.

• **Gene Expression**

Gene expression of VEGFRs is controlled by various transcription factors and regulatory elements. These include promoter regions upstream of the FLT1, KDR, and FLT4 genes that bind specific proteins to initiate transcription. Hypoxia is a significant regulator of VEGFR gene expression. Under low oxygen conditions, Hypoxia-Inducible Factor 1-alpha (HIF-1α) is stabilized and binds to hypoxia-response elements (HREs) in the promoters of VEGFR genes, upregulating their expression.

- **Receptor Synthesis**

Once transcribed, the mRNA of VEGFRs is translated into protein in the endoplasmic reticulum. These proteins undergo folding and glycosylation, which are essential for their proper function and stability. The receptors are then transported to the cell membrane, where they become functional.

- **Post-Translational Modifications**

VEGFRs undergo various post-translational modifications, such as phosphorylation, which regulate their activity, desensitization, and internalization. Phosphorylation of these receptors by kinases can lead to receptor activation, triggering downstream signaling cascades essential for angiogenesis and lymphangiogenesis.

Regulation of VEGFR

The regulation of VEGFRs involves multiple mechanisms to ensure appropriate cellular responses to VEGF ligands.

- **Desensitization and Downregulation**

Prolonged exposure to VEGF can lead to receptor desensitization, where the receptor's responsiveness is diminished. This is often followed by downregulation, where the number of receptors on the cell surface is reduced. These processes are crucial in preventing overstimulation and maintaining homeostasis. Desensitization involves receptor phosphorylation by kinases, leading to the binding of proteins that uncouple the receptors from downstream signaling pathways and target them for internalization.

- **Receptor Recycling and Degradation**

Internalized receptors can either be recycled back to the cell membrane or degraded in lysosomes. The balance between these processes determines the overall number of functional receptors on the cell surface. Recycling allows the cell to quickly restore receptor sensitivity, while degradation reduces receptor density, providing long-term regulation.

Role of Plant-Based Compounds in Regulation

Plant-based diets can influence the regulation of VEGFRs through various bioactive compounds. Phytochemicals, such as flavonoids, have been shown to modulate receptor activity and expression.

- **Flavonoids**

Flavonoids are a group of polyphenolic compounds found in fruits, vegetables, tea, and other plant-based foods. They have been reported to influence VEGFR signaling pathways. For instance, quercetin, a flavonoid found in apples, onions, and berries, can inhibit VEGFR-2-mediated angiogenesis by blocking its phosphorylation and downstream signaling.

- **Dietary Fiber**

High-fiber diets, typical of plant-based nutrition, can improve overall cardiovascular health, potentially impacting VEGFR activity. Fiber can help manage blood pressure and reduce systemic inflammation, both of which are linked to VEGFR regulation.

- **Omega-3 Fatty Acids**

Plant sources of omega-3 fatty acids, such as flaxseeds and chia seeds, have anti-inflammatory properties and can influence VEGFR function. Omega-3 fatty acids have been shown to decrease the expression of VEGFRs in endothelial cells, potentially affecting angiogenesis and lymphangiogenesis.

Plant-Based Diets and VEGFRs

Adopting a plant-based diet can have significant impacts on the regulation and function of VEGFRs. The intake of various nutrients and bioactive compounds from plants can modulate the VEGF-VEGFR system, contributing to overall health benefits.

- **Cardiovascular Health**

Plant-based diets are rich in antioxidants, dietary fiber, and healthy fats, which are beneficial for cardiovascular health. The regulation of VEGFRs in the endothelium can be positively influenced by these dietary components. For example, antioxidants can reduce oxidative stress, which is known to impair VEGFR function. Additionally, dietary fiber helps in managing blood pressure by improving endothelial function and reducing systemic inflammation.

- **Metabolic Health**

The influence of plant-based diets on VEGFRs can enhance metabolic health. Foods rich in flavonoids and omega-3 fatty acids can improve insulin sensitivity and reduce the risk of metabolic disorders such as type 2 diabetes. By modulating VEGFR activity, these diets can enhance glucose uptake and utilization, contributing to better glycemic control.

- **Cancer Prevention**

The modulation of VEGFR signaling by plant-based compounds can play a role in cancer prevention. Angiogenesis is a critical process in tumor growth and metastasis, and the inhibition of VEGFRs by plant-derived bioactive compounds can reduce tumor vascularization. Flavonoids, for instance, have been shown to inhibit VEGFR-mediated angiogenesis, thus potentially limiting cancer progression.

Vascular Endothelial Growth Factor Receptors (VEGFRs) are essential for various physiological processes, including angiogenesis, lymphangiogenesis, and vascular permeability. The production and regulation of these receptors involve complex mechanisms influenced by genetic and environmental factors, including dietary components.

Fibroblast Growth Factor Receptor (FGFR)

Fibroblast Growth Factor Receptors (FGFRs) are a family of receptor tyrosine kinases that play a pivotal role in various cellular processes including proliferation, differentiation, migration, and survival. There are four main types of FGFRs: FGFR1, FGFR2, FGFR3, and FGFR4, each with distinct functions and tissue distributions. FGFRs are activated by binding to fibroblast growth factors (FGFs), leading to the activation of downstream signaling pathways that influence cellular behavior.

Function of Fibroblast Growth Factor Receptors

- **FGFR1**

FGFR1 is widely expressed in various tissues and is involved in embryonic development, angiogenesis, wound healing, and tissue repair. Activation of FGFR1 by its ligands leads to the initiation of several signaling cascades, including the MAPK, PI3K/AKT, and PLCγ pathways. These pathways collectively contribute to cell growth, survival, and migration. FGFR1 also plays a critical role in the development of the skeletal system, influencing the differentiation and proliferation of osteoblasts and chondrocytes.

- **FGFR2**

FGFR2 is predominantly expressed in epithelial and mesenchymal tissues. It is crucial for the development of the skin, lungs, liver, and other organs. FGFR2 signaling regulates cell proliferation, differentiation, and apoptosis. Mutations in FGFR2 are associated with several craniosynostosis syndromes, where premature fusion of skull bones occurs, highlighting its importance in skeletal development.

- **FGFR3**

FGFR3 is primarily expressed in cartilage and plays a key role in regulating bone growth and development. It acts as a negative regulator of chondrocyte proliferation and differentiation, ensuring proper bone formation and maintenance. Mutations in FGFR3 are linked to skeletal disorders such as achondroplasia, characterized by shortened bones and dwarfism.

• **FGFR4**

FGFR4 is mainly found in muscle tissues and the liver. It is involved in regulating bile acid metabolism and muscle regeneration. FGFR4 activation promotes myogenesis and muscle repair processes. Additionally, it plays a role in liver development and function, influencing hepatocyte proliferation and differentiation.

Production of Fibroblast Growth Factor Receptors

The production of FGFRs involves multiple levels of regulation, including gene expression, receptor synthesis, and post-translational modifications. The genes encoding FGFR1, FGFR2, FGFR3, and FGFR4 are FGFR1, FGFR2, FGFR3, and FGFR4, respectively.

• **Gene Expression**

Gene expression of FGFRs is tightly regulated by various transcription factors and regulatory elements. Promoter regions upstream of the FGFR genes bind specific proteins that initiate transcription. Factors such as growth factors, hormones, and dietary components can influence the expression of these genes. For instance, vitamin D has been shown to upregulate FGFR expression, promoting cellular growth and differentiation.

• **Receptor Synthesis**

Once transcribed, the mRNA of FGFRs is translated into protein in the endoplasmic reticulum. These proteins undergo folding and glycosylation, which are essential for their proper function and stability. The receptors are then transported to the cell membrane, where they become functional. The folding process is assisted by molecular chaperones, ensuring that the receptors attain their correct conformation.

• **Post-Translational Modifications**

FGFRs undergo various post-translational modifications, such as phosphorylation, glycosylation, and ubiquitination, which regulate their activity, stability, and localization. Phosphorylation of FGFRs by kinases can enhance their signaling capabilities, while ubiquitination often targets the receptors for degradation, thus modulating their levels on the cell surface.

Regulation of Fibroblast Growth Factor Receptors

The regulation of FGFRs involves multiple mechanisms to ensure appropriate cellular responses to FGFs.

- **Ligand Binding and Receptor Dimerization**

FGFRs are activated by the binding of FGFs to the extracellular domain of the receptor. This binding induces dimerization of the receptors, which brings the intracellular kinase domains into close proximity, leading to their activation through autophosphorylation. This activation is essential for the initiation of downstream signaling pathways.

- **Desensitization and Downregulation**

Prolonged exposure to FGFs can lead to receptor desensitization, where the receptor's responsiveness is diminished. This is often followed by downregulation, where the number of receptors on the cell surface is reduced. These processes are crucial in preventing overstimulation and maintaining homeostasis. Desensitization involves receptor internalization and degradation in lysosomes, reducing the receptor density and ensuring controlled signaling.

- **Receptor Recycling and Degradation**

Internalized FGFRs can either be recycled back to the cell membrane or degraded in lysosomes. The balance between these processes determines the overall number of functional receptors on the cell surface. Recycling allows the cell to quickly restore receptor sensitivity, while degradation reduces the receptor density, providing long-term regulation.

Role of Plant-Based Compounds in Regulation

Plant-based diets can influence the regulation of FGFRs through various bioactive compounds. Phytochemicals, such as flavonoids, have been shown to modulate receptor activity and expression.

- **Flavonoids**

Flavonoids are a group of polyphenolic compounds found in fruits, vegetables, tea, and other plant-based foods. They have been reported to influence the FGFR signaling pathway by modulating receptor activity and expression. For instance, quercetin, a flavonoid found in apples, onions, and berries, can inhibit FGFR-mediated signaling in cancer cells, promoting apoptosis and inhibiting cell proliferation.

- **Dietary Fiber**

High-fiber diets, typical of plant-based nutrition, can improve insulin sensitivity and reduce systemic inflammation. This, in turn, may modulate the activity of FGFRs, as insulin and inflammatory cytokines are linked to receptor regulation. Soluble fiber, in particular, has been shown to influence the expression of growth factor receptors, contributing to better metabolic health.

- **Omega-3 Fatty Acids**

Plant sources of omega-3 fatty acids, such as flaxseeds and chia seeds, have anti-inflammatory properties and can influence FGFR function. Omega-3 fatty acids have been shown to modulate the expression of growth factor receptors in various tissues, potentially affecting cellular growth and differentiation.

Plant-Based Diets and Fibroblast Growth Factor Receptors

Adopting a plant-based diet can have significant impacts on the regulation and function of FGFRs. The intake of various nutrients and bioactive compounds from plants can modulate the FGFR system, contributing to overall health benefits.

- **Cardiovascular Health**

Plant-based diets are rich in antioxidants, dietary fiber, and healthy fats, which are beneficial for cardiovascular health. The regulation of FGFRs in the cardiovascular system can be positively influenced by these dietary components. For example, antioxidants can reduce oxidative stress, which is known to impair FGFR function. Additionally, dietary fiber helps in managing blood pressure by improving endothelial function and reducing systemic inflammation.

• **Metabolic Health**

The influence of plant-based diets on FGFRs can enhance metabolic health. Foods rich in flavonoids and omega-3 fatty acids can improve insulin sensitivity and reduce the risk of metabolic disorders such as type 2 diabetes. By modulating FGFR activity, these diets can enhance glucose uptake and utilization, contributing to better glycemic control.

• **Cancer Prevention**

Plant-based diets are associated with a lower risk of cancer, partly due to the modulation of FGFR signaling. Many phytochemicals found in plant foods have been shown to inhibit FGFR-mediated pathways in cancer cells, promoting apoptosis and inhibiting proliferation. For instance, curcumin, a compound found in turmeric, has been shown to inhibit FGFR signaling in various cancer models, contributing to its anti-cancer effects.

• **Bone Health**

FGFRs play a critical role in bone development and maintenance. A plant-based diet rich in vitamins, minerals, and antioxidants can support bone health by modulating FGFR activity. For example, vitamin D, found in fortified plant-based foods, can upregulate FGFR expression, promoting osteoblast differentiation and bone formation. Additionally, the anti-inflammatory properties of omega-3 fatty acids can reduce bone resorption and support overall bone health.

Plant-Based Compounds and FGFR-Related Disorders

• **Osteoporosis**

Osteoporosis is a condition characterized by weakened bones and increased fracture risk. FGFR signaling is crucial for maintaining bone density and strength. Plant-based compounds, such as isoflavones found in soy, have been shown to positively influence FGFR signaling in bone cells, promoting bone formation and reducing resorption. These effects can help mitigate the risk of osteoporosis and support bone health.

- **Cardiovascular Diseases**

Cardiovascular diseases are a leading cause of morbidity and mortality worldwide. FGFR signaling plays a role in angiogenesis and vascular repair, processes that are essential for cardiovascular health. Plant-based diets rich in antioxidants, fiber, and healthy fats can modulate FGFR activity, promoting vascular health and reducing the risk of cardiovascular diseases. For example, the anti-inflammatory effects of omega-3 fatty acids can reduce endothelial dysfunction, a key factor in cardiovascular disease development.

- **Cancer**

FGFR mutations and aberrant signaling are implicated in various cancers. Plant-based compounds have shown potential in targeting FGFR-mediated pathways in cancer cells. Curcumin, quercetin, and other phytochemicals have been studied for their ability to inhibit FGFR signaling, promote apoptosis, and inhibit proliferation in cancer cells. These compounds can be beneficial as part of a plant-based diet in reducing cancer risk and supporting cancer therapy.

- **Metabolic Disorders**

Metabolic disorders, such as type 2 diabetes, are influenced by FGFR signaling. Plant-based diets can improve metabolic health by modulating FGFR activity. For instance, high-fiber diets can enhance insulin sensitivity and reduce systemic inflammation, positively impacting FGFR signaling. Additionally, flavonoids found in fruits and vegetables can regulate glucose metabolism and support metabolic health.

Fibroblast Growth Factor Receptors (FGFRs) are crucial for various physiological processes, including cell proliferation, differentiation, and survival. The production and regulation of FGFRs involve complex mechanisms influenced by genetic and environmental factors. Plant-based diets, rich in bioactive compounds, can significantly impact the regulation and function of FGFRs, contributing to overall health benefits.

Nerve Growth Factor Receptor (NGFR)

The Nerve Growth Factor Receptor (NGFR), also known as p75^NTR, is a crucial component in the nervous system, playing an essential role in the development, survival, and apoptosis of neurons. NGFR is a member of the tumor necrosis factor receptor superfamily and interacts with neurotrophins, including nerve growth factor (NGF), brain-derived neurotrophic factor (BDNF), and others. This receptor is involved in a variety of physiological and pathological processes, making it a significant subject of study, especially in the context of neurodegenerative diseases and neural repair.

Function of Nerve Growth Factor Receptor (NGFR)

- **Neuronal Survival and Apoptosis**

NGFR has a dual role in neuronal survival and apoptosis, depending on the cellular context and the ligands involved. When bound to NGF, NGFR typically promotes cell survival and differentiation through signaling pathways that inhibit apoptosis. Conversely, in the absence of NGF or in the presence of pro-apoptotic ligands, NGFR can initiate apoptotic signaling, leading to programmed cell death.

- **Synaptic Plasticity**

NGFR is crucial for synaptic plasticity, the ability of synapses to strengthen or weaken over time, which is essential for learning and memory. By interacting with neurotrophins, NGFR influences synaptic growth and the formation of new synaptic connections.

- **Myelination**

NGFR is also involved in the myelination of neurons. It regulates the growth and differentiation of oligodendrocytes, the cells responsible for forming the myelin sheath around axons, which is critical for efficient nerve impulse transmission.

Production of Nerve Growth Factor Receptor (NGFR)

• Gene Expression

The NGFR gene, located on chromosome 17, encodes the protein p75^NTR. The expression of the NGFR gene is regulated by various transcription factors and is influenced by the cellular environment and developmental cues. Factors such as injury, inflammation, and neural activity can upregulate NGFR expression, highlighting its role in neural repair and plasticity.

• Protein Synthesis and Post-Translational Modifications

Once transcribed, the mRNA for NGFR is translated into protein in the endoplasmic reticulum. The nascent protein undergoes folding and post-translational modifications, including glycosylation and phosphorylation, which are critical for its stability, localization, and function. Glycosylation enhances the stability of NGFR on the cell surface, while phosphorylation can modulate its signaling activity.

• Transport to the Cell Membrane

After synthesis and modification, NGFR is transported to the cell membrane, where it becomes functional. The proper trafficking of NGFR is essential for its role in signaling, as it must be localized to specific regions of the cell membrane to interact with its ligands and co-receptors effectively.

Regulation of Nerve Growth Factor Receptor (NGFR)

• Ligand Binding and Signal Transduction

NGFR's activity is primarily regulated by its ligands. The binding of NGF to NGFR induces a conformational change that activates downstream signaling pathways involved in cell survival, growth, and differentiation. These pathways include the activation of nuclear factor kappa B (NF-κB) and the phosphoinositide 3-kinase (PI3K)/Akt pathway.

• Receptor Interactions

NGFR does not function in isolation; it often forms complexes with other receptors such as TrkA (tropomyosin receptor kinase A) and sortilin. The interaction between NGFR and TrkA enhances the specificity and strength of NGF signaling. Conversely, NGFR-sortilin complexes are involved in pro-apoptotic signaling, highlighting the receptor's versatility.

- **Post-Translational Modifications**

NGFR's function is further regulated by post-translational modifications, including phosphorylation and ubiquitination. Phosphorylation of NGFR by kinases can enhance or inhibit its activity, depending on the specific residues modified. Ubiquitination, on the other hand, targets NGFR for degradation, thereby modulating its levels on the cell surface.

Role of Plant-Based Compounds in Regulation

Plant-based diets, rich in bioactive compounds, can influence the regulation of NGFR and its signaling pathways. Phytochemicals such as flavonoids, polyphenols, and omega-3 fatty acids have been shown to modulate neurotrophic signaling and neuroinflammation, impacting NGFR function.

- **Flavonoids**

Flavonoids, found in various fruits, vegetables, and teas, have neuroprotective properties. For instance, quercetin, a flavonoid present in apples, onions, and berries, can enhance NGF-mediated signaling by increasing the expression of NGFR and TrkA receptors. This modulation can promote neuronal survival and differentiation.

- **Polyphenols**

Polyphenols, abundant in plant-based foods such as berries, nuts, and seeds, also play a role in NGFR regulation. Resveratrol, a polyphenol found in grapes and red wine, has been shown to activate the PI3K/Akt pathway, promoting cell survival and neuroprotection. This activation can counteract the pro-apoptotic signaling of NGFR, enhancing neuronal health.

- **Omega-3 Fatty Acids**

Omega-3 fatty acids, particularly those derived from plant sources like flaxseeds and chia seeds, have anti-inflammatory properties and can influence NGFR signaling. These fatty acids can modulate the expression of NGFR and its downstream effectors, promoting neuronal survival and reducing neuroinflammation.

Plant-Based Diets and NGFR

- **Neuroprotection**

Plant-based diets, rich in antioxidants and anti-inflammatory compounds, offer neuroprotective benefits that can positively influence NGFR signaling. The high content of vitamins, minerals, and phytochemicals in plant foods helps mitigate oxidative stress and inflammation, which are critical factors in neurodegenerative diseases.

- **Cognitive Function**

The neuroprotective and anti-inflammatory properties of plant-based diets contribute to improved cognitive function. By modulating NGFR signaling, these diets can enhance synaptic plasticity and neurogenesis, supporting learning and memory processes.

- **Neural Repair and Regeneration**

The bioactive compounds in plant-based diets promote neural repair and regeneration by modulating the expression and activity of NGFR and its co-receptors. This modulation can enhance the survival and differentiation of neural progenitor cells, facilitating recovery from neural injury.

The Nerve Growth Factor Receptor (NGFR) plays a pivotal role in the nervous system, regulating neuronal survival, apoptosis, synaptic plasticity, and myelination. Its function and regulation are influenced by a variety of factors, including ligand binding, receptor interactions, and post-translational modifications. Plant-based diets, rich in bioactive compounds such as flavonoids, polyphenols, and omega-3 fatty acids, can modulate NGFR signaling, offering neuroprotective benefits and promoting cognitive health. The integration of these dietary components into daily nutrition can enhance NGFR function and support overall neural health.

Ephrin Receptors (EphA, EphB)

Ephrin receptors (Eph receptors) are a class of receptor tyrosine kinases that play a pivotal role in cell signaling and communication. These receptors are subdivided into two main families: EphA and EphB, based on their binding preferences for ephrin-A and ephrin-B ligands, respectively. Eph receptors are crucial for various physiological processes, including cell adhesion, migration, and tissue boundary formation.

Function of Ephrin Receptors

EphA Receptors

EphA receptors primarily interact with ephrin-A ligands, which are glycosylphosphatidylinositol (GPI)-anchored to the cell membrane. The main functions of EphA receptors include:

1. **Cell-Cell Communication**: EphA receptors facilitate communication between adjacent cells, influencing cell positioning and boundary formation. This is vital during embryonic development, where precise cell positioning determines tissue and organ structure.
2. **Axon Guidance**: In the nervous system, EphA receptors guide axons to their correct targets, ensuring proper neural network formation. They achieve this by mediating repulsive or attractive signals that steer growing axons.
3. **Cell Migration and Adhesion**: EphA receptors regulate cell migration and adhesion by modulating the cytoskeleton and cell surface adhesion molecules. This function is critical in processes such as wound healing and cancer metastasis.

EphB Receptors

EphB receptors bind to ephrin-B ligands, which are transmembrane proteins. The functions of EphB receptors are diverse and include:

1. **Tissue Boundary Formation**: EphB receptors play a significant role in forming boundaries between different tissue types. This is crucial for maintaining tissue organization and function.
2. **Synaptic Plasticity**: In the brain, EphB receptors are involved in synaptic plasticity, which underlies learning and memory. They influence the formation and remodeling of synapses.
3. **Angiogenesis**: EphB receptors regulate the growth of new blood vessels (angiogenesis), which is essential for tissue growth and repair, as well as in pathological conditions like cancer.

Production of Ephrin Receptors

The production of Eph receptors involves a series of well-coordinated steps, including gene expression, receptor synthesis, and post-translational modifications.

Gene Expression

Eph receptor genes are expressed in a tissue-specific manner, regulated by various transcription factors and signaling pathways. Key factors influencing the expression of Eph receptor genes include:

1. **Developmental Signals**: During embryonic development, specific signaling molecules, such as Wnt and Notch, regulate the expression of Eph receptor genes to ensure proper tissue and organ formation.
2. **Environmental Cues**: External stimuli, such as mechanical stress and extracellular matrix components, can modulate Eph receptor gene expression. For example, in the nervous system, neuronal

activity can influence Eph receptor expression, impacting synaptic plasticity.

Receptor Synthesis

Once transcribed, the mRNA encoding Eph receptors is translated into protein in the endoplasmic reticulum (ER). The newly synthesized receptors undergo folding and glycosylation, which are crucial for their stability and function. The properly folded receptors are then transported to the Golgi apparatus for further processing before being directed to the cell membrane.

Post-Translational Modifications

Eph receptors undergo various post-translational modifications, such as phosphorylation, which regulate their activity and interactions. These modifications include:

1. **Phosphorylation**: The kinase domains of Eph receptors are phosphorylated upon ligand binding, activating downstream signaling pathways. This modification is essential for receptor function and signal transduction.
2. **Ubiquitination**: Eph receptors can be tagged with ubiquitin molecules, targeting them for degradation by the proteasome. This process helps regulate receptor levels and signaling duration.

Regulation of Ephrin Receptors

The regulation of Eph receptors is a complex process involving multiple mechanisms to ensure appropriate cellular responses.

Ligand Binding and Signal Transduction

Eph receptors are activated upon binding to their ephrin ligands, triggering bidirectional signaling—forward signaling through the Eph receptor and reverse signaling through the ephrin ligand. This bidirectional communication is crucial for coordinating cellular responses.

The binding affinity and specificity between Eph receptors and ephrin ligands are regulated by:

1. **Ligand Availability**: The expression and presentation of ephrin ligands on neighboring cells influence Eph receptor activation. Various factors, such as cell type and developmental stage, determine ligand availability.
2. **Receptor Clustering**: Upon ligand binding, Eph receptors cluster together, enhancing signal transduction. This clustering is regulated by the cytoskeletal network and membrane microdomains.

Desensitization and Downregulation

Prolonged activation of Eph receptors can lead to desensitization, where the receptor's responsiveness diminishes. This is followed by downregulation, reducing the number of receptors on the cell surface. These processes prevent overstimulation and maintain cellular homeostasis. Desensitization involves:

1. **Receptor Phosphorylation**: Specific kinases phosphorylate Eph receptors, leading to receptor desensitization. This reduces receptor activity and attenuates signaling.
2. **Endocytosis and Degradation**: Internalized receptors can either be recycled back to the cell membrane or degraded in lysosomes. The balance between these processes determines receptor levels on the cell surface.

Role of Plant-Based Compounds in Regulation

Plant-based diets can influence the regulation of Eph receptors through various bioactive compounds. Phytochemicals, such as flavonoids, have been shown to modulate receptor activity and expression.

Flavonoids

Flavonoids are a group of polyphenolic compounds found in fruits, vegetables, tea, and other plant-based foods. They have been reported to influence Eph receptor signaling pathways by modulating receptor activity. For instance, certain flavonoids can inhibit the phosphorylation of Eph receptors, thereby reducing their activation and downstream signaling.

1. **Quercetin**: Found in apples, onions, and berries, quercetin can inhibit Eph receptor-mediated signaling, impacting cell adhesion and migration.
2. **Epigallocatechin Gallate (EGCG)**: Present in green tea, EGCG has been shown to modulate Eph receptor activity, influencing processes like angiogenesis and cancer cell migration.

Dietary Fiber

High-fiber diets, typical of plant-based nutrition, can improve metabolic health and reduce inflammation, indirectly affecting Eph receptor regulation. Fiber-rich diets can modulate the gut microbiome, leading to the production of short-chain fatty acids (SCFAs) that have systemic anti-inflammatory effects. Reduced inflammation can impact the expression and function of Eph receptors, particularly in tissues prone to inflammatory signaling.

Omega-3 Fatty Acids

Plant sources of omega-3 fatty acids, such as flaxseeds and chia seeds, have anti-inflammatory properties and can influence Eph receptor function. Omega-3 fatty acids have been shown to modulate signaling pathways that interact with Eph receptor pathways, potentially affecting processes like cell migration and synaptic plasticity.

Plant-Based Diets and Ephrin Receptors

Adopting a plant-based diet can have significant impacts on the regulation and function of Eph receptors. The intake of various nutrients and bioactive compounds from plants can modulate the ephrin system, contributing to overall health benefits.

Cardiovascular Health

Plant-based diets are rich in antioxidants, dietary fiber, and healthy fats, which are beneficial for cardiovascular health. The regulation of Eph receptors in the vasculature can be positively influenced by these dietary components. For example, antioxidants can reduce oxidative stress, which is known to impair Eph receptor function. Additionally, dietary fiber helps in managing blood pressure by improving endothelial function and reducing systemic inflammation.

Neurological Health

The influence of plant-based diets on Eph receptors can enhance neurological health. Foods rich in flavonoids and omega-3 fatty acids can improve synaptic plasticity and reduce the risk of neurodegenerative diseases. By modulating Eph receptor activity, these diets can support cognitive function and protect against conditions like Alzheimer's disease.

Cancer Prevention

Eph receptors play a dual role in cancer, acting as both tumor suppressors and promoters depending on the context. Plant-based diets, which are typically high in phytochemicals, can influence Eph receptor signaling in cancer cells. Bioactive compounds from plants can modulate Eph receptor-mediated pathways, potentially inhibiting tumor growth and metastasis.

1. **Curcumin**: Found in turmeric, curcumin has been shown to inhibit Eph receptor signaling, reducing cancer cell proliferation and migration.

2. **Resveratrol**: Present in grapes and berries, resveratrol can modulate Eph receptor activity, impacting tumor progression and angiogenesis.

Ephrin receptors (EphA, EphB) are essential for various physiological processes, including cell communication, migration, and tissue organization. The production and regulation of these receptors involve complex mechanisms influenced by genetic and environmental factors. Plant-based diets, rich in bioactive compounds such as flavonoids, dietary fiber, and omega-3 fatty acids, can modulate the function and regulation of Eph receptors, contributing to overall health benefits. These dietary components can influence cardiovascular health, neurological function, and cancer prevention by impacting Eph receptor-mediated pathways.

Hepatocyte Growth Factor Receptor (HGFR/MET)

The Hepatocyte Growth Factor Receptor (HGFR), also known as MET, is a receptor tyrosine kinase that plays a vital role in various cellular processes. This receptor is encoded by the MET gene and is primarily activated by its ligand, hepatocyte growth factor (HGF). HGFR/MET is involved in cellular growth, motility, and differentiation, making it critical in embryonic development, wound healing, and tissue regeneration. However, its dysregulation is also associated with several cancers, making it a significant focus of medical research.

Function of Hepatocyte Growth Factor Receptor

The MET receptor's primary function is to mediate the effects of HGF, a multifunctional cytokine. Upon binding to HGF, MET undergoes dimerization and autophosphorylation on specific tyrosine residues within its intracellular domain, initiating a cascade of downstream signaling pathways. These pathways include the Ras-MAPK, PI3K-AKT, and STAT pathways, which collectively regulate cell proliferation, survival, migration, and morphogenesis.

Cellular Growth and Proliferation

MET signaling is crucial for cellular growth and proliferation. The activation of the Ras-MAPK pathway leads to the transcription of genes involved in cell cycle progression and DNA synthesis. This is particularly important in liver regeneration, where HGF/MET signaling promotes the rapid proliferation of hepatocytes following liver injury.

Cell Survival and Anti-Apoptosis

MET signaling also enhances cell survival and provides anti-apoptotic signals. The PI3K-AKT pathway is a major player in this aspect, promoting cellular survival by inhibiting apoptotic pathways. This function is critical in maintaining tissue integrity during repair processes and protecting cells from various forms of stress.

Cell Migration and Morphogenesis

One of the hallmark functions of MET signaling is its ability to induce cell motility and morphogenesis. This is essential during embryonic development, where MET signaling guides the migration of cells to their appropriate locations. Additionally, MET plays a role in wound healing by promoting the movement of epithelial cells to cover the wound site. The process of epithelial-mesenchymal transition (EMT), where epithelial cells acquire mesenchymal properties and become more motile, is also influenced by MET signaling.

Angiogenesis

HGF/MET signaling promotes angiogenesis, the formation of new blood vessels from existing ones. This is crucial for supplying nutrients and oxygen to growing tissues and during tissue repair. MET's role in angiogenesis is mediated through its ability to stimulate the production of angiogenic factors like vascular endothelial growth factor (VEGF).

Production of Hepatocyte Growth Factor Receptor

The production of HGFR/MET involves several steps, from gene transcription to protein processing and transportation to the cell membrane.

Gene Expression

The MET gene, located on chromosome 7q31, encodes the MET protein. The expression of this gene is regulated by various transcription factors, including SP1, AP1, and others, which bind to the promoter region of the MET gene. The regulation of MET gene expression can be influenced by multiple factors, including cellular context, external signals, and the presence of bioactive compounds in the diet.

Protein Synthesis

Once transcribed, MET mRNA is translated into a precursor protein in the endoplasmic reticulum. This precursor undergoes glycosylation, a post-translational modification essential for its stability and function. The MET precursor is then cleaved into a mature form composed of an extracellular alpha chain and a transmembrane beta chain linked by disulfide bonds.

Post-Translational Modifications

Further post-translational modifications, such as phosphorylation, are crucial for MET's activity. Autophosphorylation of specific tyrosine residues in the cytoplasmic domain of MET upon HGF binding activates its kinase activity, which is necessary for downstream signaling.

Trafficking to the Cell Membrane

The mature MET receptor is transported to the cell membrane, where it becomes functional. Proper localization of MET at the cell surface is essential for its ability to interact with HGF and initiate signaling cascades.

Regulation of Hepatocyte Growth Factor Receptor

The regulation of MET is complex and involves mechanisms at the transcriptional, post-transcriptional, and post-translational levels.

Transcriptional Regulation

The transcription of the MET gene is controlled by various factors, including growth factors, cytokines, and stress signals. For instance, hypoxia-inducible factors (HIFs) can enhance MET expression under low oxygen conditions, which is crucial for promoting angiogenesis and cell survival during hypoxic stress.

Post-Transcriptional Regulation

MicroRNAs (miRNAs) play a significant role in the post-transcriptional regulation of MET. Certain miRNAs can bind to the MET mRNA, preventing its translation and thus reducing the levels of MET protein. This regulatory mechanism ensures precise control over MET expression in response to changing cellular conditions.

Post-Translational Regulation

The activity of MET is finely tuned by post-translational modifications, including phosphorylation, ubiquitination, and glycosylation. Phosphorylation of MET on specific tyrosine residues is necessary for its activation, while ubiquitination can target MET for degradation, thus controlling the receptor's levels at the cell surface.

Internalization and Degradation

Following activation, MET is often internalized and either recycled back to the cell membrane or targeted for degradation in lysosomes. This process is crucial for terminating MET signaling and preventing excessive cellular responses.

Plant-Based Compounds and MET Regulation

Plant-based diets can influence the regulation and function of the MET receptor through various bioactive compounds. These compounds, including flavonoids, polyphenols, and other phytochemicals, can modulate MET signaling and expression, contributing to health benefits and disease prevention.

Flavonoids

Flavonoids are a diverse group of polyphenolic compounds found in fruits, vegetables, tea, and other plant-based foods. They have been shown to interact with various signaling pathways, including those involving MET. For instance, quercetin, a flavonoid found in apples, onions, and berries, can inhibit MET signaling by preventing its activation and subsequent downstream effects. This inhibition can be beneficial in preventing the excessive cell proliferation and migration associated with cancer progression.

Polyphenols

Polyphenols, abundant in foods like berries, nuts, and seeds, also play a role in modulating MET signaling. Resveratrol, a polyphenol found in grapes and red wine, has been reported to inhibit MET-mediated signaling pathways. By interfering with MET activation, resveratrol can help prevent the uncontrolled cell growth and migration seen in cancer metastasis.

Dietary Fiber

High-fiber diets, typical of plant-based nutrition, can have indirect effects on MET signaling. Dietary fiber improves gut health and reduces systemic inflammation, which can influence the expression and activity of growth factor receptors, including MET. The anti-inflammatory effects of dietary fiber may help mitigate the chronic inflammation that can lead to aberrant MET signaling in various diseases.

Omega-3 Fatty Acids

Plant sources of omega-3 fatty acids, such as flaxseeds and chia seeds, possess anti-inflammatory properties that can influence the activity of growth factor receptors. Omega-3 fatty acids have been shown to reduce the expression of pro-inflammatory cytokines and growth factors, potentially affecting MET signaling. By decreasing inflammation, omega-3 fatty acids help maintain normal MET function and prevent its dysregulation in pathological conditions.

Plant-Based Diets and MET Receptor Regulation

Adopting a plant-based diet can significantly impact the regulation and function of the MET receptor, contributing to overall health and disease prevention.

Cancer Prevention

Plant-based diets are rich in antioxidants, dietary fiber, and anti-inflammatory compounds, which collectively contribute to cancer prevention. The modulation of MET signaling by bioactive compounds in plant foods can help prevent the excessive cell proliferation and migration associated with cancer. For example, the flavonoids and polyphenols in fruits and vegetables can inhibit MET activation, reducing the risk of tumor growth and metastasis.

Cardiovascular Health

The anti-inflammatory and antioxidant properties of plant-based diets benefit cardiovascular health by maintaining normal growth factor signaling. Proper regulation of MET is essential for angiogenesis and tissue repair following cardiovascular injuries. The presence of bioactive compounds in plant foods ensures balanced MET signaling, supporting vascular health and preventing pathological angiogenesis associated with atherosclerosis and other cardiovascular diseases.

Metabolic Health

Plant-based diets can improve metabolic health by influencing the regulation of growth factor receptors, including MET. The high fiber content and presence of bioactive compounds in plant foods enhance insulin sensitivity and reduce inflammation, both of which are critical for maintaining healthy MET signaling. Improved MET function supports liver regeneration, wound healing, and metabolic processes, contributing to overall metabolic health.

Weight Management

The role of MET in regulating cell growth and metabolism makes it relevant to weight management. Plant-based diets, which are typically lower in calories and higher in fiber, can support healthy weight management by modulating MET signaling. The presence of anti-inflammatory and antioxidant compounds in plant foods helps maintain proper MET function, preventing its dysregulation in obesity and related metabolic disorders.

The Hepatocyte Growth Factor Receptor (HGFR/MET) plays a crucial role in various cellular processes, including growth, survival, migration, and morphogenesis. Its proper regulation is essential for normal cellular functions and tissue homeostasis. Plant-based diets, rich in bioactive compounds like flavonoids, polyphenols, and omega-3 fatty acids, can positively influence MET signaling, contributing to overall health benefits and disease prevention.

Tropomyosin Receptor Kinase (TRK)

Tropomyosin receptor kinases (TRKs), also known as neurotrophic tyrosine kinase receptors (NTRKs), are a family of receptor tyrosine kinases (RTKs) that play essential roles in the development, function, and survival of neurons. TRKs are involved in the mediation of neurotrophins, which are growth factors critical for the maintenance and survival of neural cells. There are three main subtypes of TRK receptors: TRKA, TRKB, and TRKC, each with distinct functions and affinities for different neurotrophins.

Function of Tropomyosin Receptor Kinases (TRKs)

TRKA

TRKA is primarily activated by nerve growth factor (NGF). This receptor is crucial for the development and maintenance of the nervous system. The activation of TRKA by NGF promotes neuronal survival, differentiation, and growth. It is particularly important for the survival of sympathetic and sensory neurons.

TRKB

TRKB is activated by brain-derived neurotrophic factor (BDNF), neurotrophin-4 (NT-4), and, to a lesser extent, neurotrophin-3 (NT-3). TRKB plays a vital role in the development and function of the central and peripheral nervous systems. It supports the survival, growth, and differentiation of various neuronal populations. TRKB signaling is also involved in synaptic plasticity, which is essential for learning and memory processes.

TRKC

TRKC is predominantly activated by neurotrophin-3 (NT-3). This receptor is involved in the development of proprioceptive neurons, which are responsible for sensing body position and movement. TRKC signaling supports neuronal survival and differentiation and is essential for the proper functioning of the nervous system.

Production of Tropomyosin Receptor Kinases

The production of TRKs is a complex process regulated at multiple levels, including gene expression, receptor synthesis, and post-translational modifications. The genes encoding TRKA, TRKB, and TRKC are NTRK1, NTRK2, and NTRK3, respectively.

Gene Expression

Gene expression of TRKs is tightly regulated by various transcription factors and regulatory elements. Promoter regions upstream of the NTRK genes bind specific proteins to initiate transcription. The expression of these genes can be influenced by several factors, including developmental signals, neuronal activity, and environmental stimuli.

Receptor Synthesis

Once transcribed, the mRNA of TRKs is translated into protein in the endoplasmic reticulum. These proteins undergo folding and glycosylation, which are essential for their proper function and stability. The receptors are then transported to the cell membrane, where they become functional.

Post-Translational Modifications

TRKs undergo various post-translational modifications, such as phosphorylation, which regulate their activity, desensitization, and internalization. Phosphorylation of these receptors by kinases can lead to receptor

activation or desensitization, modulating their responsiveness to neurotrophins.

Regulation of Tropomyosin Receptor Kinases

The regulation of TRKs involves multiple mechanisms to ensure appropriate cellular responses to neurotrophins.

Desensitization and Downregulation

Prolonged exposure to neurotrophins can lead to receptor desensitization, where the receptor's responsiveness is diminished. This is often followed by downregulation, where the number of receptors on the cell surface is reduced. These processes are crucial in preventing overstimulation and maintaining homeostasis. Desensitization involves receptor phosphorylation, which can lead to the binding of adaptor proteins that uncouple the receptors from signaling pathways and target them for internalization.

Receptor Recycling and Degradation

Internalized receptors can either be recycled back to the cell membrane or degraded in lysosomes. The balance between these processes determines the overall number of functional receptors on the cell surface. Recycling allows the cell to quickly restore receptor sensitivity, while degradation reduces the receptor density, providing long-term regulation.

Role of Plant-Based Compounds in Regulation

Plant-based diets can influence the regulation of TRKs through various bioactive compounds. Phytochemicals, such as flavonoids, have been shown to modulate receptor activity and expression.

Flavonoids

Flavonoids are a group of polyphenolic compounds found in fruits, vegetables, tea, and other plant-based foods. They have been reported to influence the TRK signaling pathway by modulating neurotrophin-induced responses. For instance, epicatechin, a flavonoid found in green tea, can enhance BDNF signaling through TRKB receptors, promoting neuronal survival and synaptic plasticity.

Curcumin

Curcumin, a polyphenolic compound found in turmeric, has been shown to upregulate the expression of BDNF and its receptor TRKB. This upregulation can enhance neurogenesis and synaptic plasticity, contributing to improved cognitive function and neuroprotection.

Omega-3 Fatty Acids

Plant sources of omega-3 fatty acids, such as flaxseeds and chia seeds, have anti-inflammatory properties and can influence TRK receptor function. Omega-3 fatty acids have been shown to increase the expression of BDNF and TRKB in the brain, promoting neuronal health and cognitive function.

Plant-Based Diets and TRK Receptors

Adopting a plant-based diet can have significant impacts on the regulation and function of TRK receptors. The intake of various nutrients and bioactive compounds from plants can modulate the neurotrophic system, contributing to overall health benefits.

Cognitive Health

Plant-based diets are rich in antioxidants, dietary fiber, and healthy fats, which are beneficial for cognitive health. The regulation of TRKB receptors in the brain can be positively influenced by these dietary components. For example, antioxidants can reduce oxidative stress, which is known to impair TRKB receptor function. Additionally, dietary fiber helps in managing blood sugar levels, which is crucial for maintaining cognitive function.

Mental Health

The influence of plant-based diets on TRKA and TRKB receptors can enhance mental health. Foods rich in flavonoids and omega-3 fatty acids can improve neurotrophin signaling and reduce the risk of mental health disorders such as depression and anxiety. By modulating TRKA and TRKB receptor activity, these diets can promote neuronal survival, neurogenesis, and synaptic plasticity, contributing to better mental health outcomes.

Neuroprotection

TRKC receptors play a crucial role in neuroprotection and the maintenance of proprioceptive neurons. Plant-based diets, which are typically lower in calories and higher in fiber, can support neuroprotection by enhancing the function of TRKC receptors. The presence of bioactive compounds in plant foods can stimulate TRKC receptor-mediated signaling, aiding in the prevention of neurodegenerative diseases and promoting healthy aging.

30

Ion Channel-Linked Receptors

Gamma-Aminobutyric Acid Receptors (GABA-A, GABA-B)

Gamma-aminobutyric acid (GABA) receptors are critical components of the central nervous system (CNS), serving as the primary inhibitory neurotransmitter receptors. There are two main types of GABA receptors: GABA-A and GABA-B, each with distinct functions, mechanisms of action, and roles in the regulation of neuronal excitability. These receptors are targets for various pharmacological agents and play a crucial role in maintaining the balance between neuronal excitation and inhibition.

Function of Gamma-Aminobutyric Acid Receptors

GABA-A Receptors

GABA-A receptors are ligand-gated ion channels that mediate fast synaptic inhibition. When GABA binds to these receptors, it triggers the opening of an intrinsic chloride ion channel, allowing chloride ions to flow into the neuron. This influx of chloride ions hyperpolarizes the neuron, making it less likely to fire an action potential.

- **Neuronal Inhibition**: The primary function of GABA-A receptors is to mediate rapid inhibitory neurotransmission in the CNS. This inhibition is essential for controlling neuronal excitability and preventing overexcitation, which can lead to conditions such as epilepsy.

- **Sedation and Anxiolysis**: Pharmacological agents that enhance GABA-A receptor activity, such as benzodiazepines and barbiturates, are commonly used for their sedative, anxiolytic, and anticonvulsant effects. These drugs bind to specific sites on the GABA-A receptor, enhancing the receptor's response to GABA.
- **Muscle Relaxation**: GABA-A receptors also play a role in muscle relaxation by inhibiting the activity of motor neurons.

GABA-B Receptors

GABA-B receptors are metabotropic receptors that mediate slow and prolonged inhibitory effects. These receptors are G protein-coupled receptors (GPCRs) that, upon activation by GABA, initiate a cascade of intracellular signaling events.

- **Neuronal Inhibition**: GABA-B receptors contribute to inhibitory neurotransmission by activating G proteins that lead to the opening of potassium channels and the inhibition of calcium channels. This results in the hyperpolarization of neurons and a decrease in neurotransmitter release.
- **Neuromodulation**: GABA-B receptors play a role in modulating synaptic transmission and plasticity. They are involved in the regulation of various neurotransmitter systems, including dopamine and serotonin, influencing mood, cognition, and pain perception.
- **Muscle Relaxation and Antispasmodic Effects**: GABA-B receptor agonists, such as baclofen, are used clinically to treat muscle spasticity and related disorders by reducing motor neuron excitability.

Production of Gamma-Aminobutyric Acid Receptors

The production of GABA receptors involves complex processes of gene expression, protein synthesis, and post-translational modifications. The genes encoding GABA-A and GABA-B receptors are GABRA, GABRB, GABRG, and GABBR1, GABBR2, respectively.

Gene Expression

The expression of GABA receptor genes is tightly regulated by various transcription factors and epigenetic mechanisms. Promoter regions upstream of the GABA receptor genes contain specific sequences that bind transcription factors, initiating the transcription of these genes into messenger RNA (mRNA).

- **Regulatory Elements**: The regulatory elements in the promoter regions can be influenced by several factors, including neuronal activity, hormones, and dietary components. For example, certain plant-derived compounds have been shown to affect the expression of genes involved in GABAergic signaling.
- **Epigenetic Modifications**: Epigenetic modifications, such as DNA methylation and histone acetylation, also play a crucial role in regulating GABA receptor gene expression. These modifications can be influenced by diet and environmental factors, highlighting the potential impact of plant-based nutrition on GABAergic function.

Receptor Synthesis

Once transcribed, the mRNA for GABA receptors is translated into protein in the rough endoplasmic reticulum (ER). The newly synthesized polypeptides undergo folding and assembly into functional receptor complexes.

- **Folding and Assembly**: Proper folding and assembly of GABA receptors are critical for their function. Chaperone proteins in the ER assist in this process, ensuring that the receptors attain the correct conformation.

- **Glycosylation**: GABA receptors undergo glycosylation, a post-translational modification that adds carbohydrate groups to the receptor protein. This modification is essential for receptor stability, trafficking, and function.

Post-Translational Modifications

GABA receptors are subject to various post-translational modifications that regulate their activity, localization, and degradation.

- **Phosphorylation**: Phosphorylation of GABA receptors by kinases can modulate receptor function, influencing their sensitivity to GABA and their desensitization rates.
- **Palmitoylation**: Palmitoylation, the addition of palmitic acid to the receptor protein, affects the receptor's localization within the cell membrane and its interaction with other proteins.

Regulation of Gamma-Aminobutyric Acid Receptors

The regulation of GABA receptors is a dynamic process that ensures appropriate inhibitory signaling in the CNS. This regulation involves mechanisms such as receptor trafficking, desensitization, and modulation by endogenous and exogenous compounds.

Desensitization and Downregulation

Prolonged exposure to GABA or pharmacological agents can lead to desensitization and downregulation of GABA receptors.

- **Desensitization**: Desensitization involves a decrease in receptor responsiveness due to prolonged agonist exposure. This process is often mediated by receptor phosphorylation and the subsequent binding of regulatory proteins.

- **Downregulation**: Downregulation refers to the reduction in the number of receptors on the cell surface. This can occur through receptor internalization followed by either recycling back to the membrane or degradation in lysosomes.

Receptor Trafficking

The trafficking of GABA receptors to and from the cell membrane is crucial for regulating their availability and function.

- **Internalization**: GABA receptors can be internalized through endocytosis, a process that removes receptors from the cell surface. This is often triggered by receptor phosphorylation and the binding of adaptor proteins.
- **Recycling and Degradation**: Internalized receptors can be recycled back to the membrane or targeted for degradation. The balance between these processes determines the overall receptor density and responsiveness.

Role of Plant-Based Compounds in Regulation

Plant-based diets can significantly influence the regulation of GABA receptors through various bioactive compounds, such as flavonoids, polyphenols, and essential fatty acids.

Flavonoids

Flavonoids are a diverse group of polyphenolic compounds found in fruits, vegetables, and other plant-based foods. They have been shown to modulate GABAergic signaling by influencing receptor function and expression.

- **Apigenin**: Apigenin, a flavonoid found in parsley, celery, and chamomile, has been shown to bind to GABA-A receptors, enhancing their inhibitory effects and producing anxiolytic and sedative effects (Viola et al., 1995).

- **Quercetin**: Quercetin, found in apples, onions, and berries, can modulate GABAergic neurotransmission by increasing GABA levels in the brain and enhancing GABA receptor function (Lee et al., 2003).

Polyphenols

Polyphenols are another class of bioactive compounds in plant-based foods that can affect GABA receptor regulation.

- **Resveratrol**: Resveratrol, a polyphenol found in grapes and red wine, has been shown to enhance GABAergic neurotransmission by modulating GABA-A receptor activity and expression (Lee et al., 2014).
- **Curcumin**: Curcumin, found in turmeric, can influence GABAergic signaling by increasing GABA levels and enhancing GABA receptor function.

Essential Fatty Acids

Omega-3 fatty acids, such as those found in flaxseeds, chia seeds, and walnuts, can also modulate GABA receptor function and expression.

- **Docosahexaenoic Acid (DHA)**: DHA, an omega-3 fatty acid, has been shown to enhance GABAergic neurotransmission by increasing the expression of GABA receptors and promoting receptor function.

Plant-Based Diets and Gamma-Aminobutyric Acid Receptors

Adopting a plant-based diet can have significant impacts on the regulation and function of GABA receptors. The intake of various nutrients and bioactive compounds from plants can modulate the GABAergic system, contributing to overall health benefits.

Mental Health

Plant-based diets rich in antioxidants, flavonoids, and essential fatty acids can enhance mental health by modulating GABAergic signaling.

- **Anxiety and Depression**: Plant-based diets have been associated with reduced symptoms of anxiety and depression, potentially through the modulation of GABA receptor activity (Davison & Kaplan, 2013). Flavonoids and polyphenols in plant foods can enhance GABAergic neurotransmission, promoting relaxation and reducing stress.
- **Cognitive Function**: The neuroprotective effects of plant-based diets can also enhance cognitive function by maintaining the balance between excitation and inhibition in the brain. Compounds like resveratrol and curcumin have been shown to improve cognitive performance and protect against neurodegenerative diseases.

Neurological Health

Plant-based diets can support neurological health by influencing GABA receptor regulation and function.

- **Epilepsy**: GABAergic dysfunction is a key factor in epilepsy, and enhancing GABAergic signaling through dietary means can help manage this condition. Flavonoids and polyphenols have anticonvulsant properties and can enhance the inhibitory effects of GABA.
- **Neuroprotection**: Antioxidants in plant-based foods can protect neurons from oxidative stress, a major contributor to neurodegenerative diseases. By maintaining GABAergic function, plant-based diets can provide neuroprotection and support brain health.

Muscle Health

GABA receptors play a role in muscle relaxation, and plant-based diets can support muscle health by modulating GABAergic signaling.

- **Muscle Relaxation**: Plant-based compounds like apigenin and quercetin can enhance GABAergic inhibition, promoting muscle relaxation and reducing spasticity.
- **Antispasmodic Effects**: GABA-B receptor agonists like baclofen are used clinically for their antispasmodic effects. Plant-based diets can enhance the function of these receptors, providing natural support for muscle relaxation and spasm reduction.

Gamma-aminobutyric acid (GABA) receptors are essential for regulating neuronal excitability and maintaining the balance between excitation and inhibition in the CNS. The production and regulation of GABA-A and GABA-B receptors involve complex processes influenced by genetic, environmental, and dietary factors.

Glycine Receptors (GlyRs)

Glycine receptors (GlyRs) are ligand-gated ion channels that mediate inhibitory neurotransmission in the central nervous system (CNS). These receptors play critical roles in motor control, sensory processing, and various CNS functions. The GlyR family includes multiple subtypes, each with unique functions and tissue distributions.

Function of Glycine Receptors

GlyRs are predominantly found in the spinal cord, brainstem, and other regions of the brain. Their activation by the amino acid glycine results in an influx of chloride ions into neurons, leading to hyperpolarization and inhibition of neuronal firing. This inhibitory action is essential for maintaining the balance between excitation and inhibition within the CNS.

GlyR Subtypes

There are four main subtypes of GlyRs, designated as α1, α2, α3, and α4, along with a β subunit. Each subtype has distinct functional roles and developmental patterns.

α1 GlyR

The α1 GlyR subtype is the most abundant in adult neurons. It is primarily involved in mediating fast synaptic inhibition in the spinal cord and brainstem. The proper function of α1 GlyRs is crucial for motor coordination and preventing hyperexcitability that can lead to conditions like spasticity and epilepsy.

α2 GlyR

The α2 GlyR subtype is predominantly expressed during early development. It plays a key role in the formation and maturation of neuronal circuits. As development progresses, the expression of α2 GlyRs decreases, and they are gradually replaced by α1 GlyRs in adult neurons.

α3 GlyR

The α3 GlyR subtype is involved in modulating sensory processing, particularly in the spinal cord's dorsal horn. It contributes to the inhibition of pain pathways and has been implicated in the regulation of inflammatory pain.

β GlyR

The β subunit of GlyRs does not form functional channels on its own but co-assembles with α subunits to form heteromeric receptors.

These heteromeric GlyRs exhibit distinct pharmacological and functional properties compared to homomeric α subunit receptors.

Production of Glycine Receptors

The production of GlyRs is a tightly regulated process involving gene expression, protein synthesis, and post-translational modifications. The genes encoding the GlyR subunits are GLRA1, GLRA2, GLRA3, and GLRB, which correspond to the α1, α2, α3, and β subunits, respectively.

Gene Expression

Gene expression of GlyR subunits is controlled by various transcription factors and regulatory elements. These include promoter regions upstream of the GLRA and GLRB genes that bind specific proteins to initiate transcription. The expression of these genes can be influenced by several factors, including neural activity, developmental signals, and dietary components.

Receptor Synthesis

Once transcribed, the mRNA of GlyR subunits is translated into protein in the endoplasmic reticulum. These proteins undergo folding and assembly into pentameric structures, either as homomeric α subunit receptors or heteromeric α/β receptors. Proper folding and assembly are critical for the receptors' functionality and stability.

Post-Translational Modifications

GlyRs undergo various post-translational modifications, such as glycosylation and phosphorylation, which regulate their activity, trafficking, and degradation. Glycosylation of GlyR subunits is essential for their proper folding, cell surface expression, and stability. Phosphorylation can modulate receptor sensitivity and responsiveness to glycine.

Regulation of Glycine Receptors

The regulation of GlyRs involves multiple mechanisms to ensure appropriate inhibitory neurotransmission.

Synaptic Localization and Trafficking

The localization and trafficking of GlyRs to synaptic sites are crucial for their function. GlyRs are anchored at inhibitory synapses by the scaffolding protein gephyrin, which interacts with the receptors and cytoskeletal elements. This anchoring ensures the precise localization of GlyRs to postsynaptic sites where they can effectively mediate inhibition.

Desensitization and Internalization

Prolonged activation of GlyRs can lead to receptor desensitization, where the receptor's responsiveness is diminished. This is often followed by internalization, where receptors are removed from the cell surface. These processes are crucial in preventing overstimulation and maintaining homeostasis. Internalized receptors can either be recycled back to the cell membrane or degraded in lysosomes.

Role of Plant-Based Compounds in Regulation

Plant-based diets can influence the regulation of GlyRs through various bioactive compounds. Phytochemicals, such as flavonoids and polyphenols, have been shown to modulate receptor activity and expression.

Flavonoids

Flavonoids are a group of polyphenolic compounds found in fruits, vegetables, tea, and other plant-based foods. They have been reported to influence the glycinergic signaling pathway by modulating GlyR activity. For instance, quercetin, a flavonoid found in apples, onions, and berries, can enhance GlyR-mediated chloride currents, potentially enhancing inhibitory neurotransmission.

Polyphenols

Polyphenols, abundant in plant-based foods such as berries, nuts, and seeds, have antioxidant and anti-inflammatory properties. These compounds can modulate GlyR function by influencing receptor expression and sensitivity. Resveratrol, a polyphenol found in grapes and red wine, has been shown to enhance GlyR function and improve inhibitory signaling.

Omega-3 Fatty Acids

Plant sources of omega-3 fatty acids, such as flaxseeds and chia seeds, have neuroprotective properties and can influence GlyR function. Omega-3 fatty acids have been shown to modulate the expression of GlyRs and enhance their inhibitory effects, contributing to improved neuronal function and reduced excitotoxicity.

Plant-Based Diets and Glycine Receptors

Adopting a plant-based diet can have significant impacts on the regulation and function of GlyRs. The intake of various nutrients and bioactive compounds from plants can modulate the glycinergic system, contributing to overall health benefits.

Neurological Health

Plant-based diets are rich in antioxidants, polyphenols, and omega-3 fatty acids, which are beneficial for neurological health. The regulation of GlyRs in the CNS can be positively influenced by these dietary components. For example, antioxidants can reduce oxidative stress, which is known to impair GlyR function. Additionally, polyphenols can enhance inhibitory neurotransmission, supporting cognitive function and reducing the risk of neurological disorders.

Pain Management

The influence of plant-based diets on $\alpha 3$ GlyRs can enhance pain management. Foods rich in flavonoids and polyphenols can modulate GlyR activity in the spinal cord, contributing to the inhibition of pain pathways. This can be particularly beneficial in managing inflammatory pain and conditions such as chronic pain syndromes.

Muscle Relaxation and Motor Control

GlyRs play a crucial role in motor control and muscle relaxation. Plant-based diets, which are typically high in nutrients and low in pro-inflammatory compounds, can support muscle relaxation and improve motor coordination. The presence of bioactive compounds in plant foods can enhance GlyR-mediated inhibition, aiding in the prevention of muscle spasms and promoting smooth motor function.

Mental Health

The regulation of GlyRs is also essential for mental health. Plant-based diets, rich in omega-3 fatty acids and polyphenols, can support the function of GlyRs in the brain, contributing to improved inhibitory signaling and reduced neuronal hyperexcitability. This can have positive effects on mood regulation and the prevention of mental health disorders such as anxiety and depression.

Glycine receptors are essential for various physiological processes, including motor control, sensory processing, and pain modulation. The production and regulation of these receptors involve complex mechanisms influenced by genetic and environmental factors.

Glutamate Receptors (NMDA, AMPA, Kainate)

Glutamate receptors are a critical component of the central nervous system, playing a vital role in synaptic transmission, plasticity, and neurodegenerative processes. These receptors, which include NMDA (N-Methyl-D-Aspartate), AMPA (α-Amino-3-Hydroxy-5-Methyl-4-Isoxazolepropionic Acid), and Kainate receptors, are ionotropic receptors that mediate excitatory synaptic transmission.

Function of Glutamate Receptors

NMDA Receptors

NMDA receptors are known for their involvement in synaptic plasticity, which is crucial for learning and memory. These receptors are highly permeable to calcium ions (Ca2+) and are unique in requiring the binding of glutamate and a co-agonist, typically glycine, to activate.

NMDA receptors also need membrane depolarization to relieve the magnesium (Mg2+) block in their ion channel.

Key Functions:

- **Synaptic Plasticity:** NMDA receptors play a crucial role in long-term potentiation (LTP), a cellular mechanism underlying learning and memory.
- **Calcium Signaling:** The influx of Ca2+ through NMDA receptors triggers various intracellular signaling pathways essential for synaptic plasticity and neuroprotection.
- **Development:** NMDA receptors are vital for the development of the nervous system, influencing neuronal growth and differentiation.

AMPA Receptors

AMPA receptors are responsible for fast excitatory synaptic transmission in the central nervous system. They are tetrameric structures composed of different subunits (GluA1-4), which determine their permeability and kinetics.

Key Functions:

- **Rapid Synaptic Transmission:** AMPA receptors mediate quick, transient excitatory synaptic currents, essential for normal brain function.
- **Synaptic Plasticity:** They contribute to synaptic plasticity by trafficking to and from the synaptic membrane, thereby regulating synaptic strength.
- **Neuronal Communication:** AMPA receptors ensure efficient neuronal communication, which is critical for processing sensory information and executing motor functions.

Kainate Receptors

Kainate receptors are less understood compared to NMDA and AMPA receptors but are known to play roles in both presynaptic and postsynaptic modulation of synaptic transmission.

Key Functions:

- **Modulation of Synaptic Transmission:** Kainate receptors modulate neurotransmitter release, affecting both excitatory and inhibitory synaptic transmission.
- **Neurodevelopment:** They are involved in the regulation of neuronal network formation during development.
- **Plasticity and Excitability:** Kainate receptors contribute to synaptic plasticity and neuronal excitability, influencing processes such as learning and memory.

Production of Glutamate Receptors

Gene Expression

The genes encoding NMDA, AMPA, and Kainate receptors are regulated at the transcriptional level by various transcription factors and promoter regions.

NMDA Receptors:

- **NR1 Subunit:** Encoded by the GRIN1 gene, essential for the formation of functional NMDA receptors.
- **NR2 Subunits (A-D):** Encoded by GRIN2A-D genes, these subunits confer different properties to the NMDA receptors.
- **NR3 Subunits (A-B):** Encoded by GRIN3A-B genes, these subunits modulate the receptor's properties and functions.

AMPA Receptors:

- **GluA1-4 Subunits:** Encoded by the GRIA1-4 genes, these subunits form the functional AMPA receptors with diverse kinetic properties.

Kainate Receptors:

- **GluK1-5 Subunits:** Encoded by the GRIK1-5 genes, these subunits determine the receptor's properties and distribution in the nervous system.

Receptor Synthesis

The synthesis of glutamate receptors involves transcription, translation, and post-translational modifications.

- **Transcription:** The receptor genes are transcribed into mRNA in the cell nucleus.
- **Translation:** The mRNA is translated into protein in the ribosomes, primarily associated with the rough endoplasmic reticulum.
- **Post-Translational Modifications:** The newly synthesized receptors undergo folding, glycosylation, and assembly into functional units.

Trafficking and Assembly

After synthesis, glutamate receptors are transported to the Golgi apparatus for further processing and then to the cell membrane where they are inserted into the synaptic and extrasynaptic sites.

- **Trafficking:** The receptors are trafficked along the cytoskeleton to their target destinations in the neuronal membrane.

- **Assembly:** Subunits assemble into tetrameric structures for AMPA and Kainate receptors or into more complex structures for NMDA receptors.

Regulation of Glutamate Receptors

Synaptic Activity

The regulation of glutamate receptors is closely tied to synaptic activity and neuronal signaling.

- **Synaptic Insertion:** Activity-dependent insertion of AMPA receptors into the synapse is crucial for synaptic strengthening during LTP.
- **Endocytosis:** Receptors can be internalized through endocytosis in response to prolonged activation, leading to synaptic weakening or long-term depression (LTD).

Phosphorylation

Phosphorylation of glutamate receptors by various kinases modulates their activity, localization, and interaction with other proteins.

- **NMDA Receptors:** Phosphorylation by protein kinases such as CaMKII and PKC enhances NMDA receptor function and synaptic plasticity.
- **AMPA Receptors:** Phosphorylation of GluA1 subunits by PKA and CaMKII increases receptor insertion into the synapse and synaptic strength.
- **Kainate Receptors:** Less is known, but phosphorylation likely influences their trafficking and function.

Interaction with Auxiliary Proteins

Auxiliary proteins such as TARPs (Transmembrane AMPA Receptor Regulatory Proteins) and MAGUKs (Membrane-Associated

Guanylate Kinases) interact with glutamate receptors to regulate their trafficking, localization, and function.

- **TARPs:** Regulate AMPA receptor trafficking and gating.
- **MAGUKs:** Scaffold proteins that anchor NMDA and AMPA receptors at synaptic sites.

Role of Plant-Based Compounds in Regulation

Plant-based diets can influence the regulation of glutamate receptors through various bioactive compounds, impacting brain health and neuroprotection.

Flavonoids

Flavonoids are polyphenolic compounds found in fruits, vegetables, tea, and other plant-based foods. They have neuroprotective properties and can modulate glutamate receptor activity.

- **Quercetin:** Found in apples, onions, and berries, quercetin has been shown to protect neurons by modulating NMDA and AMPA receptor activity and reducing excitotoxicity.
- **Epigallocatechin Gallate (EGCG):** Present in green tea, EGCG can inhibit NMDA receptor-mediated neurotoxicity and support neuronal health.

Omega-3 Fatty Acids

Omega-3 fatty acids, such as those found in flaxseeds, chia seeds, and walnuts, are crucial for maintaining neuronal membrane integrity and function.

- **Docosahexaenoic Acid (DHA):** DHA modulates NMDA receptor function and enhances synaptic plasticity, supporting cognitive function and protecting against neurodegenerative diseases.

Curcumin

Curcumin, the active compound in turmeric, has anti-inflammatory and antioxidant properties, which can benefit brain health by modulating glutamate receptor activity.

- **Neuroprotection:** Curcumin has been shown to protect against NMDA receptor-mediated excitotoxicity and support synaptic plasticity, making it beneficial for conditions like Alzheimer's disease.

Polyphenols

Polyphenols found in a variety of plant-based foods have been shown to interact with glutamate receptors, influencing their function and protecting against neurodegenerative processes.

- **Resveratrol:** Found in grapes and berries, resveratrol can modulate NMDA receptor activity and protect neurons from oxidative stress and excitotoxicity.

Plant-Based Diets and Glutamate Receptors

Cognitive Health

A plant-based diet rich in antioxidants, flavonoids, and omega-3 fatty acids supports cognitive health by modulating glutamate receptor activity and promoting synaptic plasticity.

- **Antioxidants:** Reduce oxidative stress, which can impair glutamate receptor function and lead to neurodegeneration.
- **Flavonoids and Polyphenols:** Enhance synaptic plasticity and protect against excitotoxicity, contributing to improved learning and memory.

Neuroprotection

Plant-based diets offer neuroprotection by reducing inflammation, oxidative stress, and excitotoxicity, which are critical factors in neurodegenerative diseases.

- **Anti-Inflammatory Compounds:** Such as curcumin and omega-3 fatty acids, reduce neuroinflammation and support neuronal health.
- **Reduced Excitotoxicity:** Compounds like EGCG and resveratrol modulate glutamate receptor activity, protecting neurons from excessive glutamate-induced damage.

Mood and Mental Health

Dietary components of a plant-based diet can influence mood and mental health by modulating neurotransmitter systems, including glutamate receptors.

- **Serotonin and Dopamine Pathways:** Nutrients and bioactive compounds in plant-based foods can influence serotonin and dopamine pathways, indirectly affecting glutamate receptor function and mood regulation.
- **Stress Reduction:** Plant-based diets are associated with lower stress levels, which can positively impact glutamate receptor regulation and mental health.

Glutamate receptors, including NMDA, AMPA, and Kainate receptors, play crucial roles in synaptic transmission, plasticity, and neuroprotection. The production and regulation of these receptors involve complex genetic and molecular mechanisms. A plant-based diet rich in antioxidants, flavonoids, omega-3 fatty acids, and polyphenols supports the function and regulation of glutamate receptors, promoting cognitive health, neuroprotection, and mental well-being. The bioactive compounds in plant-based foods can modulate receptor activity, reduce oxidative stress, and protect against excitotoxicity, offering a natural approach to maintaining brain health.

Purinergic Receptors (P2X, P2Y)

Purinergic receptors are a diverse group of cell surface receptors activated by purine nucleotides such as ATP (adenosine triphosphate). These receptors are categorized into two main families: P2X and P2Y receptors. P2X receptors are ligand-gated ion channels, whereas P2Y receptors are G protein-coupled receptors (GPCRs). Purinergic receptors play critical roles in numerous physiological processes, including neurotransmission, inflammation, and immune responses.

Function of Purinergic Receptors

P2X Receptors

P2X receptors are trimeric ATP-gated ion channels that allow the flow of cations such as Na+, K+, and Ca2+ across the cell membrane. There are seven known P2X receptor subtypes (P2X1-7), each with distinct tissue distributions and functions.

P2X1 Receptors

P2X1 receptors are predominantly expressed in smooth muscle tissues and are crucial for muscle contraction. Activation of P2X1 receptors by ATP leads to rapid depolarization and subsequent muscle contraction. These receptors are vital in the vas deferens for sperm ejaculation and in blood vessels for regulating vascular tone.

P2X2 Receptors

P2X2 receptors are found mainly in the nervous system, including the central and peripheral neurons. They mediate fast synaptic transmission and are involved in sensory signal processing, such as pain and taste perception.

P2X3 Receptors

P2X3 receptors are primarily located in sensory neurons, where they play a key role in nociception (pain perception). These receptors are activated by ATP released from damaged or stressed cells, contributing to the sensation of pain.

P2X4 Receptors

P2X4 receptors are widely expressed in the brain, heart, and immune cells. They are involved in regulating vascular function, synaptic plasticity, and immune responses. P2X4 receptors are also implicated in the release of pro-inflammatory cytokines, which are crucial in immune modulation.

P2X5 Receptors

P2X5 receptors are less well characterized but are known to be expressed in various tissues, including skeletal muscle and the nervous system. They are believed to play a role in muscle function and development.

P2X6 Receptors

P2X6 receptors are predominantly found in the central nervous system. Their exact physiological role remains unclear, but they are thought to participate in neuronal signaling and synaptic function.

P2X7 Receptors

P2X7 receptors are mainly expressed in immune cells, including macrophages and microglia. They are involved in the regulation of inflammatory responses, cell death, and the release of cytokines. P2X7 receptors play a critical role in the immune system's response to infection and tissue injury.

P2Y Receptors

P2Y receptors are GPCRs that respond to nucleotides like ATP, ADP, UTP, and UDP. There are eight known P2Y receptor subtypes (P2Y1, P2Y2, P2Y4, P2Y6, P2Y11-14), each mediating various cellular responses.

P2Y1 Receptors

P2Y1 receptors are widely distributed in the cardiovascular system and platelets. They are involved in platelet aggregation, vascular tone regulation, and neurotransmission. Activation of P2Y1 receptors by ADP is essential for platelet plug formation during blood clotting.

P2Y2 Receptors

P2Y2 receptors are expressed in epithelial cells, endothelial cells, and smooth muscle cells. They mediate inflammatory responses, cell proliferation, and fluid secretion. P2Y2 receptors play a significant role in wound healing and tissue regeneration.

P2Y4 Receptors

P2Y4 receptors are found in various tissues, including the intestine and the central nervous system. They are involved in regulating ion transport, fluid secretion, and gastrointestinal motility.

P2Y6 Receptors

P2Y6 receptors are expressed in immune cells, including macrophages and dendritic cells. They mediate immune responses, including the release of cytokines and chemokines, and play a role in inflammation and immune cell migration.

P2Y11 Receptors

P2Y11 receptors are found in the heart, pancreas, and immune cells. They are involved in the regulation of immune responses, insulin secretion, and cardiac function. P2Y11 receptors mediate the release of ATP and other nucleotides, which act as signaling molecules in various physiological processes.

P2Y12 Receptors

P2Y12 receptors are predominantly expressed in platelets and are crucial for platelet aggregation and thrombosis. They are the target of antiplatelet drugs like clopidogrel, which are used to prevent heart attacks and strokes.

P2Y13 Receptors

P2Y13 receptors are expressed in the liver, spleen, and immune cells. They play a role in lipid metabolism, immune regulation, and the clearance of cholesterol.

P2Y14 Receptors

P2Y14 receptors are found in various tissues, including the brain, immune cells, and gastrointestinal tract. They are involved in the regulation of immune responses, inflammation, and mucosal secretion.

Production of Purinergic Receptors

The production of purinergic receptors involves gene expression, receptor synthesis, and post-translational modifications. The genes encoding P2X and P2Y receptors are transcribed and translated into proteins, which undergo various modifications to become functional receptors.

Gene Expression

The expression of purinergic receptor genes is regulated by transcription factors and promoter regions specific to each receptor subtype. Factors such as tissue type, developmental stage, and physiological conditions influence gene expression. For instance, the P2X1 receptor gene (P2RX1) is highly expressed in smooth muscle cells, while the P2Y12 receptor gene (P2RY12) is predominantly expressed in platelets.

Receptor Synthesis

Purinergic receptor proteins are synthesized in the endoplasmic reticulum (ER) and undergo folding and glycosylation. Proper folding is essential for receptor function, and chaperone proteins in the ER assist in this process. Glycosylation, the addition of carbohydrate moieties, is crucial for receptor stability, trafficking, and ligand binding.

Post-Translational Modifications

Purinergic receptors undergo several post-translational modifications, including phosphorylation, ubiquitination, and palmitoylation. These modifications regulate receptor activity, desensitization, internalization, and degradation. Phosphorylation of P2X and P2Y receptors by kinases can modulate their responsiveness to ligands, while ubiquitination often targets receptors for degradation.

Regulation of Purinergic Receptors

The regulation of purinergic receptors involves mechanisms that control receptor sensitivity, density, and signaling efficacy. These mechanisms include desensitization, internalization, recycling, and degradation.

Desensitization and Downregulation

Prolonged exposure to agonists can lead to receptor desensitization, reducing receptor sensitivity and preventing overstimulation. This process often involves receptor phosphorylation and the binding of regulatory proteins such as β-arrestins, which uncouple receptors from their associated G proteins. Downregulation, the reduction of receptor density on the cell surface occurs through receptor internalization and degradation.

Receptor Recycling and Degradation

Internalized purinergic receptors can be either recycled back to the cell surface or targeted for degradation in lysosomes. Recycling allows receptors to be quickly reused, maintaining receptor availability and responsiveness. Degradation reduces receptor numbers, providing long-term regulation of receptor activity.

Role of Plant-Based Compounds in Regulation

Plant-based diets can influence the regulation of purinergic receptors through bioactive compounds such as flavonoids, polyphenols, and dietary fibers.

Flavonoids

Flavonoids are a group of polyphenolic compounds found in fruits, vegetables, tea, and other plant-based foods. They have been reported to modulate purinergic signaling pathways. For example, quercetin, a flavonoid found in apples and onions, can inhibit ATP-induced responses in P2X7 receptors, reducing inflammation and cell death.

Polyphenols

Polyphenols, found in a variety of plant-based foods, have antioxidant and anti-inflammatory properties. They can modulate purinergic receptor activity and expression. For instance, resveratrol, a polyphenol found in grapes and berries, can inhibit P2Y12 receptor-mediated platelet aggregation, providing cardiovascular benefits.

Dietary Fiber

High-fiber diets, typical of plant-based nutrition, can influence purinergic signaling indirectly by improving gut health and reducing systemic inflammation. Fiber fermentation by gut microbiota produces short-chain fatty acids (SCFAs) that can modulate immune responses and purinergic receptor activity.

Plant-Based Diets and Purinergic Receptors

Adopting a plant-based diet can significantly impact the regulation and function of purinergic receptors, contributing to overall health benefits.

Cardiovascular Health

Plant-based diets rich in antioxidants, dietary fiber, and healthy fats can improve cardiovascular health by modulating purinergic receptor function. For instance, the regulation of P2Y12 receptors in platelets can be positively influenced by dietary polyphenols, reducing the risk of thrombosis and cardiovascular diseases.

Immune and Inflammatory Responses

The anti-inflammatory properties of plant-based diets can modulate the activity of P2X7 receptors in immune cells, reducing inflammation and promoting immune health. Bioactive compounds in plant foods, such as flavonoids and polyphenols, can inhibit P2X7 receptor-mediated release of pro-inflammatory cytokines, contributing to the resolution of chronic inflammation.

Metabolic Health

Plant-based diets can enhance metabolic health by influencing purinergic receptors involved in energy homeostasis and lipid metabolism. For example, P2Y13 receptors in the liver regulate cholesterol clearance, and their activity can be modulated by dietary components such as polyphenols and fibers, improving lipid profiles and reducing the risk of metabolic disorders.

Neurological Health

Purinergic receptors in the nervous system, such as P2X2 and P2X4, are involved in synaptic transmission and plasticity. Plant-based diets rich in antioxidants and anti-inflammatory compounds can support neurological health by modulating purinergic signaling pathways, potentially protecting against neurodegenerative diseases.

Purinergic receptors, including P2X and P2Y subtypes, are essential for various physiological processes, including neurotransmission, inflammation, and immune responses. The production and regulation of these receptors involve complex mechanisms influenced by genetic and environmental factors, including dietary components.

31

Nuclear Receptors

Estrogen Receptors (ERα, ERβ)

Estrogen receptors (ERs) are a group of proteins found within cells, crucial for mediating the physiological effects of estrogens, primarily 17β-estradiol (E2). There are two main types of estrogen receptors: ERα and ERβ. These receptors are part of the nuclear receptor family of intracellular receptors and are involved in various biological processes, including reproduction, cardiovascular health, bone integrity, and behavior.

Function of Estrogen Receptors

ERα

ERα is predominantly expressed in reproductive tissues such as the uterus, mammary glands, and ovaries. It plays a significant role in the regulation of reproductive functions and development. Activation of ERα leads to:

1. **Gene Transcription:** ERα binds to estrogen response elements (EREs) on DNA, influencing the transcription of genes involved in cell proliferation, differentiation, and survival.
2. **Reproductive Health:** ERα regulates the growth and development of reproductive tissues and is essential for fertility.

3. **Bone Health:** It contributes to bone density maintenance by promoting osteoblast activity and inhibiting osteoclast formation, reducing the risk of osteoporosis.

ERβ

ERβ is primarily found in non-reproductive tissues such as the prostate, lungs, gastrointestinal tract, and central nervous system. It has distinct functions compared to ERα, including:

1. **Anti-Proliferative Effects:** ERβ generally acts to inhibit cell proliferation, counteracting the proliferative actions of ERα in certain tissues.
2. **Neuroprotection:** ERβ is involved in protecting neurons against injury and degeneration, playing a role in brain health and function.
3. **Cardiovascular Health:** It helps in maintaining vascular function and integrity, contributing to cardiovascular protection.

Production of Estrogen Receptors

The production of estrogen receptors involves multiple stages, from gene transcription to protein synthesis and post-translational modifications.

Gene Expression

The genes encoding ERα and ERβ are ESR1 and ESR2, respectively. Their expression is regulated by various factors, including hormones, growth factors, and environmental influences.

1. **Promoter Regions:** The promoter regions upstream of ESR1 and ESR2 genes contain binding sites for transcription factors that regulate their expression.

2. **Hormonal Regulation:** Estrogens and other hormones like progesterone and androgens can modulate the expression of ERs through feedback mechanisms.
3. **Environmental Factors:** Phytoestrogens and other dietary components can influence ER gene expression by mimicking or blocking the effects of endogenous estrogens.

Receptor Synthesis

After transcription, the mRNA of estrogen receptors is translated into protein in the endoplasmic reticulum.

1. **Folding and Glycosylation:** Proper folding and glycosylation are essential for the stability and function of ERs. Misfolded proteins are usually targeted for degradation.
2. **Transport to Nucleus:** ERs are transported to the nucleus where they bind to DNA and regulate gene expression upon activation by estrogen.

Post-Translational Modifications

Estrogen receptors undergo various post-translational modifications that influence their activity and stability.

1. **Phosphorylation:** Phosphorylation by kinases can alter the activity, localization, and degradation of ERs.
2. **Ubiquitination:** Ubiquitination tags ERs for proteasomal degradation, regulating their levels within the cell.
3. **Acetylation:** Acetylation can enhance the DNA-binding ability of ERs, increasing their transcriptional activity.

Regulation of Estrogen Receptors

The regulation of estrogen receptors involves complex mechanisms to ensure appropriate responses to estrogenic signals.

Ligand Binding

The binding of estrogens or other ligands to ERs induces conformational changes that enable the receptors to interact with coactivators or corepressors, influencing gene transcription.

1. **Agonists and Antagonists:** Natural estrogens and synthetic compounds can act as agonists (activators) or antagonists (inhibitors) of ERs, modulating their activity.
2. **Selective Estrogen Receptor Modulators (SERMs):** These compounds can act as agonists or antagonists in a tissue-specific manner, providing targeted therapeutic effects.

Coactivators and Corepressors

ERs interact with coactivators and corepressors to modulate gene transcription.

1. **Coactivators:** These proteins enhance the transcriptional activity of ERs by facilitating the assembly of the transcriptional machinery.
2. **Corepressors:** Corepressors inhibit the transcriptional activity of ERs by recruiting histone deacetylases, leading to chromatin condensation and transcriptional repression.

Receptor Recycling and Degradation

The balance between recycling and degradation of ERs determines their cellular levels and responsiveness to estrogens.

1. **Receptor Recycling:** Internalized receptors can be recycled back to the nucleus or cell membrane, allowing rapid reactivation.
2. **Proteasomal Degradation:** Ubiquitinated ERs are targeted for degradation in the proteasome, reducing their levels and preventing overstimulation.

Role of Plant-Based Compounds in Regulation

Plant-based diets and compounds can significantly influence the regulation and function of estrogen receptors.

Phytoestrogens

Phytoestrogens are plant-derived compounds that structurally resemble estrogens and can bind to ERs, modulating their activity.

1. **Isoflavones:** Found in soybeans and other legumes, isoflavones like genistein and daidzein can mimic or antagonize the effects of estrogens, depending on the tissue context.
2. **Lignans:** Present in flaxseeds, lignans are metabolized into enterolignans in the gut, which have estrogenic and antiestrogenic effects.
3. **Coumestans:** Found in clover and alfalfa, coumestans also exhibit estrogenic activity, influencing ER-mediated processes.

Flavonoids

Flavonoids are a diverse group of polyphenolic compounds found in fruits, vegetables, and tea, known for their antioxidant and estrogenic/antiestrogenic properties.

1. **Quercetin:** This flavonoid, abundant in apples, onions, and berries, can modulate ER activity by inhibiting or enhancing estrogenic signaling.
2. **Apigenin:** Found in parsley, celery, and chamomile, apigenin has been shown to inhibit ERα activity while promoting ERβ-mediated effects, providing a balanced estrogenic response.

Dietary Fiber

High-fiber diets, typical of plant-based nutrition, can influence estrogen metabolism and ER regulation.

1. **Gut Microbiota Modulation:** Dietary fiber promotes a healthy gut microbiota, which can metabolize estrogens and phytoestrogens into active or inactive forms, affecting their availability and action.
2. **Estrogen Excretion:** Fiber binds to estrogens in the gut, facilitating their excretion and reducing reabsorption, which can lower circulating estrogen levels and modulate ER activity.

Plant-Based Diets and Estrogen Receptors

Adopting a plant-based diet can have significant impacts on the regulation and function of estrogen receptors, contributing to various health benefits.

Reproductive Health

Plant-based diets rich in phytoestrogens and antioxidants can support reproductive health by modulating ER activity.

1. **Menstrual Health:** Phytoestrogens can help balance estrogen levels, reducing symptoms of menstrual disorders such as dysmenorrhea and menorrhagia.
2. **Menopause:** During menopause, declining estrogen levels can lead to various symptoms. Phytoestrogens can provide mild estrogenic effects, alleviating symptoms such as hot flashes and osteoporosis.

Bone Health

ERs play a critical role in bone density maintenance, and plant-based diets can support this through various mechanisms.

1. **Osteoblast Activation:** Phytoestrogens can enhance osteoblast activity, promoting bone formation and reducing the risk of osteoporosis.

2. **Calcium Absorption:** Plant-based diets rich in calcium and vitamin D from sources like leafy greens and fortified plant milks can support bone health by ensuring adequate calcium absorption.

Cardiovascular Health

ERβ is involved in maintaining cardiovascular health, and plant-based diets can positively influence this receptor.

1. **Antioxidant Effects:** Antioxidants in plant foods reduce oxidative stress, which can damage blood vessels and impair ERβ function.
2. **Cholesterol Management:** Plant-based diets are typically low in saturated fats and high in fiber, helping to manage cholesterol levels and support cardiovascular health.

Cancer Prevention

Estrogen receptors are implicated in various cancers, and plant-based diets can play a role in cancer prevention through ER modulation.

1. **Breast Cancer:** Phytoestrogens can act as weak estrogens or anti-estrogens, potentially reducing the risk of hormone-dependent breast cancers by competing with stronger endogenous estrogens for receptor binding.
2. **Prostate Cancer:** ERβ has anti-proliferative effects in the prostate, and plant-based diets rich in phytoestrogens and antioxidants can support prostate health and reduce cancer risk.

Estrogen receptors (ERα and ERβ) are crucial for mediating the effects of estrogens in various tissues, influencing processes such as reproduction, bone health, cardiovascular function, and cancer prevention. The production and regulation of these receptors involve complex mechanisms influenced by genetic, hormonal, and environmental factors.

Androgen Receptors (AR)

Androgen receptors (AR) are a class of nuclear receptors that are activated by binding any of the androgenic hormones, such as testosterone and dihydrotestosterone (DHT). These receptors play pivotal roles in the development and maintenance of male characteristics and reproductive activity. In addition to their critical functions in males, androgen receptors are also present in females and play roles in a variety of tissues, including muscle, liver, and the central nervous system.

Function of Androgen Receptors

Development and Maintenance of Male Characteristics

The primary function of androgen receptors is to mediate the effects of androgens, which are essential for the development of male primary and secondary sexual characteristics. This includes the development of the male reproductive organs, such as the testes and prostate, and secondary sexual characteristics, such as facial hair, deepening of the voice, and increased muscle mass.

Muscle Growth and Maintenance

Androgen receptors are highly expressed in skeletal muscle tissue, where they promote muscle growth and maintenance. The binding of androgens to AR in muscle cells stimulates protein synthesis and inhibits protein breakdown, leading to muscle hypertrophy. This anabolic effect of androgens is one reason why they are often misused in the form of anabolic steroids in sports to enhance performance.

Bone Density Regulation

Androgen receptors play a significant role in maintaining bone density. Androgens stimulate bone formation and inhibit bone resorption, thereby increasing bone density. This function is crucial in preventing osteoporosis, particularly in aging men, but also plays a role in bone health in women.

Central Nervous System Effects

In the central nervous system, androgen receptors are involved in regulating mood, cognition, and libido. The exact mechanisms are complex and involve interactions with various neurotransmitter systems. Androgens have been shown to have neuroprotective effects, which may be mediated through their receptors.

Production of Androgen Receptors

The production of androgen receptors involves multiple steps, including gene expression, receptor synthesis, and post-translational modifications. The gene encoding the androgen receptor is AR, located on the X chromosome.

Gene Expression

The expression of the AR gene is regulated by various transcription factors and hormonal signals. Promoter regions upstream of the AR gene bind specific proteins that initiate transcription. Factors such as age, sex, and hormonal status can influence the expression levels of AR.

Receptor Synthesis

Once transcribed, the mRNA of the androgen receptor is translated into protein in the ribosomes. This protein then undergoes folding and glycosylation in the endoplasmic reticulum, which are crucial for its proper function and stability. The receptor is then transported to the cell membrane or nuclear membrane, where it becomes functional.

Post-Translational Modifications

Androgen receptors undergo various post-translational modifications, such as phosphorylation, acetylation, and ubiquitination, which regulate their activity, stability, and localization. Phosphorylation can activate or deactivate the receptor, acetylation can enhance DNA binding, and ubiquitination often marks the receptor for degradation.

Regulation of Androgen Receptors

The regulation of androgen receptors involves several mechanisms to ensure appropriate cellular responses to androgens.

Ligand Binding and Activation

The primary mechanism of androgen receptor activation is through the binding of androgens. Once bound, the receptor undergoes a conformational change, allowing it to translocate to the nucleus, where it binds to androgen response elements (AREs) in the DNA, thereby regulating the transcription of target genes.

Desensitization and Downregulation

Prolonged exposure to high levels of androgens can lead to desensitization of androgen receptors. This involves reducing the receptor's responsiveness to prevent overstimulation. Downregulation involves decreasing the number of receptors on the cell surface or within the cell, usually through internalization and degradation.

Receptor Recycling and Degradation

Internalized receptors can either be recycled back to the cell membrane or degraded in lysosomes. The balance between these processes determines the overall number of functional receptors. Recycling allows the cell to quickly restore receptor sensitivity, while degradation reduces the receptor density, providing long-term regulation.

Role of Plant-Based Compounds in Regulation

Plant-based diets can influence the regulation of androgen receptors through various bioactive compounds. Phytochemicals, such as flavonoids and lignans, have been shown to modulate receptor activity and expression.

Flavonoids

Flavonoids are a group of polyphenolic compounds found in fruits, vegetables, tea, and other plant-based foods. They have been reported to influence androgen receptor signaling pathways. For example, quercetin, a flavonoid found in apples, onions, and berries, can modulate

AR activity and inhibit androgen-induced responses in prostate cancer cells.

Lignans

Lignans are phytoestrogens found in seeds, whole grains, and vegetables. They can influence androgen metabolism and receptor activity. Lignans have been shown to inhibit the conversion of testosterone to DHT, thus reducing the activation of androgen receptors.

Dietary Fiber

High-fiber diets, typical of plant-based nutrition, can improve insulin sensitivity and reduce systemic inflammation. This can indirectly modulate the activity of androgen receptors, as insulin and inflammation are linked to androgen receptor regulation.

Omega-3 Fatty Acids

Plant sources of omega-3 fatty acids, such as flaxseeds and chia seeds, have anti-inflammatory properties and can influence androgen receptor function. Omega-3 fatty acids have been shown to modulate lipid metabolism and reduce the expression of AR in certain tissues.

Plant-Based Diets and Androgen Receptors

Adopting a plant-based diet can have significant impacts on the regulation and function of androgen receptors. The intake of various nutrients and bioactive compounds from plants can modulate androgen signaling, contributing to overall health benefits.

Prostate Health

Plant-based diets are rich in antioxidants, dietary fiber, and healthy fats, which are beneficial for prostate health. The regulation of AR in the prostate can be positively influenced by these dietary components. For example, antioxidants can reduce oxidative stress, which is known to impair AR function and contribute to prostate cancer progression. Additionally, dietary fiber helps in managing hormone levels and reducing systemic inflammation, which can affect AR activity.

Metabolic Health

The influence of plant-based diets on AR can enhance metabolic health. Foods rich in flavonoids and omega-3 fatty acids can improve insulin sensitivity and reduce the risk of metabolic disorders such as type 2 diabetes. By modulating AR activity, these diets can enhance muscle growth and maintenance, contributing to better metabolic health.

Cardiovascular Health

Androgen receptors play a role in cardiovascular health, influencing vascular function and lipid metabolism. Plant-based diets, which are typically lower in saturated fats and higher in polyunsaturated fats, can support cardiovascular health by modulating AR activity. The presence of bioactive compounds in plant foods can reduce the risk of cardiovascular diseases by influencing lipid profiles and vascular function.

Cancer Prevention

Plant-based diets have been associated with a reduced risk of various cancers, including prostate cancer. Phytochemicals in plant foods can modulate AR signaling pathways and inhibit cancer cell proliferation. For example, lignans and flavonoids have been shown to interfere with AR-mediated transcription in cancer cells, thereby reducing their growth and survival.

Androgen receptors are essential for various physiological processes, including the development and maintenance of male characteristics, muscle growth, bone density regulation, and central nervous system effects. The production and regulation of these receptors involve complex mechanisms influenced by genetic and environmental factors.

Glucocorticoid Receptors (GR)

Glucocorticoid receptors (GR) are a type of nuclear receptor that mediate the effects of glucocorticoids, which are steroid hormones involved in the regulation of various physiological processes, including metabolism, immune response, and stress response. These receptors are critical for maintaining homeostasis within the body and are implicated in numerous health conditions when dysregulated.

Function of Glucocorticoid Receptors

GRs function primarily by acting as transcription factors that regulate the expression of specific genes. When glucocorticoids bind to GRs, the receptor-hormone complex translocates to the nucleus, where it binds to glucocorticoid response elements (GREs) in the DNA to modulate gene expression. This process affects a wide range of biological activities:

Immune Response Modulation

GRs play a crucial role in suppressing inflammation and modulating the immune response. Upon activation by glucocorticoids, GRs inhibit the transcription of pro-inflammatory genes, such as cytokines and chemokines, and promote the expression of anti-inflammatory genes. This immunosuppressive effect is essential for preventing overactive immune responses and is utilized therapeutically in conditions like asthma and autoimmune diseases.

Metabolic Regulation

GRs are involved in the regulation of glucose, lipid, and protein metabolism. They stimulate gluconeogenesis in the liver, leading to increased blood glucose levels, and promote the breakdown of fats and proteins to provide energy substrates. This metabolic effect ensures that the body has sufficient energy during periods of stress or fasting.

Stress Response

GRs are integral to the body's stress response system. In response to stress, the hypothalamus-pituitary-adrenal (HPA) axis is activated, leading to the release of glucocorticoids from the adrenal cortex. These hormones bind to GRs, facilitating the physiological changes necessary to cope with stress, such as increasing blood pressure and mobilizing energy stores.

Production of Glucocorticoid Receptors

The production of GRs involves several steps, from gene expression to protein synthesis and post-translational modifications. The gene encoding the glucocorticoid receptor is NR3C1.

Gene Expression

The expression of the NR3C1 gene is regulated by various transcription factors and hormonal signals. The promoter region of NR3C1 contains binding sites for transcription factors like NF-κB and AP-1, which can either enhance or repress gene transcription in response to cellular signals.

Receptor Synthesis

Following transcription, the NR3C1 mRNA is translated into protein in the cytoplasm. The newly synthesized GR protein undergoes folding and post-translational modifications, such as phosphorylation and ubiquitination, which are crucial for its proper function and regulation.

Post-Translational Modifications

GRs undergo several post-translational modifications that influence their activity and stability. Phosphorylation, for example, can modulate the receptor's ability to bind glucocorticoids and interact with other proteins. Ubiquitination often targets the receptor for degradation, thereby regulating the levels of functional GRs in the cell.

Regulation of Glucocorticoid Receptors

The regulation of GRs is complex and involves multiple mechanisms to ensure appropriate cellular responses to glucocorticoids.

Ligand-Induced Downregulation

Prolonged exposure to high levels of glucocorticoids can lead to downregulation of GRs. This process involves the internalization and degradation of the receptor, reducing the cell's sensitivity to glucocorticoids. This mechanism helps prevent excessive glucocorticoid signaling, which can be detrimental.

Receptor Recycling and Degradation

After internalization, GRs can be either recycled back to the cell membrane or targeted for degradation. The balance between these processes determines the overall number of functional receptors on the cell surface. Recycling allows the cell to quickly restore receptor sensitivity, while degradation reduces receptor density, providing long-term regulation.

Role of Plant-Based Compounds in Regulation

Plant-based diets can influence the regulation of GRs through various bioactive compounds. Phytochemicals, such as flavonoids, have been shown to modulate receptor activity and expression.

Flavonoids

Flavonoids are a group of polyphenolic compounds found in fruits, vegetables, tea, and other plant-based foods. They have been reported to influence GR signaling pathways. For instance, quercetin, a flavonoid found in apples, onions, and berries, can modulate the activity of GRs by affecting their expression and signaling pathways.

Dietary Fiber

High-fiber diets, typical of plant-based nutrition, can improve insulin sensitivity and reduce systemic inflammation. This, in turn, may modulate the activity of GRs, as inflammation and metabolic status are closely linked to receptor regulation.

Omega-3 Fatty Acids

Plant sources of omega-3 fatty acids, such as flaxseeds and chia seeds, have anti-inflammatory properties and can influence GR function. Omega-3 fatty acids have been shown to modulate the expression of genes regulated by GRs, potentially affecting inflammatory and metabolic processes.

Plant-Based Diets and Glucocorticoid Receptors

Adopting a plant-based diet can have significant impacts on the regulation and function of GRs. The intake of various nutrients and bioactive compounds from plants can modulate glucocorticoid signaling, contributing to overall health benefits.

Anti-Inflammatory Effects

Plant-based diets are rich in anti-inflammatory compounds, such as flavonoids, carotenoids, and omega-3 fatty acids. These compounds can enhance the anti-inflammatory effects of GRs, helping to prevent and manage chronic inflammatory conditions. For example, a diet high in fruits and vegetables has been associated with lower levels of inflammatory markers and improved inflammatory profiles.

Metabolic Health

The influence of plant-based diets on GRs can enhance metabolic health. Foods rich in dietary fiber and antioxidants can improve insulin sensitivity and reduce the risk of metabolic disorders, such as type 2 diabetes. By modulating GR activity, these diets can help regulate glucose and lipid metabolism, contributing to better overall metabolic control.

Stress Resilience

A plant-based diet may also enhance the body's resilience to stress by modulating GR function. Nutrients and phytochemicals in plant foods can support the optimal functioning of the HPA axis, ensuring appropriate glucocorticoid signaling during stress. This can help mitigate the adverse effects of chronic stress on health.

Cardiovascular Health

Plant-based diets are beneficial for cardiovascular health, partly due to their effects on GR regulation. By reducing inflammation and improving metabolic health, these diets can help maintain healthy blood pressure and reduce the risk of cardiovascular diseases. The anti-inflammatory and antioxidant properties of plant-based foods play a crucial role in protecting cardiovascular health.

Weight Management

GRs are involved in the regulation of body weight and adipose tissue distribution. Plant-based diets, which are typically lower in calories and higher in fiber, can support weight management by modulating GR activity. The presence of bioactive compounds in plant foods can influence GR-mediated metabolic processes, aiding in the reduction of fat stores and promoting healthy weight loss.

Chronic Disease Prevention

By modulating the activity of GRs, plant-based diets can help prevent and manage various chronic diseases. The anti-inflammatory, antioxidant, and metabolic benefits of plant-based nutrition can reduce the risk of conditions such as type 2 diabetes, cardiovascular diseases, and certain cancers.

Glucocorticoid receptors are essential for various physiological processes, including immune response modulation, metabolic regulation, and stress response. The production and regulation of these receptors involve complex mechanisms influenced by genetic and environmental factors. Plant-based diets, rich in bioactive compounds such as flavonoids, dietary fiber, and omega-3 fatty acids, can modulate GR activity and contribute to overall health benefits. By enhancing the anti-inflammatory effects of GRs, improving metabolic health, supporting stress resilience, and promoting weight management, plant-based diets offer a holistic approach to maintaining and improving health.

Progesterone Receptors (PR)

Progesterone receptors (PR) are a class of intracellular receptors that are activated by the steroid hormone progesterone. They play a crucial role in various physiological processes, including reproductive function, cellular proliferation, and differentiation. There are two main isoforms of progesterone receptors: PR-A and PR-B, each with distinct functions and tissue distributions.

Function of Progesterone Receptors

PR-A and PR-B Isoforms

Progesterone receptors exist in two isoforms, PR-A and PR-B, which arise from the same gene but differ in their N-terminal regions due to alternative promoter usage and translational initiation. These isoforms have distinct roles and regulatory functions in various tissues.

PR-A

PR-A acts primarily as a repressor of other steroid hormone receptors, including estrogen receptors. It is crucial for the inhibitory effects of progesterone on uterine contraction and immune modulation during pregnancy. PR-A's role is particularly significant in maintaining uterine quiescence and preventing preterm labor.

PR-B

PR-B is a full-length receptor and functions as a transcriptional activator. It is essential for the proliferative and differentiative effects of progesterone in the mammary gland, facilitating breast development and differentiation during pregnancy. PR-B also plays a role in the regulation of gene expression in response to progesterone in other reproductive tissues.

Production of Progesterone Receptors

The production of progesterone receptors is a complex process involving gene expression, receptor synthesis, and post-translational modifications. The gene encoding PR is PGR, located on chromosome 11q22.

Gene Expression

The expression of the PGR gene is regulated by multiple transcription factors and regulatory elements. Estrogen, through its receptor ERα, is a major regulator, enhancing the transcription of the PGR gene. This interplay between estrogen and progesterone signaling is crucial for the coordinated regulation of reproductive processes.

Receptor Synthesis

Once transcribed, the mRNA of progesterone receptors is translated into protein in the cytoplasm. The receptors undergo folding and post-translational modifications, including phosphorylation, which are essential for their functional activity and stability. After these modifications, the receptors translocate to the nucleus, where they bind to specific DNA sequences known as progesterone response elements (PREs) to regulate target gene expression.

Post-Translational Modifications

Progesterone receptors undergo several post-translational modifications, such as phosphorylation, acetylation, and ubiquitination, which modulate their activity, stability, and subcellular localization. Phosphorylation by kinases like CDK2 and MAPKs enhances receptor activity and promotes transcriptional activation. Ubiquitination regulates receptor turnover and degradation, maintaining cellular receptor levels.

Regulation of Progesterone Receptors

The regulation of progesterone receptors involves multiple mechanisms to ensure appropriate cellular responses to progesterone.

Ligand-Dependent Regulation

Progesterone binding to its receptors induces conformational changes that activate the receptors, enabling them to bind DNA and regulate gene transcription. This ligand-dependent activation is a primary regulatory mechanism, ensuring that receptor activity is tightly controlled by progesterone levels.

Receptor Phosphorylation

Phosphorylation of progesterone receptors by kinases such as CDK2 and MAPKs can modulate receptor activity. Phosphorylation enhances receptor stability, transcriptional activity, and interaction with co-regulators, facilitating effective gene regulation in response to progesterone.

Co-Regulators and Transcriptional Machinery

Progesterone receptors interact with various co-regulators, including co-activators and co-repressors, which modulate their transcriptional activity. These co-regulators influence receptor binding to DNA, chromatin remodeling, and recruitment of the transcriptional machinery, fine-tuning gene expression.

Receptor Degradation

Progesterone receptors are subject to ubiquitin-mediated proteasomal degradation, a key regulatory mechanism that controls receptor levels and prevents prolonged or excessive signaling. Ubiquitination tags the receptors for degradation, ensuring timely receptor turnover and maintaining cellular homeostasis.

Role of Plant-Based Compounds in Regulation

Plant-based diets can influence the regulation of progesterone receptors through various bioactive compounds. Phytochemicals, such as flavonoids, have been shown to modulate receptor activity and expression.

Phytoestrogens

Phytoestrogens are plant-derived compounds with estrogenic activity, found in foods like soy, flaxseeds, and legumes. They can modulate progesterone receptor expression and activity by interacting with estrogen receptors, which regulate PGR gene transcription. For example, genistein, a phytoestrogen in soy, can enhance progesterone receptor expression by activating ERα.

Flavonoids

Flavonoids, a group of polyphenolic compounds found in fruits, vegetables, and tea, can influence progesterone receptor signaling. Quercetin, a flavonoid found in apples, onions, and berries, has been shown to inhibit the proliferation of breast cancer cells by modulating PR expression and activity. Flavonoids can affect receptor phosphorylation and interaction with co-regulators, impacting receptor function.

Dietary Fiber

High-fiber diets, typical of plant-based nutrition, can improve insulin sensitivity and reduce systemic inflammation. These effects can indirectly influence progesterone receptor regulation, as insulin and inflammatory cytokines are linked to receptor modulation. Improved metabolic health and reduced inflammation can enhance receptor function and stability.

Omega-3 Fatty Acids

Plant sources of omega-3 fatty acids, such as flaxseeds and chia seeds, have anti-inflammatory properties and can influence steroid hormone receptor function. Omega-3 fatty acids have been shown to decrease the expression of inflammatory cytokines, which can modulate progesterone receptor activity. Reduced inflammation can enhance receptor function and improve cellular responses to progesterone.

Plant-Based Diets and Progesterone Receptors

Adopting a plant-based diet can have significant impacts on the regulation and function of progesterone receptors. The intake of various nutrients and bioactive compounds from plants can modulate steroid hormone signaling, contributing to overall health benefits.

Reproductive Health

Plant-based diets rich in phytoestrogens, flavonoids, and omega-3 fatty acids can positively influence reproductive health by modulating progesterone receptor activity. These dietary components can enhance receptor expression and function, supporting reproductive processes and potentially reducing the risk of hormone-related disorders. For example, phytoestrogens can improve menstrual cycle regularity and alleviate menopausal symptoms by modulating estrogen and progesterone receptor signaling.

Breast Health

Progesterone receptors play a crucial role in breast development and differentiation. Plant-based diets, which are rich in antioxidants and anti-inflammatory compounds, can support breast health by modulating receptor activity. Flavonoids like quercetin can inhibit the proliferation of breast cancer cells by affecting progesterone receptor signaling, highlighting the potential protective effects of plant-based diets against breast cancer.

Metabolic Health

The influence of plant-based diets on progesterone receptors can enhance metabolic health. Improved insulin sensitivity and reduced inflammation, promoted by high-fiber and omega-3-rich diets, can positively impact progesterone receptor function. Enhanced receptor activity can support metabolic processes, contributing to better glycemic control and reduced risk of metabolic disorders such as type 2 diabetes.

Cardiovascular Health

Plant-based diets are rich in antioxidants, dietary fiber, and healthy fats, which are beneficial for cardiovascular health. Progesterone receptors have been implicated in cardiovascular function, including the regulation of vascular tone and endothelial function. The regulation of progesterone receptors in the cardiovascular system can be positively influenced by dietary components, supporting cardiovascular health and reducing the risk of cardiovascular diseases.

Progesterone receptors are essential for various physiological processes, including reproductive function, cellular proliferation, and differentiation. The production and regulation of these receptors involve complex mechanisms influenced by genetic and environmental factors. Plant-based diets, rich in phytoestrogens, flavonoids, dietary fiber, and omega-3 fatty acids, can modulate the activity and expression of progesterone receptors, contributing to overall health benefits.

Thyroid Hormone Receptors (TRα, TRβ)

Thyroid hormone receptors (TRα and TRβ) are nuclear receptors that mediate the effects of thyroid hormones, primarily triiodothyronine (T3) and thyroxine (T4). These receptors play vital roles in regulating the metabolism, development, and differentiation of cells. TRα and TRβ are encoded by separate genes, THRA and THRB, respectively, and they exhibit tissue-specific expression and distinct physiological functions.

Function of Thyroid Hormone Receptors

TRα

TRα receptors are predominantly expressed in cardiac and skeletal muscle tissues, as well as in the central nervous system. Their activation by thyroid hormones influences several critical functions:

1. **Cardiac Function**: TRα receptors regulate heart rate and cardiac output. They modulate the expression of genes involved in cardiac contractility, leading to increased heart rate and enhanced force of contraction. This is crucial for maintaining cardiovascular homeostasis.
2. **Skeletal Muscle Metabolism**: In skeletal muscles, TRα receptors influence the basal metabolic rate and energy expenditure. Activation of these receptors enhances oxidative metabolism and mitochondrial biogenesis, promoting efficient energy utilization and muscle function.
3. **Neuronal Development**: In the central nervous system, TRα receptors are essential for brain development and function. They regulate the differentiation and maturation of neurons, synaptogenesis, and myelination, impacting cognitive functions and neurological health.

TRβ

TRβ receptors are mainly found in the liver, kidneys, and hypothalamus. Their functions include:

1. **Metabolic Regulation**: TRβ receptors in the liver play a critical role in regulating lipid and carbohydrate metabolism. They influence the expression of genes involved in gluconeogenesis, cholesterol synthesis, and lipid metabolism, thereby maintaining metabolic homeostasis.
2. **Thermoregulation**: In the hypothalamus, TRβ receptors contribute to the regulation of body temperature. They modulate the set point for thermogenesis and energy expenditure, helping the body adapt to changes in environmental temperature.
3. **Development and Growth**: TRβ receptors are also involved in the growth and development of various tissues, including bones and the reproductive system. They ensure proper developmental processes by regulating gene expression during critical periods of growth.

Production of Thyroid Hormone Receptors

The production of thyroid hormone receptors involves a series of steps from gene expression to protein synthesis and post-translational modifications.

Gene Expression

The genes encoding TRα and TRβ receptors, THRA and THRB, are located on chromosomes 17 and 3, respectively. Their expression is regulated by various transcription factors and signaling pathways:

1. **Transcriptional Regulation**: The promoters of THRA and THRB genes contain binding sites for transcription factors such as thyroid hormone response elements (TREs), which facilitate the transcriptional activation in response to thyroid hormones.

Additionally, factors like Sp1 and NF-κB can modulate the transcription of these genes.

2. **Epigenetic Modifications**: Histone modifications and DNA methylation also play a role in regulating the expression of TR genes. These epigenetic changes can influence the accessibility of the promoter regions to transcriptional machinery.

Receptor Synthesis

Once transcribed, the mRNA of TRα and TRβ receptors is translated into proteins in the cytoplasm. These proteins undergo folding and assembly to attain their functional conformation:

1. **Protein Folding**: The newly synthesized TR proteins fold into their functional three-dimensional structures with the help of molecular chaperones. Proper folding is crucial for their stability and function.
2. **Post-Translational Modifications**: TR proteins undergo various post-translational modifications, such as phosphorylation and acetylation, which regulate their activity and interaction with other cellular components. These modifications can affect the receptor's ability to bind to DNA and interact with coactivators or corepressors.

Localization and Activation

The mature TR proteins are transported to the nucleus, where they bind to TREs on target genes. Activation of these receptors by thyroid hormones triggers the transcription of downstream genes involved in metabolism, growth, and development.

Regulation of Thyroid Hormone Receptors

The regulation of thyroid hormone receptors involves multiple mechanisms to ensure appropriate cellular responses to thyroid hormones.

Hormonal Feedback Mechanisms

Thyroid hormone levels are tightly regulated by feedback mechanisms involving the hypothalamus-pituitary-thyroid axis:

1. **Hypothalamic Regulation**: The hypothalamus secretes thyrotropin-releasing hormone (TRH), which stimulates the pituitary gland to produce thyroid-stimulating hormone (TSH). TSH, in turn, promotes the synthesis and release of thyroid hormones (T3 and T4) from the thyroid gland.
2. **Negative Feedback**: Elevated levels of T3 and T4 inhibit the release of TRH and TSH, creating a negative feedback loop that maintains thyroid hormone levels within a physiological range. This feedback mechanism ensures that TR activation is balanced and prevents excessive or insufficient thyroid hormone activity.

Receptor Sensitivity and Availability

The sensitivity and availability of TRs are modulated through various processes:

1. **Receptor Isoforms**: Alternative splicing of TR genes generates different receptor isoforms with distinct tissue distribution and functional properties. This diversity allows fine-tuning of thyroid hormone responses in different tissues.
2. **Coactivators and Corepressors**: The activity of TRs is influenced by their interaction with coactivators and corepressors. Coactivators, such as steroid receptor coactivators (SRCs) and thyroid hormone receptor-associated proteins (TRAPs), enhance TR-mediated transcription, while corepressors, like nuclear receptor corepressor (NCoR) and silencing mediators of retinoic acid and thyroid hormone receptors (SMRT), inhibit it.

Role of Plant-Based Compounds in Regulation

Plant-based diets can influence the regulation of thyroid hormone receptors through various bioactive compounds. Phytochemicals, such as flavonoids, and other dietary components can modulate TR activity and expression.

Flavonoids

Flavonoids are a group of polyphenolic compounds found in fruits, vegetables, tea, and other plant-based foods. They have been reported to influence thyroid hormone signaling pathways:

1. **Quercetin**: Quercetin, found in apples, onions, and berries, has been shown to inhibit the activity of deiodinase enzymes, which convert T4 to the more active T3. This can modulate the availability of T3 for TR activation.
2. **Genistein**: Genistein, an isoflavone present in soy products, can interact with TRs and alter their transcriptional activity. It has been demonstrated to bind to TRs and inhibit their ability to activate gene expression, potentially affecting thyroid hormone signaling.

Dietary Fiber

High-fiber diets, typical of plant-based nutrition, can improve thyroid function and hormone regulation:

1. **Gut Health**: Dietary fiber supports gut health by promoting the growth of beneficial gut bacteria. A healthy gut microbiota can enhance the enterohepatic circulation of thyroid hormones, improving their bioavailability and function.
2. **Insulin Sensitivity**: Improved insulin sensitivity, resulting from high-fiber diets, can positively influence thyroid hormone metabolism. Insulin resistance has been linked to altered thyroid hormone levels and impaired TR function.

Omega-3 Fatty Acids

Plant sources of omega-3 fatty acids, such as flaxseeds and chia seeds, have anti-inflammatory properties and can influence thyroid hormone receptor function:

1. **Anti-Inflammatory Effects**: Omega-3 fatty acids can reduce systemic inflammation, which is known to affect thyroid function and hormone levels. By mitigating inflammation, omega-3s help maintain proper thyroid hormone signaling.
2. **Lipid Metabolism**: Omega-3 fatty acids can modulate lipid metabolism, which is closely linked to thyroid hormone action. Enhanced lipid profiles resulting from omega-3 intake can support optimal TR function and metabolic regulation.

Plant-Based Diets and Thyroid Hormone Receptors

Adopting a plant-based diet can have significant impacts on the regulation and function of thyroid hormone receptors. The intake of various nutrients and bioactive compounds from plants can modulate thyroid hormone signaling, contributing to overall health benefits.

Cardiovascular Health

Plant-based diets are rich in antioxidants, dietary fiber, and healthy fats, which are beneficial for cardiovascular health:

1. **Antioxidants**: Antioxidants from plant foods can reduce oxidative stress, which impairs TR function. By protecting against oxidative damage, these compounds support proper thyroid hormone signaling in cardiovascular tissues.
2. **Dietary Fiber**: High-fiber diets help manage blood pressure and reduce systemic inflammation, improving cardiovascular health and supporting the function of TRα receptors in the heart.

Metabolic Health

The influence of plant-based diets on TRβ receptors can enhance metabolic health:

1. **Flavonoids**: Foods rich in flavonoids can improve insulin sensitivity and reduce the risk of metabolic disorders. By modulating TRβ receptor activity, these diets can enhance glucose uptake and utilization, contributing to better glycemic control.
2. **Omega-3 Fatty Acids**: Plant-based omega-3s can improve lipid metabolism and reduce inflammation, supporting the function of TRβ receptors in metabolic tissues.

Weight Management

TRα and TRβ receptors play crucial roles in energy metabolism and weight regulation:

1. **Caloric Density**: Plant-based diets, typically lower in calories and higher in fiber, can support weight management by enhancing the function of TRα receptors in skeletal muscle and TRβ receptors in metabolic tissues.
2. **Bioactive Compounds**: The presence of bioactive compounds in plant foods can stimulate thyroid hormone receptor-mediated thermogenesis and lipolysis, aiding in the reduction of fat stores and promoting healthy weight loss.

Thyroid hormone receptors (TRα and TRβ) are essential for various physiological processes, including cardiovascular function, metabolic regulation, and development. The production and regulation of these receptors involve complex mechanisms influenced by genetic and environmental factors.

Vitamin D Receptors (VDR)

Vitamin D receptors (VDR) are crucial components in the regulation of calcium and phosphate homeostasis in the human body. These receptors are a type of nuclear receptor that mediates the effects of vitamin D by regulating the expression of specific genes.

Function of Vitamin D Receptors (VDR)

Vitamin D receptors are involved in various physiological functions, primarily related to calcium and bone metabolism, immune response, and cell proliferation.

Calcium and Bone Metabolism

VDRs play a central role in maintaining calcium and phosphate levels in the blood, which are essential for healthy bone formation and maintenance. Upon activation by its ligand, 1,25-dihydroxyvitamin D (calcitriol), the VDR forms a complex with the retinoid X receptor (RXR). This complex binds to vitamin D response elements (VDREs) in the DNA, regulating the transcription of target genes involved in calcium absorption in the intestines, reabsorption in the kidneys, and mobilization from bones.

Immune Response

Vitamin D receptors are also expressed in various immune cells, including T cells, B cells, and macrophages. Activation of VDR in these cells modulates the immune response, enhancing the pathogen-fighting capabilities while also exerting anti-inflammatory effects. This regulatory role of VDR in the immune system is critical for maintaining immune homeostasis and preventing chronic inflammatory diseases.

Cell Proliferation and Differentiation

VDR activation influences cell proliferation and differentiation, processes crucial for tissue development and repair. In various tissues, including the skin, breast, and prostate, VDR activation can inhibit cell proliferation and induce differentiation, thereby playing a potential role in cancer prevention and treatment.

Production of Vitamin D Receptors

The production of VDR involves gene expression, protein synthesis, and post-translational modifications. The gene encoding the VDR is known as VDR, located on chromosome 12.

Gene Expression

The expression of the VDR gene is tightly regulated by various factors, including hormones, dietary components, and environmental stimuli. Promoter regions upstream of the VDR gene contain binding sites for transcription factors such as SP1, C/EBP, and VDRE-binding proteins. These factors can either upregulate or downregulate VDR gene expression depending on the physiological needs.

Protein Synthesis

After transcription, the mRNA of VDR is translated into a protein in the endoplasmic reticulum. The VDR protein then undergoes folding and post-translational modifications such as phosphorylation, which are crucial for its proper function and stability. These modifications can affect the receptor's ability to bind to vitamin D and its interaction with other cellular proteins.

Regulation of Vitamin D Receptors

The regulation of VDR is multifaceted, involving transcriptional control, ligand availability, and post-translational modifications.

Transcriptional Control

Transcriptional regulation of VDR involves the interaction of various transcription factors with the VDR gene promoter. Factors such as 1,25-dihydroxyvitamin D, parathyroid hormone (PTH), and certain cytokines can influence VDR expression. For example, 1,25-dihydroxyvitamin D, the active form of vitamin D, can induce its own receptor's expression in a feedback loop, ensuring adequate levels of VDR are available for optimal physiological function.

Ligand Availability

The availability of 1,25-dihydroxyvitamin D is crucial for VDR activation. This ligand is synthesized in the skin from 7-dehydrocholesterol upon exposure to UVB radiation or obtained from dietary sources. It is then converted in the liver and kidneys to its active form. Factors affecting the synthesis and availability of 1,25-dihydroxyvitamin D, such as sunlight exposure, skin pigmentation, and dietary intake, indirectly regulate VDR activity.

Post-Translational Modifications

Post-translational modifications of VDR, such as phosphorylation, acetylation, and ubiquitination, play significant roles in regulating its function. Phosphorylation by kinases can enhance or inhibit VDR's ability to bind DNA and interact with other proteins, thereby modulating its transcriptional activity.

Plant-Based Diets and Vitamin D Receptors

Adopting a plant-based diet can significantly influence the regulation and function of VDR through various nutrients and bioactive compounds.

Sources of Vitamin D in Plant-Based Diets

Vitamin D is primarily obtained from sunlight exposure and animal-based foods. However, plant-based sources of vitamin D include fortified foods and certain mushrooms exposed to UV light. Fortified plant milk, cereals, and orange juice can provide vitamin D2 (ergocalciferol), which can be converted to the active form of vitamin D in the body.

Bioactive Compounds and VDR Regulation

Plant-based diets are rich in bioactive compounds such as polyphenols, flavonoids, and carotenoids, which can modulate VDR activity.

Flavonoids Flavonoids, found in fruits, vegetables, tea, and soy products, have been shown to influence the VDR pathway. For instance, quercetin, a flavonoid present in apples and onions, can enhance VDR expression and activity, potentially enhancing the immune response and reducing inflammation.

Polyphenols Polyphenols, such as resveratrol found in grapes and peanuts, can modulate VDR activity by influencing the expression of VDR and its target genes. These compounds can enhance the transcriptional activity of VDR, contributing to improved calcium absorption and bone health.

Carotenoids Carotenoids, like beta-carotene in carrots and sweet potatoes, can also affect VDR regulation. Beta-carotene, as a precursor of vitamin A, plays a role in maintaining immune function and can interact with the VDR pathway to modulate immune responses.

Impact on Calcium and Bone Health

Plant-based diets, when appropriately planned, can support calcium and bone health. Foods rich in calcium, such as leafy greens (e.g., kale, bok choy), fortified plant milk, and tofu, along with vitamin D from fortified sources, ensure adequate calcium absorption and bone maintenance through VDR-mediated pathways.

Immune Modulation

The anti-inflammatory and antioxidant properties of plant-based foods can support VDR function in immune regulation. Diets high in fruits, vegetables, nuts, and seeds provide essential nutrients and bioactive compounds that can enhance the immune-modulating effects of VDR.

Vitamin D receptors play a vital role in regulating calcium and phosphate homeostasis, immune response, and cell proliferation. The production and regulation of VDR are complex processes influenced by genetic and environmental factors, including diet.

Retinoic Acid Receptors (RARα, RARβ, RARγ)

Retinoic Acid Receptors (RARs) are nuclear receptors that mediate the biological effects of retinoic acid (RA), a metabolite of vitamin A. These receptors are crucial for various physiological processes, including cell differentiation, proliferation, and apoptosis. There are three main subtypes of RARs: RARα, RARβ, and RARγ, each with distinct roles and tissue distributions.

Function of Retinoic Acid Receptors

RARα (Retinoic Acid Receptor Alpha)

RARα is widely expressed in various tissues, including the liver, spleen, and hematopoietic cells. Its primary function is to regulate gene expression involved in cell growth and differentiation. In hematopoiesis, RARα plays a critical role in the differentiation of myeloid cells. It also influences the development and function of the immune system, particularly T cells and dendritic cells.

RARβ (Retinoic Acid Receptor Beta)

RARβ is predominantly found in the brain, spinal cord, and developing limbs. It is essential for the proper development of the nervous system. RARβ regulates genes involved in neuronal differentiation, axonal growth, and synaptic plasticity. Additionally, it plays a role in maintaining the homeostasis of epithelial tissues by promoting differentiation and inhibiting proliferation.

RARγ (Retinoic Acid Receptor Gamma)

RARγ is highly expressed in the skin, lungs, and skeletal tissues. It is crucial for skeletal development and homeostasis, regulating the expression of genes involved in chondrocyte differentiation and cartilage formation. RARγ also contributes to skin health by modulating keratinocyte proliferation and differentiation, thus playing a role in the treatment of skin disorders such as acne and psoriasis.

Production of Retinoic Acid Receptors

The production of Retinoic Acid Receptors is a multi-step process involving gene expression, receptor synthesis, and post-translational modifications.

Gene Expression

The genes encoding RARα, RARβ, and RARγ are RARA, RARB, and RARG, respectively. The expression of these genes is tightly regulated by various transcription factors and regulatory elements. Retinoic acid itself can influence the expression of its receptors through feedback mechanisms. Promoter regions upstream of the RAR genes contain retinoic acid response elements (RAREs), which bind to retinoic acid-bound RARs to initiate transcription.

Receptor Synthesis

Once transcribed, the mRNA of RARs is translated into protein in the endoplasmic reticulum. These proteins undergo proper folding and post-translational modifications, such as phosphorylation, which are essential for their function and stability. The receptors are then transported to the nucleus, where they exert their effects on gene expression.

Post-Translational Modifications

RARs undergo various post-translational modifications that regulate their activity. Phosphorylation is one such modification that can influence the receptor's ability to bind DNA and interact with other proteins. Additionally, acetylation and ubiquitination can modulate the stability and degradation of RARs, thereby affecting their cellular levels and activity.

Regulation of Retinoic Acid Receptors

The regulation of Retinoic Acid Receptors involves multiple mechanisms to ensure appropriate cellular responses to retinoic acid.

Ligand Availability

The availability of retinoic acid, the ligand for RARs, is a key regulatory factor. Retinoic acid is derived from dietary vitamin A (retinol) through a series of enzymatic reactions. The cellular levels of retinoic acid are tightly regulated by the balance between its synthesis and degradation. Enzymes such as retinaldehyde dehydrogenases (RALDHs) and cytochrome P450 enzymes (CYP26) play crucial roles in this process.

Coactivators and Corepressors

RARs interact with coactivators and corepressors to regulate gene transcription. In the absence of retinoic acid, RARs are bound to corepressors, which inhibit transcription. Upon binding to retinoic acid, RARs undergo a conformational change that leads to the dissociation of corepressors and recruitment of coactivators, thereby activating transcription. Examples of coactivators include steroid receptor coactivators (SRCs) and p300/CBP, while corepressors include nuclear receptor corepressors (NCoR) and silencing mediators for retinoid and thyroid hormone receptors (SMRT).

Phosphorylation

Phosphorylation of RARs by kinases such as MAPKs and CDKs can modulate their activity. Phosphorylation can influence the receptor's ability to bind to DNA, interact with other proteins, and be degraded. For instance, phosphorylation of RARα can enhance its transcriptional activity, while phosphorylation of RARβ and RARγ can affect their stability and function.

Plant-Based Compounds in Regulation

Plant-based diets can influence the regulation of Retinoic Acid Receptors through various bioactive compounds. Phytochemicals, such as carotenoids and flavonoids, have been shown to modulate RAR activity and expression.

Carotenoids

Carotenoids are precursors of retinoic acid and are abundant in plant-based foods such as carrots, sweet potatoes, and leafy greens. β-carotene, a prominent carotenoid, is converted into retinoic acid in the body, thereby influencing RAR activity. Studies have shown that carotenoid-rich diets can enhance the expression of RARs and promote their beneficial effects on cell differentiation and proliferation.

Flavonoids

Flavonoids, found in fruits, vegetables, tea, and other plant-based foods, have been reported to interact with the retinoic acid signaling pathway. For instance, quercetin, a flavonoid present in apples and onions, can modulate the activity of RARs by influencing the availability of retinoic acid and interacting with receptor signaling.

Plant-Based Diets and Retinoic Acid Receptors

Adopting a plant-based diet can have significant impacts on the regulation and function of Retinoic Acid Receptors. The intake of various nutrients and bioactive compounds from plants can modulate the retinoic acid signaling pathway, contributing to overall health benefits.

Skin Health

Plant-based diets are rich in carotenoids, which are crucial for skin health. Retinoic acid, derived from carotenoids, regulates the expression of genes involved in keratinocyte proliferation and differentiation. This helps maintain skin integrity and can be beneficial in treating skin disorders such as acne and psoriasis. Studies have shown that a diet rich in β-carotene can improve skin health by enhancing the activity of RARγ in the skin.

Immune Function

The influence of plant-based diets on RARα can enhance immune function. Retinoic acid regulates the differentiation and function of T cells and dendritic cells, which are critical for immune responses. Plant-based foods rich in vitamin A and carotenoids can support the immune system by modulating RARα activity. For instance, studies have shown that carotenoid supplementation can improve immune responses by enhancing RARα-mediated gene expression in immune cells.

Bone Health

RARγ plays a crucial role in bone health by regulating chondrocyte differentiation and cartilage formation. Plant-based diets, which are typically rich in antioxidants and anti-inflammatory compounds, can support bone health by modulating RARγ activity. For example, flavonoids such as quercetin and resveratrol have been shown to influence bone metabolism by interacting with RARγ signaling pathways.

Retinoic Acid Receptors (RARα, RARβ, RARγ) are essential for various physiological processes, including cell differentiation, proliferation, and apoptosis. The production and regulation of these receptors involve complex mechanisms influenced by genetic and environmental factors.

32

Cytokine Receptors

Interleukin Receptors (IL-1R, IL-2R, IL-6R, IL-10R)

Interleukin receptors (IL-1R, IL-2R, IL-6R, IL-10R) are critical components of the immune system, responsible for mediating the effects of their respective interleukins, which are key cytokines in the regulation of immune responses, inflammation, and hematopoiesis.

Function of Interleukin Receptors

IL-1R (Interleukin-1 Receptor)

IL-1R is the receptor for interleukin-1 (IL-1), which exists in two forms: IL-1α and IL-1β. Both forms bind to IL-1R and are involved in the initiation of inflammatory responses. IL-1R is found on a variety of cell types, including immune cells, endothelial cells, and fibroblasts.

Key Functions:

- **Inflammatory Response:** IL-1R activation leads to the production of pro-inflammatory cytokines, chemokines, and adhesion molecules, facilitating the recruitment of immune cells to sites of infection or injury.
- **Fever Induction:** IL-1R signaling in the hypothalamus induces fever, a common response to infection.

- **Cell Proliferation and Differentiation:** IL-1R plays a role in the proliferation and differentiation of T cells and B cells, essential for adaptive immunity.

IL-2R (Interleukin-2 Receptor)

IL-2R is the receptor for interleukin-2 (IL-2), a cytokine crucial for the growth, proliferation, and survival of T cells. IL-2R is composed of three subunits: IL-2Rα (CD25), IL-2Rβ (CD122), and IL-2Rγ (CD132).

Key Functions:

- **T Cell Proliferation:** IL-2R signaling promotes the clonal expansion of activated T cells, essential for mounting effective immune responses.
- **Regulatory T Cells (Tregs):** IL-2R is critical for the development and function of Tregs, which help maintain immune tolerance and prevent autoimmune responses.
- **B Cell Differentiation:** IL-2R also supports the differentiation of B cells into antibody-producing plasma cells.

IL-6R (Interleukin-6 Receptor)

IL-6R is the receptor for interleukin-6 (IL-6), a cytokine involved in both pro-inflammatory and anti-inflammatory responses. IL-6R is expressed on immune cells, hepatocytes, and some stromal cells.

Key Functions:

- **Acute Phase Response:** IL-6R activation in the liver leads to the production of acute-phase proteins, such as C-reactive protein (CRP), which are important markers of inflammation.
- **B Cell Maturation:** IL-6R signaling promotes the differentiation of B cells and the production of antibodies.

- **T Cell Activation:** IL-6R is involved in the differentiation of T cells into Th17 cells, a subset of T cells that play a role in autoimmune diseases.

IL-10R (Interleukin-10 Receptor)

IL-10R is the receptor for interleukin-10 (IL-10), an anti-inflammatory cytokine that helps regulate immune responses to prevent excessive inflammation and tissue damage. IL-10R is found on various immune cells, including macrophages, dendritic cells, and T cells.

Key Functions:

- **Anti-inflammatory Effects:** IL-10R signaling suppresses the production of pro-inflammatory cytokines and inhibits the activation of macrophages and dendritic cells.
- **Immune Regulation:** IL-10R helps maintain immune homeostasis by promoting the survival and function of Tregs.
- **Inhibition of Autoimmunity:** IL-10R is crucial in preventing autoimmune responses by limiting the activation and proliferation of autoreactive T cells.

Production of Interleukin Receptors

Gene Expression

The genes encoding interleukin receptors are tightly regulated and influenced by various transcription factors and signaling pathways. Each receptor's gene expression can be modulated by cytokines, growth factors, and environmental factors, including diet.

Key Genes:

- **IL1R1:** The gene encoding IL-1R.
- **IL2RA, IL2RB, IL2RG:** The genes encoding the α, β, and γ subunits of IL-2R, respectively.
- **IL6R:** The gene encoding IL-6R.

- **IL10RA and IL10RB:** The genes encoding the α and β subunits of IL-10R, respectively.

Receptor Synthesis

Interleukin receptors are synthesized in the endoplasmic reticulum, where they undergo proper folding and post-translational modifications, such as glycosylation. These processes are essential for the stability and functionality of the receptors.

Receptor Assembly:

- **IL-1R:** Assembled as a single-chain receptor.
- **IL-2R:** Assembled from three subunits, with the β and γ subunits being crucial for signal transduction.
- **IL-6R:** Assembled as a complex with the signal-transducing subunit gp130.
- **IL-10R:** Assembled from two subunits, IL-10RA and IL-10RB, both required for functional signaling.

Post-Translational Modifications

Post-translational modifications, such as phosphorylation and ubiquitination, play critical roles in regulating the activity and stability of interleukin receptors. These modifications can affect receptor localization, signaling capacity, and degradation.

Regulation of Interleukin Receptors

Signaling Pathways

Interleukin receptors activate various intracellular signaling pathways upon ligand binding, leading to diverse biological effects.

Key Pathways:

- **NF-κB Pathway:** Activated by IL-1R and involved in the transcription of pro-inflammatory genes.

- **JAK/STAT Pathway:** Activated by IL-2R, IL-6R, and IL-10R, crucial for the transcription of genes involved in cell proliferation, survival, and differentiation.
- **MAPK Pathway:** Activated by IL-1R and IL-6R, involved in cell proliferation and differentiation.

Receptor Desensitization and Downregulation

Prolonged exposure to interleukins can lead to receptor desensitization, reducing cellular responsiveness. This is often followed by receptor downregulation, where receptor levels on the cell surface are decreased to prevent overstimulation.

Mechanisms:

- **Desensitization:** Involves receptor phosphorylation and internalization, reducing receptor availability at the cell surface.
- **Downregulation:** Involves the degradation of internalized receptors in lysosomes.

Receptor Recycling

Internalized receptors can be recycled back to the cell membrane or targeted for degradation. The balance between these processes determines the number of functional receptors available for signaling.

Role of Plant-Based Compounds in Regulation

Phytochemicals

Plant-based diets provide various bioactive compounds, such as flavonoids, polyphenols, and carotenoids, which can modulate the activity and expression of interleukin receptors.

Key Compounds:

- **Flavonoids:** Found in fruits, vegetables, and tea, flavonoids like quercetin and epigallocatechin gallate (EGCG) can inhibit inflammatory signaling pathways, reducing the expression and activity of IL-1R and IL-6R.

- **Polyphenols:** Found in berries, nuts, and seeds, polyphenols can modulate cytokine production and receptor signaling, potentially enhancing the anti-inflammatory effects of IL-10R.
- **Carotenoids:** Found in carrots, sweet potatoes, and leafy greens, carotenoids like beta-carotene can reduce oxidative stress and inflammation, influencing the activity of IL-6R and IL-1R.

Dietary Fiber

High-fiber diets, typical of plant-based nutrition, can improve gut health and modulate immune responses. Dietary fiber promotes the production of short-chain fatty acids (SCFAs) by gut microbiota, which have anti-inflammatory effects and can influence interleukin receptor activity.

Effects:

- **SCFAs:** SCFAs like butyrate can inhibit the expression of pro-inflammatory cytokines and receptors, enhancing the anti-inflammatory effects of IL-10R and reducing the activity of IL-1R and IL-6R.
- **Gut Microbiota:** A healthy gut microbiota supported by dietary fiber can modulate systemic inflammation and immune responses, indirectly affecting interleukin receptor signaling.

Omega-3 Fatty Acids

Plant sources of omega-3 fatty acids, such as flaxseeds, chia seeds, and walnuts, have anti-inflammatory properties and can influence interleukin receptor function.

Effects:

- **Anti-inflammatory:** Omega-3 fatty acids can reduce the production of pro-inflammatory cytokines and inhibit the activation of IL-1R and IL-6R.
- **Immune Regulation:** Omega-3 fatty acids can enhance the function of IL-10R, promoting anti-inflammatory responses and immune tolerance.

Plant-Based Diets and Interleukin Receptors

Inflammation Modulation

Plant-based diets are rich in anti-inflammatory compounds, which can modulate the activity of interleukin receptors and reduce chronic inflammation.

Key Benefits:

- **Reduced IL-1R and IL-6R Activity:** By decreasing the levels of pro-inflammatory cytokines, plant-based diets can lower the activity of IL-1R and IL-6R, reducing the risk of chronic inflammatory diseases.
- **Enhanced IL-10R Function:** The anti-inflammatory properties of plant-based diets can enhance the activity of IL-10R, promoting immune regulation and preventing excessive inflammation.

Immune System Support

A diet rich in fruits, vegetables, nuts, and seeds can support the immune system by providing essential nutrients and bioactive compounds that influence interleukin receptor signaling.

Key Benefits:

- **Enhanced T Cell Function:** Plant-based diets can support the proliferation and differentiation of T cells, essential for effective immune responses and regulated by IL-2R.
- **Improved Antibody Production:** Nutrients from plant-based foods can support B cell function and antibody production, mediated by IL-6R.

Disease Prevention and Management

Adopting a plant-based diet can help prevent and manage various diseases by modulating interleukin receptor activity and reducing inflammation.

Key Benefits:

- **Autoimmune Diseases:** By enhancing the function of IL-10R and reducing pro-inflammatory signaling, plant-based diets can help prevent and manage autoimmune diseases.
- **Cardiovascular Diseases:** Reduced IL-6R activity and lower systemic inflammation from plant-based diets can decrease the risk of cardiovascular diseases.
- **Metabolic Disorders:** Improved insulin sensitivity and reduced inflammation can result from plant-based diets, influencing IL-1R and IL-6R activity and lowering the risk of metabolic disorders.

Interleukin receptors play essential roles in immune responses, inflammation, and disease regulation.

Tumor Necrosis Factor Receptors (TNFR1, TNFR2)

Tumor necrosis factor receptors (TNFR1 and TNFR2) are critical components of the immune system, playing significant roles in inflammation, cell survival, apoptosis, and immunity. These receptors are part of the larger tumor necrosis factor receptor superfamily, which includes various receptors involved in immune responses. TNFR1 and TNFR2, specifically, bind to tumor necrosis factor-alpha (TNF-α), a cytokine involved in systemic inflammation and immune system regulation.

Function of Tumor Necrosis Factor Receptors

TNFR1

TNFR1 (Tumor Necrosis Factor Receptor 1), also known as p55 or CD120a, is ubiquitously expressed in most tissues and is the primary mediator of TNF-α signaling. TNFR1 activation can lead to several cellular responses depending on the cellular context and the presence of other signaling molecules. The primary functions of TNFR1 include:

1. **Induction of Apoptosis**: TNFR1 can trigger programmed cell death (apoptosis) through its death domain, which recruits adaptor proteins like TRADD (TNFR1-associated death domain protein) and FADD (Fas-associated death domain protein). This pathway is crucial for eliminating damaged or infected cells.
2. **Inflammatory Response**: Activation of TNFR1 can lead to the activation of the NF-κB (nuclear factor kappa-light-chain-enhancer of activated B cells) pathway, resulting in the transcription of pro-inflammatory genes. This pathway is essential for mounting an effective immune response against pathogens.
3. **Cell Survival and Proliferation**: TNFR1 signaling can also promote cell survival and proliferation through the activation of various downstream kinases and transcription factors, such as JNK (c-Jun N-terminal kinase) and AP-1 (activator protein-1).

TNFR2

TNFR2 (Tumor Necrosis Factor Receptor 2), also known as p75 or CD120b, is primarily expressed in immune cells, endothelial cells, and certain neuronal populations. The functions of TNFR2 include:

1. **Immune Regulation**: TNFR2 plays a crucial role in modulating immune responses by promoting the activation and proliferation of regulatory T cells (Tregs), which are essential for maintaining immune tolerance and preventing autoimmune diseases.
2. **Tissue Regeneration and Repair**: TNFR2 activation can enhance tissue regeneration and repair by promoting the survival and proliferation of endothelial cells and other cell types involved in tissue homeostasis.
3. **Neuroprotection**: In the nervous system, TNFR2 can mediate neuroprotective effects by promoting the survival and regeneration of neurons and glial cells.

Production of Tumor Necrosis Factor Receptors

The production of TNFR1 and TNFR2 involves complex regulatory mechanisms at the genetic, transcriptional, and post-transcriptional levels.

Gene Expression

The genes encoding TNFR1 and TNFR2 are TNFRSF1A and TNFRSF1B, respectively. The expression of these genes is regulated by various transcription factors and signaling pathways. For instance, NF-κB, AP-1, and STAT (signal transducer and activator of transcription) proteins can bind to the promoter regions of TNFRSF1A and TNFRSF1B, influencing their transcription.

1. **TNFRSF1A (TNFR1)**: The expression of TNFR1 is constitutive in most tissues, meaning it is continuously expressed at

a baseline level. However, its expression can be upregulated in response to inflammatory cytokines like TNF-α, IL-1 (interleukin-1), and IFN-γ (interferon-gamma).

2. **TNFRSF1B (TNFR2)**: TNFR2 expression is more restricted and inducible. It is primarily upregulated in immune cells such as T cells, B cells, and macrophages upon activation. Additionally, various stress signals and growth factors can enhance TNFR2 expression.

Receptor Synthesis and Post-Translational Modifications

Once transcribed, the mRNA of TNFR1 and TNFR2 is translated into proteins in the endoplasmic reticulum (ER). The receptors undergo several post-translational modifications, including glycosylation, which are essential for their stability, folding, and function.

1. **Glycosylation**: Glycosylation of TNFR1 and TNFR2 occurs in the ER and Golgi apparatus, where sugar moieties are added to specific asparagine residues. This modification is crucial for the proper folding and surface expression of the receptors.
2. **Cleavage and Shedding**: TNFR1 and TNFR2 can be cleaved by metalloproteases, resulting in the release of soluble forms of the receptors (sTNFR1 and sTNFR2) into the extracellular space. These soluble receptors can bind to TNF-α, acting as decoys to modulate TNF-α signaling.

Regulation of Tumor Necrosis Factor Receptors

The regulation of TNFR1 and TNFR2 is complex and involves multiple mechanisms to ensure precise control of TNF-α signaling.

Receptor Desensitization and Downregulation

Prolonged exposure to TNF-α can lead to receptor desensitization and downregulation. This process involves the internalization of the receptors from the cell surface and their subsequent degradation or recycling.

1. **Internalization**: Upon TNF-α binding, TNFR1 and TNFR2 can be internalized via clathrin-mediated endocytosis. This internalization is crucial for terminating the signaling and preventing excessive inflammatory responses.
2. **Receptor Recycling and Degradation**: Internalized receptors can be recycled back to the cell surface or targeted for degradation in lysosomes. The balance between recycling and degradation determines the overall number of functional receptors available for signaling.

Role of Plant-Based Compounds in Regulation

Plant-based diets can influence the regulation of TNFR1 and TNFR2 through various bioactive compounds. Phytochemicals, antioxidants, and anti-inflammatory agents found in plant foods can modulate TNF-α signaling pathways.

1. **Flavonoids**: Flavonoids are polyphenolic compounds found in fruits, vegetables, tea, and other plant-based foods. They have been shown to modulate TNF-α signaling by inhibiting the activation of NF-κB and reducing the expression of TNFR1 and TNFR2. For example, quercetin, a flavonoid found in apples, onions, and berries, can inhibit TNF-α-induced NF-κB activation, thereby reducing inflammation.
2. **Curcumin**: Curcumin, the active component of turmeric, has potent anti-inflammatory properties. It can downregulate the expression of TNFR1 and TNFR2 by inhibiting the transcriptional activity of NF-κB and other pro-inflammatory transcription factors.
3. **Resveratrol**: Resveratrol, a polyphenol found in grapes, berries, and peanuts, can inhibit TNF-α signaling by reducing the

expression of TNFR1 and TNFR2. Resveratrol has been shown to modulate various signaling pathways, including NF-κB, AP-1, and STAT3, contributing to its anti-inflammatory effects.

Plant-Based Diets and Tumor Necrosis Factor Receptors

Adopting a plant-based diet can have significant impacts on the regulation and function of TNFR1 and TNFR2. The intake of various nutrients and bioactive compounds from plants can modulate TNF-α signaling, contributing to overall health benefits.

Cardiovascular Health

Plant-based diets are rich in antioxidants, dietary fiber, and healthy fats, which are beneficial for cardiovascular health. The regulation of TNFR1 and TNFR2 in endothelial cells can be positively influenced by these dietary components. For example, antioxidants can reduce oxidative stress, which is known to impair TNFR function and contribute to endothelial dysfunction.

1. **Polyphenols**: Polyphenols, such as those found in green tea, cocoa, and berries, can enhance endothelial function by reducing TNF-α-induced inflammation and oxidative stress. These compounds can inhibit the expression of TNFR1 and TNFR2, thereby reducing the inflammatory response in blood vessels.
2. **Dietary Fiber**: High-fiber diets can improve vascular health by reducing systemic inflammation and improving endothelial function. Soluble fiber, in particular, can lower circulating levels of TNF-α, which in turn can modulate the expression of TNFR1 and TNFR2.

Immune System Modulation

The influence of plant-based diets on TNFR2 can enhance immune system function. Foods rich in flavonoids and other anti-inflammatory compounds can promote the activation and proliferation of regulatory

T cells (Tregs), which are essential for maintaining immune balance and preventing autoimmune diseases.

1. **Flavonoids**: Flavonoids like quercetin and catechins can enhance Treg function by modulating TNF-α signaling and reducing the expression of TNFR2 on immune cells. This modulation can help in maintaining immune tolerance and preventing chronic inflammatory conditions.
2. **Omega-3 Fatty Acids**: Plant sources of omega-3 fatty acids, such as flaxseeds and chia seeds, have anti-inflammatory properties and can influence TNF-α signaling. Omega-3 fatty acids can reduce the expression of TNFR2 on immune cells, thereby modulating the inflammatory response.

Neuroprotection

Plant-based diets can also have neuroprotective effects by modulating TNF-α signaling in the nervous system. Bioactive compounds in plant foods can reduce neuroinflammation and promote the survival of neurons and glial cells.

1. **Curcumin**: Curcumin can protect against neurodegenerative diseases by inhibiting TNF-α-induced inflammation and reducing the expression of TNFR1 and TNFR2 in neuronal cells. This neuroprotective effect can help in maintaining cognitive function and preventing diseases like Alzheimer's.
2. **Resveratrol**: Resveratrol has been shown to protect against neuroinflammation and oxidative stress by modulating TNF-α signaling pathways. Its ability to reduce the expression of TNFR1 and TNFR2 in the brain can contribute to its neuroprotective properties.

Tumor necrosis factor receptors (TNFR1 and TNFR2) are essential for various physiological processes, including immune regulation, inflammation, cell survival, and apoptosis. The production and regulation of these receptors involve complex mechanisms influenced by genetic and environmental factors.

Interferon Receptors (IFNAR1, IFNAR2)

Interferon receptors (IFNAR1 and IFNAR2) are integral components of the immune system's response to viral infections and other immune challenges. They belong to the class of cytokine receptors and play a pivotal role in the cellular response to interferons (IFNs), which are critical signaling proteins. These receptors are essential for initiating the antiviral, antiproliferative, and immunomodulatory actions of interferons.

Function of Interferon Receptors

Interferon receptors, specifically IFNAR1 and IFNAR2, mediate the effects of type I interferons (IFN-α and IFN-β). These receptors are present on nearly all cell types and initiate a signaling cascade crucial for antiviral defense, regulation of cell growth, and modulation of the immune response.

IFNAR1

IFNAR1 is one of the two subunits that form the interferon-α/β receptor complex. It is primarily responsible for binding to the interferon ligands and initiating the signal transduction pathways. Upon binding of IFN-α or IFN-β to IFNAR1, conformational changes facilitate the recruitment and activation of associated signaling molecules, such as Janus kinases (JAKs) and signal transducers and activators of transcription (STATs).

IFNAR2

IFNAR2 serves as the second subunit of the interferon receptor complex. It exists in three isoforms: a short soluble form (IFNAR2a), a transmembrane form with a truncated intracellular domain (IFNAR2b), and a full-length transmembrane form (IFNAR2c). The full-length IFNAR2c is crucial for signal transduction, whereas the soluble form can act as a decoy receptor, modulating the availability of interferons and their ability to signal through cell surface receptors.

Production of Interferon Receptors

The production of interferon receptors involves a sophisticated interplay of genetic regulation, protein synthesis, and post-translational modifications.

Gene Expression

The genes encoding IFNAR1 and IFNAR2 are IFNAR1 and IFNAR2, respectively. Their expression is tightly regulated by various transcription factors, including those activated by interferons themselves. This creates a feedback loop where interferon signaling can enhance the expression of its receptors, thus amplifying the cellular response to interferons.

Receptor Synthesis

Once the genes are transcribed, the mRNA of IFNAR1 and IFNAR2 is translated into proteins within the endoplasmic reticulum (ER). These proteins undergo proper folding and glycosylation, which are crucial for their stability and function. The glycosylated receptors are then transported to the Golgi apparatus for further processing and finally to the cell membrane.

Post-Translational Modifications

Interferon receptors undergo several post-translational modifications, including phosphorylation and ubiquitination. Phosphorylation of specific tyrosine residues on IFNAR1 and IFNAR2 is essential for the activation of downstream signaling pathways. Ubiquitination can regulate receptor turnover and degradation, thus controlling the duration and intensity of interferon signaling.

Regulation of Interferon Receptors

The regulation of interferon receptors is a multi-faceted process involving feedback mechanisms, receptor internalization, and modulation by various factors, including diet.

Feedback Mechanisms

Interferon signaling itself regulates the expression of IFNAR1 and IFNAR2. For instance, the activation of interferon-stimulated genes (ISGs) can enhance the transcription of interferon receptors, thereby promoting a sustained antiviral response. Conversely, negative regulators such as suppressors of cytokine signaling (SOCS) proteins can inhibit the signaling pathways, preventing excessive inflammation and tissue damage.

Receptor Internalization and Recycling

After ligand binding, interferon receptors undergo internalization through endocytosis. The receptors can either be recycled back to the cell surface or targeted for degradation in lysosomes. The balance between these pathways determines the cellular sensitivity to interferons. Efficient recycling can maintain a high level of receptor availability, whereas degradation reduces receptor numbers, thus attenuating the response.

Plant-Based Compounds in Regulation

Plant-based diets, rich in various bioactive compounds, can influence the regulation of interferon receptors. Phytochemicals such as flavonoids, polyphenols, and other antioxidants play a role in modulating immune responses and receptor functions.

Flavonoids

Flavonoids, found in abundance in fruits and vegetables, can modulate the immune response by affecting cytokine production and signaling pathways. For instance, quercetin has been shown to enhance the antiviral response by upregulating the expression of interferon receptors and promoting the activation of downstream signaling pathways.

Polyphenols

Polyphenols, such as resveratrol and curcumin, exhibit anti-inflammatory and immunomodulatory properties. These compounds can enhance the expression and function of interferon receptors by reducing oxidative stress and modulating signaling pathways. For example, resveratrol has been reported to increase the sensitivity of cells to interferon-induced antiviral responses by upregulating IFNAR1 and IFNAR2 expression.

Dietary Fiber

High-fiber diets typical of plant-based nutrition can improve gut health and modulate immune function. Soluble fibers, such as beta-glucans, have been shown to enhance the immune response by increasing the expression of interferon receptors and promoting the activation of interferon-stimulated genes.

Plant-Based Diets and Interferon Receptors

Adopting a plant-based diet can significantly impact the regulation and function of interferon receptors, contributing to enhanced antiviral defense and overall immune health.

Enhanced Antiviral Defense

Plant-based diets rich in vitamins, minerals, and antioxidants support the optimal function of interferon receptors. Vitamin C and E, for example, can protect interferon receptors from oxidative damage, thus maintaining their functionality during viral infections. Additionally, selenium, found in nuts and seeds, is crucial for the proper functioning of the immune system and can enhance the expression of interferon receptors.

Reduced Inflammation

Chronic inflammation can impair the function of interferon receptors. Plant-based diets, which are anti-inflammatory, help in reducing systemic inflammation and thereby support the proper functioning of interferon receptors. Omega-3 fatty acids from flaxseeds and chia seeds can reduce the production of pro-inflammatory cytokines, thus maintaining a balanced immune response.

Improved Immune Modulation

Bioactive compounds in plant foods can modulate the immune system and enhance the response to interferons. For instance, compounds like curcumin and green tea polyphenols have been shown to enhance the antiviral response by modulating the expression and function of interferon receptors.

Interferon receptors, particularly IFNAR1 and IFNAR2, are crucial for the immune system's ability to combat viral infections and regulate immune responses. The production and regulation of these receptors involve complex genetic and biochemical processes that can be influenced by various factors, including diet.

Growth Hormone Receptors (GHR)

Growth Hormone Receptors (GHR) are crucial components of the body's endocrine system, mediating the effects of growth hormone (GH). These receptors play significant roles in growth, metabolism, and overall homeostasis.

Function of Growth Hormone Receptors

Growth Hormone Receptors are found on the surface of various cell types and are responsible for mediating the actions of growth hormone, which is secreted by the pituitary gland. When GH binds to GHR, it triggers a cascade of intracellular signaling pathways that lead to various physiological responses.

Growth and Development

GHRs are integral to growth and development, especially during childhood and adolescence. When GH binds to GHR, it activates the JAK2-STAT5 signaling pathway, promoting the expression of insulin-like growth factor 1 (IGF-1) in the liver. IGF-1 then acts on various tissues to stimulate growth, including bone elongation and muscle mass increase.

Metabolism

GHRs also play a crucial role in regulating metabolism. Activation of GHR influences carbohydrate, lipid, and protein metabolism. GH promotes lipolysis, the breakdown of triglycerides into free fatty acids and glycerol, enhancing fat utilization as an energy source. It also impacts glucose metabolism by promoting gluconeogenesis in the liver and reducing insulin sensitivity, which can increase blood glucose levels.

Immune Function

Growth hormone and its receptor also have roles in modulating the immune system. GH can enhance the function of various immune cells, including T cells and natural killer cells, thereby contributing to the body's defense mechanisms.

Production of Growth Hormone Receptors

The production of Growth Hormone Receptors involves several stages, including gene expression, protein synthesis, and post-translational modifications.

Gene Expression

The GHR gene is located on chromosome 5 in humans. Its expression is regulated by various transcription factors and hormonal signals. Nutritional status, including the intake of certain plant-based nutrients, can influence the expression of the GHR gene. For example, certain polyphenols found in plant foods can modulate gene expression through epigenetic mechanisms.

Protein Synthesis

Once the GHR gene is transcribed into mRNA, it is translated into protein in the endoplasmic reticulum. The nascent GHR protein undergoes folding and glycosylation, which are essential for its proper function and stability. These processes ensure that the receptor attains the correct conformation to effectively bind growth hormone.

Post-Translational Modifications

GHRs undergo various post-translational modifications that regulate their activity and stability. Phosphorylation of GHR by kinases such as JAK2 is a key step in the receptor's activation and signal transduction. Additionally, ubiquitination can target GHRs for degradation, thereby modulating receptor levels on the cell surface.

Regulation of Growth Hormone Receptors

The regulation of Growth Hormone Receptors involves complex mechanisms to maintain appropriate cellular responses to growth hormone. These mechanisms include receptor desensitization, internalization, recycling, and degradation.

Desensitization and Downregulation

Prolonged exposure to GH can lead to GHR desensitization, where the receptor's responsiveness is diminished. This process involves the phosphorylation of GHR and the binding of regulatory proteins such as SOCS (Suppressor of Cytokine Signaling), which inhibit further signaling. Downregulation involves the reduction of GHR numbers on the cell surface, often through receptor internalization and degradation.

Receptor Recycling and Degradation

Internalized GHRs can be recycled back to the cell membrane or targeted for degradation in lysosomes. The balance between these processes determines the overall number of functional receptors available for GH binding. Recycling allows the cell to quickly restore receptor sensitivity, while degradation reduces receptor density, providing long-term regulation.

Plant-Based Diets and Regulation of Growth Hormone Receptors

Plant-based diets can influence the regulation of Growth Hormone Receptors through various bioactive compounds. These compounds can modulate receptor activity, expression, and the overall endocrine environment.

Phytochemicals

Phytochemicals, such as flavonoids, are abundant in plant-based diets and have been shown to modulate GHR activity. For instance, quercetin, a flavonoid found in apples, onions, and berries, can influence the signaling pathways activated by GHR, potentially enhancing or inhibiting its effects depending on the context.

Dietary Fiber

High-fiber diets, typical of plant-based nutrition, can improve insulin sensitivity and reduce systemic inflammation. These effects can indirectly influence GHR function, as insulin and inflammatory cytokines are linked to GH signaling. Improved insulin sensitivity can enhance the anabolic effects of GH, while reduced inflammation can prevent the desensitization of GHR.

Omega-3 Fatty Acids

Plant sources of omega-3 fatty acids, such as flaxseeds and chia seeds, have anti-inflammatory properties and can modulate endocrine functions. Omega-3 fatty acids have been shown to influence the expression of various receptors, including GHR, by altering membrane fluidity and signaling pathways.

Plant-Based Diets and Growth Hormone Receptors

Adopting a plant-based diet can have significant impacts on the regulation and function of Growth Hormone Receptors. The intake of various nutrients and bioactive compounds from plants can modulate the endocrine system, contributing to overall health benefits.

Cardiovascular Health

Plant-based diets are rich in antioxidants, dietary fiber, and healthy fats, which are beneficial for cardiovascular health. The regulation of GHR in various tissues can be positively influenced by these dietary components. For example, antioxidants can reduce oxidative stress, which is known to impair GH signaling. Additionally, dietary fiber helps in managing blood pressure and improving endothelial function, which can enhance the cardiovascular benefits of GH.

Metabolic Health

The influence of plant-based diets on GHR can enhance metabolic health. Foods rich in flavonoids and omega-3 fatty acids can improve insulin sensitivity and reduce the risk of metabolic disorders such as type 2 diabetes. By modulating GHR activity, these diets can enhance glucose uptake and utilization, contributing to better glycemic control.

Weight Management

Growth hormone plays a crucial role in fat metabolism and lean body mass maintenance. Plant-based diets, which are typically lower in calories and higher in fiber, can support weight management by enhancing the function of GHR. The presence of bioactive compounds in plant foods can stimulate GH-mediated lipolysis, aiding in the reduction of fat stores and promoting healthy weight loss.

Case Studies and Research on Plant-Based Diets and GHR

Research has demonstrated the beneficial effects of plant-based diets on the endocrine system, including the regulation of GHR. Studies have shown that individuals following plant-based diets have improved metabolic profiles, reduced inflammation, and better cardiovascular health, all of which are linked to GH signaling.

Study on Flavonoids and GHR

A study investigated the impact of quercetin on GH signaling in muscle cells. The results indicated that quercetin enhanced the phosphorylation of GHR, leading to improved muscle protein synthesis.

This suggests that the inclusion of flavonoid-rich foods in the diet can potentiate the anabolic effects of GH.

Dietary Fiber and GH Sensitivity

Research has shown that high-fiber diets can improve GH sensitivity in obese individuals. The study found that dietary fiber reduced systemic inflammation and improved insulin sensitivity, which in turn enhanced GH signaling. This highlights the importance of dietary fiber in maintaining healthy GH receptor function.

Omega-3 Fatty Acids and GH Signaling

A study examined the effects of omega-3 fatty acids on GH signaling in adipose tissue. The findings revealed that omega-3 fatty acids reduced the expression of inflammatory cytokines and enhanced GHR expression, promoting better GH-mediated lipolysis and fat metabolism. This underscores the role of plant-based sources of omega-3 in supporting healthy GH function.

Practical Implications for Plant-Based Nutrition

Understanding the relationship between plant-based diets and Growth Hormone Receptors can inform dietary recommendations and interventions aimed at optimizing health.

Dietary Recommendations

To support healthy GHR function, it is beneficial to include a variety of plant-based foods rich in antioxidants, dietary fiber, and omega-3 fatty acids. Foods such as berries, leafy greens, whole grains, flaxseeds, and chia seeds should be staples in the diet. These foods provide essential nutrients and bioactive compounds that can enhance GH signaling and overall endocrine health.

Lifestyle Interventions

In addition to dietary choices, lifestyle interventions such as regular physical activity, stress management, and adequate sleep are important for maintaining healthy GH levels and GHR function. Exercise, in particular, can stimulate GH secretion and improve receptor sensitivity, while stress management and sleep are crucial for hormonal balance.

Growth Hormone Receptors are vital for mediating the effects of growth hormone on growth, metabolism, and immune function. The production and regulation of GHR are influenced by genetic and environmental factors, including dietary choices.

www.ingramcontent.com/pod-product-compliance
Lightning Source LLC
LaVergne TN
LVHW052203200926
848481LV00001B/16